Men's
Health
Today

Men's Health Today

THE HOTTEST NEW DISCOVERIES ABOUT

SEX, FITNESS AND STRESS-FREE LIVING

AND HOW TO MAKE THEM WORK FOR YOU

Edited by Michael Lafavore, Men'sHealth Magazine

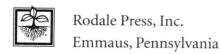

Rodale Press, Inc.
Emmaus, Pennsylvania

This book is being published simultaneously by Rodale Press as *Men's Health Today 1997*.

Men's Health is a registered trademark of Rodale Press, Inc.

Printed in the United States of America on acid-free ∞, recycled paper ♻

Library of Congress Cataloging-in-Publication Data

        Men's health today : the hottest new discoveries about sex, fitness and stress-free living and how to make them work for you / edited by Michael Lafavore.
           p.   cm.
        Includes index.
        ISBN 0–87596–417–6 paperback
        1. Men—health and hygiene.   I. Lafavore, Michael.
RA777.8.M474   1997
613'.04234—dc21   96–48142

Distributed in the book trade by St. Martin's Press

2   4   6   8   10   9   7   5   3   1   paperback

—— OUR PURPOSE ——

"We inspire and enable people to improve their lives and the world around them."

Notice

This book is intended as a reference volume only, not as a medical manual. The information given here is designed to help you make informed decisions about your health. It is not intended as a substitute for any treatment that may have been prescribed by your doctor. If you suspect that you have a medical problem, we urge you to seek competent medical help.

MEN'S HEALTH TODAY EDITORIAL STAFF

Executive Editor, *Men's Health* Magazine: Michael Lafavore

Senior Managing Editor, *Men's Health* Books: Neil Wertheimer

Editor: John D. Reeser

Contributing Writers: Alisa Bauman, K. Winston Caine, Brian Chichester, Doug Dollemore, Perry Garfinkel, Stephen C. George, Brian Paul Kaufman, Cathy Raymond, Wendy Wetherbee

Researchers and Fact Checkers: Tanya H. Bartlett, Susan E. Burdick, Valerie Edwards-Paulik, Jan Eickmeier, Jane Unger Hahn, Sally A. Reith

Permissions: Tanya H. Bartlett

Copy Editor: David R. Umla

Art Director: Jane Colby Knutila

Book Designer: Charles Beasley

Cover Designer: Vic Mazurkiewicz

Photo Editor: Susan Pollack

Photographer: Mitch Mandel

Illustrator: Chris Gall

Studio Manager: Stefano Carbini

Layout Artist: Joe Golden

Manufacturing Coordinator: Patrick T. Smith

Office Staff: Roberta Mulliner, Julie Kehs, Bernadette Sauerwine, Mary Lou Stephen

RODALE HEALTH AND FITNESS BOOKS

Vice-President and Editorial Director: Debora T. Yost

Design and Production Director: Michael Ward

Research Manager: Ann Gossy Yermish

Copy Manager: Lisa D. Andruscavage

Book Manufacturing Director: Helen Clogston

Contents

Introduction xiii

FITNESS

Benchmarks .2
Vital Reading
  Reaching for the Next Level 3
  Limber Up Fast 4
  Total-Body Exercises 7
  Seven Boredom Busters 13
  Mastering a Classic 17
  Build Powerful Legs 18
Best Reads
  Strength-Training Myths 23
  How to Get Fit Fast 25
Interviews
  Louis Garcia on
  Freestyle Jump Roping 27
  Carlos DeJesus on
  Faster, Better Workouts 29
News Flashes 32
Soon to Be News 34
Fad Alerts .35
New Tools .36
Resources 38
Actions 39

EATING

Benchmarks 44
Vital Reading
  Another Look at Salt 45
Best Reads
  A Plateful of Miracles 47

A Man's Kitchen 48
Quality Counts 53
Interviews
  Mary Friesz on
  Eating Strategies for Men 55
  Doreen Virtue on
  Having a Romantic Dinner 57
News Flashes 59
Soon to Be News 60
Fad Alerts .61
New Tools .63
Resources 65
Actions 66

SEX

Benchmarks 72
Vital Reading
  Herbs for Better Erections 73
  Slip Sliding Away 74
Best Reads
  Peak Erotic Experiences 76
  Breasts .79
  Aphrodisiacs 82
Interviews
  Richard A. Carroll on Making Love
  through the Ages 84
  Marilyn K. Volker on
  Foreplay: The Big Buildup 87
News Flashes 90
Soon to Be News 91
Fad Alerts .92
New Tools .94
Resources 96
Actions 97

WEIGHT LOSS

Benchmarks **102**

Vital Reading
 A New Angle on Weight Loss **103**

Best Reads
 Our Obsession with Fat **106**
 The Failure of the Low-Fat,
 High-Carbohydrate Diet **107**

Interviews
 Kelly Brownell on
 The Sociology of Weight Loss **111**
 Daniel Kosich on
 Weight Management **113**

News Flashes **115**

Soon to Be News **117**

Fad Alerts **118**

New Tools **120**

Resources **121**

Actions **122**

DISEASE-PROOF

Benchmarks **126**

Vital Reading
 Beneficial Bacteria **127**
 The Heart-Helping Big Four **129**
 Unheralded Minerals **131**
 Nipping Melanoma in the Bud **132**
 The Magic of Garlic **133**

Best Reads
 Aging: It's a State of Mind **135**

Interviews
 Robert Carney on
 The Mind-Disease Connection **139**
 Harinder Garewal on
 Understanding Antioxidants **141**

News Flashes **145**

Soon to Be News **147**

Fad Alerts **148**

New Tools **150**

Resources **152**

Actions **153**

MENTAL TOUGHNESS

Benchmarks **158**

Best Reads
 Emotions **159**
 The Law of Lifetime Growth **162**

Interviews
 Phil Jackson on
 Building Personal and Team
 Mental Toughness **165**
 James Loehr on
 Toughening Your Mental Muscles . . .**167**

News Flashes **169**

Soon to Be News **171**

Fad Alerts **172**

Resources **175**

Actions **176**

CURES

Benchmarks **182**

Vital Reading
 The Virility Robbers **183**
 Nature's Cure for a Prostate Problem **186**
 Exterminating a Pesky Bug **187**

Best Reads
 Optimizing Your Healing System **189**

Interviews
 Thomas Platts-Mills on
 Asthma Causes and Cures **193**
 Edward Laskowski on
 Knee Pain Causes and Cures **195**

News Flashes 199
Soon to Be News 201
Fad Alerts .202
New Tools .203
Resources .205
Actions 206

SLEEP

Benchmarks 210
Vital Reading
The Importance of a Good Bed **211**
Best Reads
What Your Dreams
May Be Telling You **214**
Interview
Alex Clerk and Jack Coleman on
Apnea and Snoring **217**
News Flashes 219
Soon to Be News 220
Fad Alerts .221
New Tools .222
Resources .223
Actions 224

HEALTH MANAGEMENT

Benchmarks 228
Best Reads
Facing the Facts 229
Choosing Your Doctor 234
Interviews
Mike Magee on
A Positive Approach to Medicine **240**
John J. Connolly on
Sorting Out the ABCs of HMOs **244**
News Flashes 247
Soon to Be News 249
Fad Alerts .250
New Tools .251
Resources .253
Actions 254

Credits 259
Index 261

Introduction

Getting What You Wish For

This book was not our idea.

It was yours.

You see, we at *Men's Health* routinely ask the men of America what information and products they would most like us to provide. Not long ago we asked specifically about health books. And the answer we received, with a clarity and fervency that surprised us, was for a compilation of the best, most current thinking about leading a stronger, healthier life. You wanted tons of tips, and you wanted them to reflect the cutting edge of scientific research.

So what did we do first? Complain, of course. That's a lot of work, you know. Although men's health is still a relatively new area of interest in the health field, the body of material is growing by leaps and bounds every year. Just look at the health section of a bookstore. Whereas five years ago, you would have been hard-pressed to see anything on men's health, today's shelves contain books for men on a whole slew of topics—from breakthroughs in prostate cancer research to the new science of mental-toughness training for athletes.

Maybe that's why you wanted a book like *Men's Health Today*. With the flood of information out there, it's hard to tell what's worthwhile and what's not. And besides, who has the time to sift through all that stuff?

We do, of course. So we plowed through stacks of books, magazines and studies. We conducted interviews and searched the World Wide Web. We read it all with a discriminating eye, then came up with the most essential knowledge out there.

We came across the raging debate over melatonin. You've probably heard that taking supplements of this hormone is effective against jet lag, but is the new claim that melatonin slows the aging process valid? You'll find the answer in these pages. And we happened upon coenzyme Q_{10}, an antioxidant that could very well take away the limelight from vitamin E and beta-carotene. One doctor we talked to calls it "the biggest medical discovery of the twentieth century, bigger than the Salk polio vaccine." We tell you why he thinks it could change the health industry and, if you believe him, where to get it.

Gathering this information was one thing; organizing it was another. So we put our heads together and came up with what we think is an innovative solution. *Men's Health Today* is written in a chapterless format where the information is presented in short, fact-filled bursts. No 20-page dissertations on herbal enemas here. To keep things organized, we split the information into nine topics: areas such as sex, mental toughness, disease prevention, fitness. Within each of these topic areas are a number of different elements to showcase the wide range of advice and insight we wanted to provide.

Here's what you'll find inside.

Benchmarks. What percentage of his body weight can an average guy lift? How many sex partners does he have in a lifetime? What man doesn't want to know how he stands up against the average guy? These standards, averages and extremes allow you to see how you fare.

Vital Reading. Out of the mountain of magazines we perused comes the best of what's out there. The majority of these articles ended up being from *Men's Confidential*, a newsletter that provides the latest health, sex and fitness news for men and comes from the publisher of *Men's Health* magazine.

Best Reads. These excerpts are from the best, and most controversial, books on men's health and the changing role of men in today's culture.

Interviews. Hear it right from the horse's mouth as we talk with the leading researchers, experts and doctors who are shaping the landscape of men's health.

News Flashes. Roundups of recent findings that you need to know, from what vitamin will improve your memory to what vegetable will cause your prostate cancer risk to plummet.

Soon to Be News. Ongoing studies and developments that might just make the headlines in the months ahead. Topics range from the near-completion of a drug that could be up to 85 percent effective in treating impotence to the search for safer, more effective diet pills.

Fad Alerts. These look at the latest trends, how they started and whether they are legitimate. For example, do "smart" drinks really enhance your mental performance?

New Tools. Guys love toys, and these collections won't disappoint you. We've assembled some low- and high-tech gizmos that can make a difference in your life.

Resources. Need more information or help?

We point you toward the best Web sites, organizations and associations.

Actions. Each of the nine parts ends with actions you can take right now to never miss a day to sickness, injury or lethargy.

Writing this book turned out to be an eye-opening experience. It forced us to take a step back and truly see the burgeoning amount of men's health literature in today's marketplace. It's been a long time coming. And it's the right time for a book that separates the wheat from the chaff.

So go ahead. Dive right in and take a look at what we have put together. After all, you asked for it.

Michael Lafavore
Executive Editor, *Men's Health* Magazine

1

FITNESS

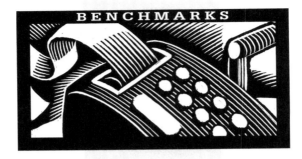

AVERAGES

■ Number of people who exercised at least 100 times in 1995: 52.7 million, or about one-fifth of the U.S. population

■ Percentage of adults who say that they "never exercise": 25

■ Number of people who learn to scuba dive each year: more than 200,000

■ Number of calories a 175-pound man burns per hour playing touch football: 630

■ Percentage longer a man will stay on a stationary bike if he listens to music: 30

■ Amount of muscle on a man: 70 to 80 pounds

■ Number of minutes it takes a man to run a mile: 12

■ Number of sit-ups a man can do in a minute: 33.5

■ Percentage decrease since 1980 in the number of Americans who belong to a bowling league: 44

■ Rank of golf among sports generating the largest number of patents: 1

■ Estimated number of cricket players in the United States: 5,500

■ Percentage of Americans who own running shoes but don't run: 87

■ Time of day when a man's hand-eye coordination is at its peak: between 2:30 P.M. and 4:00 P.M.

■ Rank of badminton among racket sports causing the largest number of eye injuries: 1

■ Number of times in 30 seconds a 40-year-old male can curl a five-pound dumbbell: at least 30 times

EXTREMES

■ Largest biceps: 30¾ inches

■ Largest chest: 74¹⁄₁₆ inches

■ Most consecutive one-finger push-ups: 124

■ Most sit-ups performed in 24 hours: 70,715

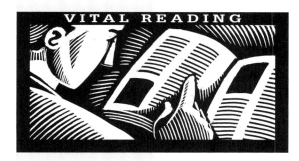

Reaching for the Next Level

A few adjustments may be all you need to improve your sports performance.

Sometimes a slight turn of the wrist or a different placement of your feet can bump you from B league right on up to A. We asked pros in three sports to offer their best game-winning advice.

Sink More Baskets

Forty percent of good basketball shooting is attitude and confidence, says David Jensen, a winning player in the 1993 Hoop-It-Up 3-on-3 street ball world championship. Still, that leaves 60 percent skill and mechanics. To hit the bucket, try these tips.

Face the basket. "Get your chest and feet square to the basket," says Jensen. Fancy sidelong shots may look good, but you won't make them as often.

Favor your strong hand. Bring the ball up with both hands, but if you're right-handed, take the left one off the ball before you release. You'll get better control and speed.

Let go from the wrist. Propelling the ball solely with the arms hinders your aim. Let the ball roll off your fingertips, sliding off the index and middle fingers last.

Improve Your Serve

Because tennis rackets are more powerful, "recreational players are playing 20 percent worse than they were 20 years ago," says Dennis Van der Meer, who coaches pros and club players at his Tennis University on Hilton Head Island, South Carolina. The problems created by the new rackets are control and poor mechanics. Here's how to get more.

Hit up on the ball. A lot of people think that they can add velocity by using more power coming down on the ball, but that'll just put it into the net.

Cut down on extra motion. It's common for players to deliberately jump on the swing, thinking that will impart energy to the ball, but it actually hinders a fluid swing, robbing you of power.

Follow through the swing. Many players want to cut their serve swing short to get ready for the serve return, but by cutting it short, you are actually putting on the brakes at the time of the hit.

Adjust Your Golf Swing

There are two basic problems: slicing to the right and hooking to the left. Both can often be solved with simple grip adjustments, says Hank Haney, Professional Golfers' Association 1993 Teacher of the Year.

To fix a slice, turn your grip slightly so that the Vs formed by your thumbs and forefingers point more toward your right shoulder. That'll help your hands square the club face and eliminate the slice.

To fix a hook, move those same Vs to point more toward your chin.

Finally, amateur players always think that they'll hit farther than they do, Haney says. Pick a club that's one lower than you think you need. "You won't go over as many times as you'd otherwise go short," he adds.

Limber Up Fast

In five minutes you can stretch your
entire body to warm up your muscles
and cut down on injuries. Here's how.

You don't stretch. You know you're supposed
to. You know it warms up your muscles, protects
you from injury, blah blah blah, but you don't do
it. It takes too long. It's boring. It looks funny.
You want to go out and play, not sit on the side-
lines and twist yourself into a pretzel.

You're a busy man, so we're not going to
waste our time or yours by beating you over the
head with all the reasons you should stretch
more. In fact, we're here to save you a little time.
We've found a way for you to stretch your entire
body, even muscles you've never heard of, in four
simple moves. We're going to call it the five-
minute total-body stretch. But you can probably
do it in less than three.

As a bonus, we've simplified these stretches
by eliminating your wristwatch. Simply hold
each stretch for ten breaths. This will not only
ensure that you've held the stretch long enough
but also prevent you from holding your breath
during each exercise, says Larry Payne, Ph.D., director of the Samata Yoga Center in Los Angeles
and creator of the audiotape *Breathe Stretch
Relax.*

Slow, controlled breathing can actually help
your body relax more. Add a ten-second rest in
between stretches and you've given yourself a
complete tune-up in less time than it takes to
lace your sneakers.

THE TRIANGLE (stretches the muscles of the upper back, chest, hips, shoulders and neck)

1. Take a wide stance, placing your feet about twice your shoulder-width apart. Your legs should be loose with your knees unlocked, feet parallel to each other. (Your feet will naturally point outward a bit. Try to keep them pointing straight ahead throughout the exercise, but don't force it.) Rest your left hand on the side of your left thigh and raise your right hand straight over your head.
2. Keeping your right arm straight, slowly lean to-

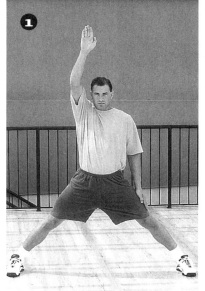 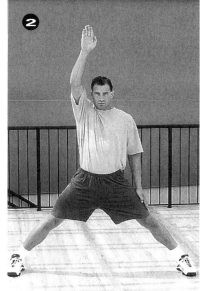

ward your left side as far as you can, letting your left hand slide down your leg. (This helps support the body but can also help you gauge how far you're stretching.) Hold for ten breaths, then slowly bend back into the starting position. Now switch your hand position and stretch to the right side. (*Tip:* If you have back problems, you can bend your knees slightly. This will help take pressure off your back.)

THE QUAD-BUSTER (stretches the quadriceps and the muscles of the back, abdomen and neck)

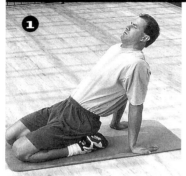
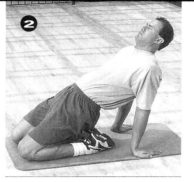
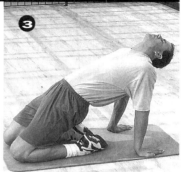

1. Sit on your heels with the tops of your feet flat on the floor. Place your hands flat on the floor a few inches behind your butt. Your thumbs should be pointing out to each side with your fingertips pointing away from you.

2. Keeping your hands pressed to the floor, tilt your pelvis upward, tucking your tailbone underneath you. You should feel a slight stretch in the front of your thighs. Slowly raise your hips as high as they will comfortably go and lift your chest as high as you can.

3. Slowly lower your head back, stretching the front of the neck. (If you feel any pain in your back or neck, skip this part.) Hold for ten breaths, then slowly lift your head into alignment with your back, and lower your chest and hips until you are once again sitting on your heels.

THE LUNGE (stretches the muscles of the legs and groin)

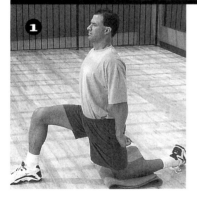
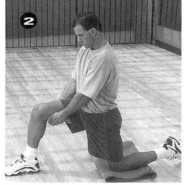
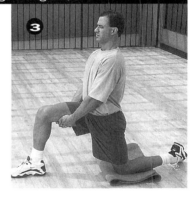

1. Stand with your feet hip-width apart and take a large step forward with your right foot, so your leg forms a right angle. (Make sure that your right knee doesn't extend past your right foot.) Lower your left knee until it rests on the floor. (You can use a pillow for comfort.)

2. Link your hands under the back of your supporting leg, just behind your right knee.

3. Lift your chest. Gently rotate your left thigh inward; you'll feel a stretch in your lower back. Hold for ten breaths, rotate your left thigh back into its natural position, let go of your knee and step back into a standing position. Repeat, with your left foot.

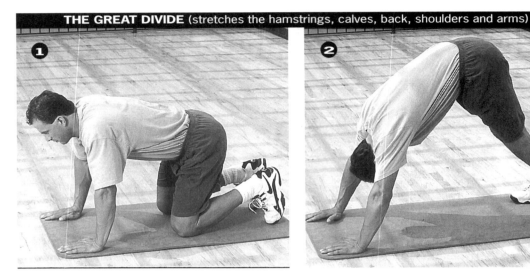
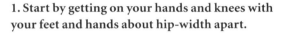
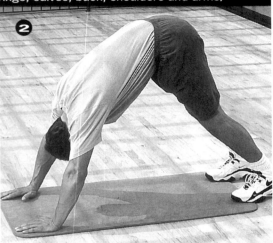

THE GREAT DIVIDE (stretches the hamstrings, calves, back, shoulders and arms)

1. Start by getting on your hands and knees with your feet and hands about hip-width apart.

2. Without moving your feet, gently raise your buttocks into the air, straightening your legs without locking your knees. Keep your feet and hands as flat as possible on the floor. Your body should now be shaped like an upside-down V with your butt in the air. Gently lower your head as far as you can and hold for ten breaths.

Total-Body Exercises

In a hurry and want to get as complete a workout as possible in a short time? These three power moves will keep you fit in five minutes a day or less.

Versatility is one of those manly traits that most of us want to possess. We like to think that we can do it all: We can bring home the bacon, fry it up in a pan and use the leftover grease to oil the new trail bike/baby carriage combo we soldered together in the home workshop.

And because we want ourselves to be multi-faceted, we appreciate this quality in other things. We like switch-hitters, Swiss Army knives and pretty much anything else that can satisfy more than one of our needs at a time.

Yet when we get into the gym, the whole idea of versatility goes out the window. There's one machine to exercise our latissimus dorsi, another for our gluteus maximus—a guy could spend all day in the weight room trying to put together a full-body workout.

Wouldn't it be better to have one exercise to shore up as many muscle groups as possible—one exercise that acts like a relentless drill instructor, commanding almost every muscle in your body to come to attention? And, while we're at it, one that takes only five minutes to complete? Sound beyond the realm of reason? It's not.

"The secret to shaving time off your workout involves 'compound' exercises," says John Arce, strength and conditioning coordinator at Purdue University in West Lafayette, Indiana. Compound exercises are exactly what they sound like: a combination of two or more exercises rolled into one. A single exercise can work five to ten muscle groups at once.

Even if you're among the dedicated and always find time to work out, these exercises can still give your program a jolt. A compound exer-cise acts like a penny-pinching boss, forcing your body to work harder than ever. "The end results are well worth the effort, with your body adapting by building larger, more powerful muscles," says Michael Stone, Ph.D., president of the National Strength and Conditioning Association.

By working several muscle groups simultaneously, your body will use greater amounts of stored calories for fuel, and you'll also burn more fat. If you feel strange hitting the gym for only 5 minutes, relax. Chances are that you'll be burning more calories in those 5 minutes than most people burn in 10 or 15.

There's another benefit, too. The exercises shown on these pages may even help you avoid injury. Regular exercises strengthen individual muscles, but they don't train the surrounding muscles to work in relation to that muscle. You might build a strong hamstring muscle, for example, but if the other muscles of the leg aren't developed enough to support it, you may still be at risk for a sprain or other injuries. By comparison, compound exercises are the United Nations of weight training. They pull your muscles together to accomplish a feat and, in the meantime, teach your muscle groups to work as a team.

So you're eager to get started, right? Okay, just three words of caution: Use light weights—at least at first. We know, you're a big, tough guy and all that. But form is critical here. So start light until you feel confident that you've mastered the moves. Then you can start adding weight. "But never add so much weight that you sacrifice technique," reminds Arce.

Choose one of the exercises and do eight repetitions. That's one set. Rest about 60 seconds between sets. Because the average set takes about 45 to 60 seconds to complete, you'll perform a set every two minutes. Use a bit of math and that's three sets in five minutes or less. There's only one downside: You'll never again be able to use the excuse that you don't have time to exercise.

POWER CLEAN AND PRESS (works the shoulders, triceps, chest, back, abdominals and legs)

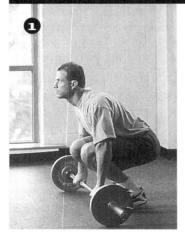

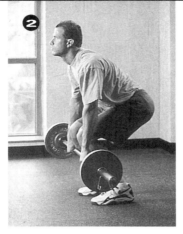

1. Place a barbell on the floor in front of you and stand with your feet about shoulder-width apart. Bend down and grab the bar with an overhand grip, hands slightly wider than shoulder width. Before lifting, make sure your back is straight and your shoulders are not arched forward. Your butt should be lower than your chest.

2. With your arms straight and head facing forward, slowly stand using only your leg muscles.

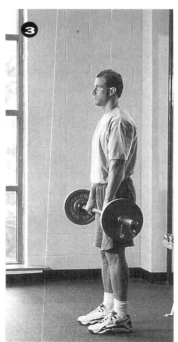

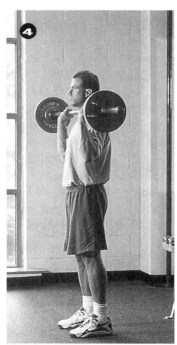

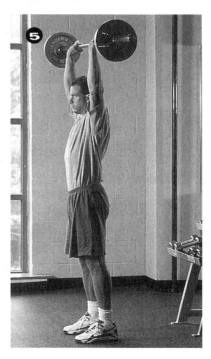

3. Your arms and back should be straight as the bar passes your knees and comes to rest against your thighs.

4. Next, swing the barbell upward, bending only at the elbows, until the bar rests directly in front of your chest.

5. Now, with your back straight, use your shoulders and arms to press the barbell directly overhead. Hold a moment. Then, keeping your abdominal muscles tight to support your lower back, lower the weight to the floor.

POWER LUNGE (works the legs, calves, shoulders, lower and upper back, biceps and forearms)

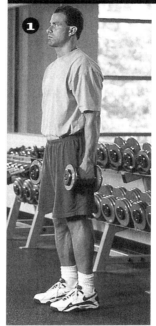

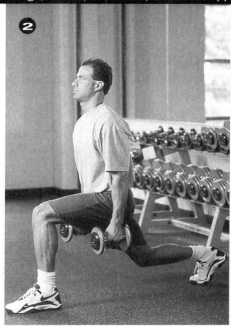

1. Stand with a light dumbbell in each hand, palms facing your thighs. Space your feet six to eight inches apart. (This will allow for better balance throughout the exercise.) Your back should be straight, your face forward.
2. Take a large step forward with your left foot until your left leg forms a 90-degree angle. Your upper left thigh should be almost parallel to the floor. (*Note:* Your left knee should never extend beyond the toes of your left foot, since that can stress the knee joint.)

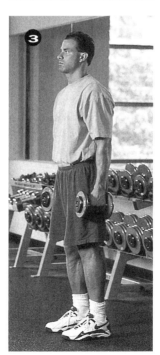

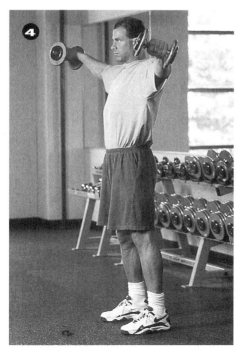

3. Reverse the motion, lightly pushing off with your left foot, until you're back in a standing position.
4. Next, bend your elbows slightly and slowly raise your arms from your sides until they are parallel to the floor. (Your palms should face down.) You'll resemble the letter T.

(continued)

POWER LUNGE—CONTINUED

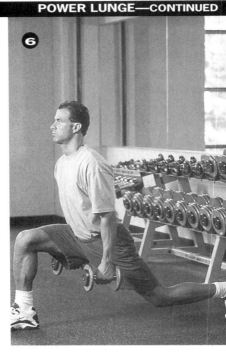

5. Hold for a second, then lower the weights to your sides.

6. Repeat the lunge again, this time with the right leg.

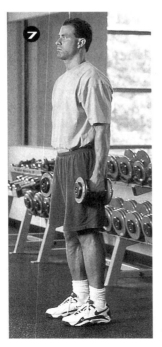

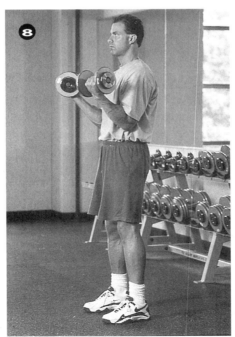

7. Step back into an upright position.

8. Immediately curl the weights to your armpits, with your palms facing upward as you do so. Slowly lower the weights to your sides.

SUPER SQUAT (works the legs, lower back, arms, shoulders, chest, abdominals and calves)

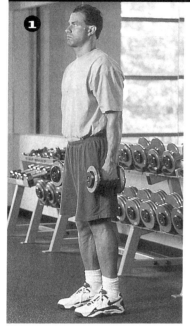
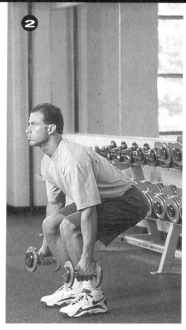

1. Stand with a dumbbell in each hand and with your feet about shoulder-width apart. Your palms should be facing your thighs.

2. Keeping your back straight, squat until your thighs are almost parallel to the floor. Try to keep your feet flat and your knees from extending beyond the front of your toes.

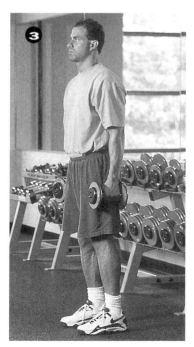
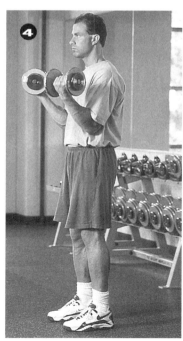

3. Slowly return to the starting position.

4. Now slowly curl both dumbbells to your shoulders, rotating your wrists outward as you go. Your palms should end up facing your shoulders.

(continued)

SUPER SQUAT—CONTINUED

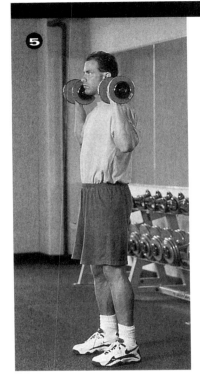

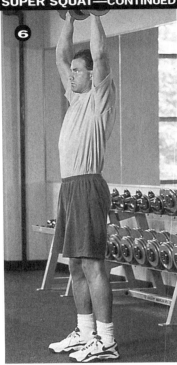

5. Next, turn your palms outward so they face away from you.

6. Now press both weights overhead. Lower the weights to your shoulders, then turn your wrists inward so your palms face you again. Finally, curl the weights back down to your sides, rotating your hands inward so your palms again face your thighs.

Seven Boredom Busters

If you're in need of a new and invigorating weight-room routine, here are some unique exercises to give your regimen a lift.

The problem isn't you, really. You know, the whole get-back-in-shape psychodrama that comes up every year. You envision yourself six months from now, shorn of bulky clothing and that girdle of gelatinous flesh around your belly. But six months later, well, you'd best keep your shirt on to hide evidence of yet another plan gone the way of the British Empire.

Here's the good news. It's not your willpower that needs an overhaul. It's your workout.

"The reason most people can't stick to resolutions is that they fall back on their old routines," says Eric Ludlow, senior trainer for World Gym in New York City.

To solve the problem, we've combed the globe for seven unique exercises that even some personal trainers we spoke with hadn't heard of. "They may be unknown to many, but each is an effective muscle builder," says Ludlow. Even if you're dedicated to your workouts, one or two of these could be just the thing to pump new life into a stale routine. But combined, these magnificent seven form a full-body workout unlike any you've ever tried before. Complete the routine twice a week for starters, working up to three times a week when you feel comfortable.

LOW PULLEY CABLE FLY (works the upper chest)

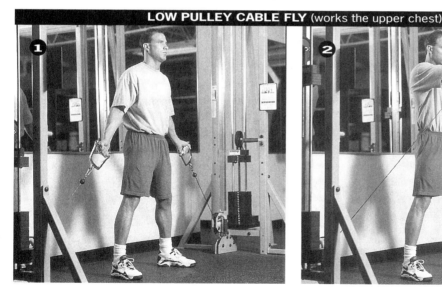
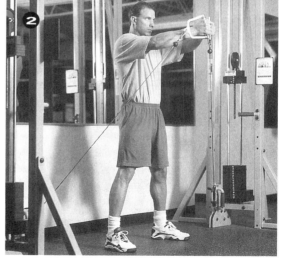

1. Stand between two low pulley stations with your feet about hip-width apart and grab a pulley in each hand. Let the resistance of the pulleys extend your arms from your body. Your hands should be about 18 to 20 inches from your sides.

2. With your arms straight (elbows unlocked), slowly raise your fists in front of you in a curved motion until your fists are together at about eye level. Your arms should be about parallel to the floor. Squeeze your chest muscles for two seconds, then slowly reverse the motion. Do three sets of eight to ten repetitions.

STANDING STRAIGHT-BAR PULLDOWN (works the back and triceps)

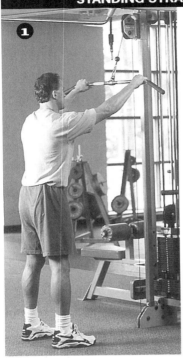 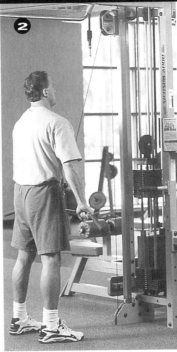

1. Attach a long bar to a high pulley. Grab the bar with your hands palms down and shoulder-width apart. Move back a step or two from the machine until your arms are extended in front of you, slightly higher than parallel with the floor.
2. Slowly pull the bar down in a sweeping motion, keeping your arms straight as you go, until the bar touches the front of your thighs. Be sure to keep your back straight throughout the exercise. Reverse the motion by slowly allowing the bar to return to the starting position, maintaining resistance as you go. Do three sets of 12 to 15 repetitions.

LYING DUMBBELL CURL (works the biceps)

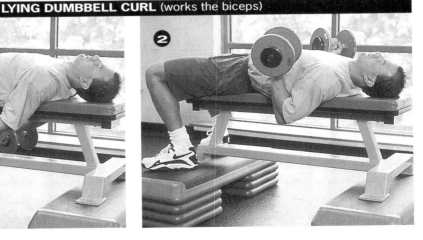

1. Lie on your back on a flat bench with a dumbbell in each hand. Let your arms hang, palms facing inward. (You may need to raise the bench on some stable aerobic steps to do so; or use an incline bench.)

2. With your head flat on the bench, slowly curl both weights upward until they reach your armpits. Squeeze your biceps for a second, then slowly lower the weights until your arms are again hanging. Do three sets of 10 to 12 repetitions.

KNEELING CLOSE-GRIP TRICEPS EXTENSION (works the triceps)

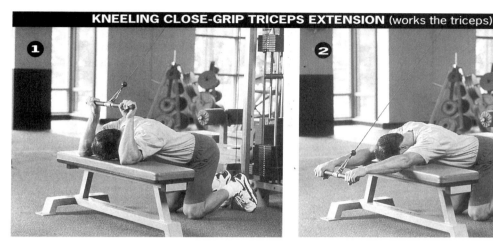

1. Attach a short bar to a high cable pulley and place a flat bench sideways about three feet in front of it. With your back to the pulley, reach up and grab the bar overhead, your hands four to six inches apart. Kneel in front of the bench, lean forward and rest your forehead and elbows flat on the bench.

2. Slowly pull the bar forward until your arms are extended. Squeeze your triceps muscles for two seconds, then slowly bring the bar back to the starting position, resisting the pull of the cable as you go. Do three sets of 12 to 15 repetitions.

INCLINE ONE-ARM LATERAL RAISE (works the sides and back of shoulders)

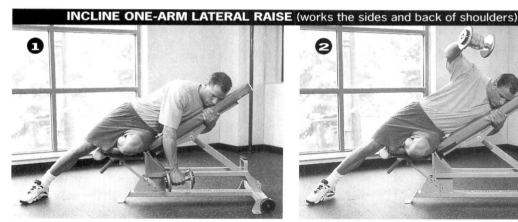

1. Lie on your left side on an incline bench. To do this, bend your left leg and rest it on the seat. Allow your right leg to extend toward the floor in front of the bench. Hold a light dumbbell in your right hand and let your right arm hang in front of you, palm facing the bench. Loop your left arm around the bench to help you stay balanced.

2. With a slight bend in your right elbow, slowly raise the dumbbell as high as you can. Slowly bring the weight down until it again hangs below you. Do 10 to 12 repetitions for the right shoulder, then turn around and lie on your right side to work the left shoulder. Do three sets for each side.

BACK SQUAT (works the legs)

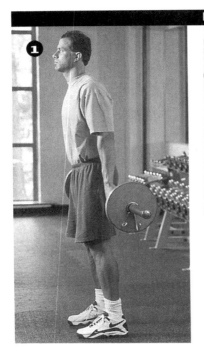
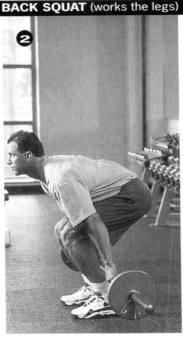

1. Stand straight with your feet shoulder-width apart. Your arms should be at your sides, hands behind your thighs, palms out. Have a partner hand you a barbell from behind so that you're holding the weight in back of you, hands spaced about shoulder-width apart. This is the starting position.
2. With your back straight, slowly squat until your thighs are almost parallel to the floor. Push yourself up until you are back in the starting position. Do four sets of 12 to 15 repetitions.

STANDING SINGLE-KNEE RAISE (works the obliques, hip flexors and abdominals)

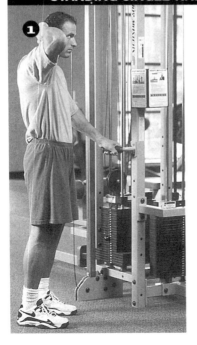
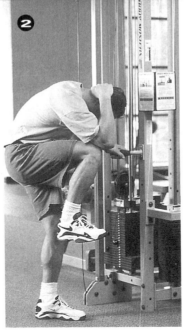

1. Stand to the right of a chair (or something supportive) and place your left hand on it for balance. Put your right hand behind your head, with your right arm bent and your right elbow pointing forward.
2. Slowly raise your right knee as high as possible in front of you and simultaneously curl your torso toward your right knee. Hold this position for a second, then slowly bring your right leg down and return to a standing position. Do 20 repetitions, then repeat with the left side. Do two sets for both the left and the right sides.

Mastering a Classic

What's the true measure of a man? His IQ? The horsepower on his boat? His credit limit? Nah. It's how much he benches. Find out how to master this simple yet powerful exercise.

The bench press is a classic exercise, a time-saving move that works the chest, shoulders and triceps. It's the best upper-body strength builder there is. Plus, it's a measure of manhood.

Think about it: When was the last time somebody asked you how much you can wrist-curl? Never, right? "The bench press has become a measurement of strength among men," says Ken Sprague, author of *The Gold's Gym Weight Training Book*.

Everybody knows how to do a bench press, even guys who don't exercise regularly. And everyone has his ideas on what constitutes proper technique. Chances are that you learned your technique from a friend who learned from a friend and so on. The rules start looking like an urban legend.

As the previous owner of Gold's Gym, Sprague has seen a lot of guys misusing the bench press and welcomed the chance to set things straight. And if this move is the measure of a man, you should strive for perfection.

So follow the rules we've set out here. Sprague recommends doing three sets of 8 to 12 repetitions twice a week (three times a week after about two months of solid training). He also suggests putting your pride in check and never lifting without a spotter. Get a friend to help, or ask a weight-room staffer to assist you. Your rib cage will thank you for it.

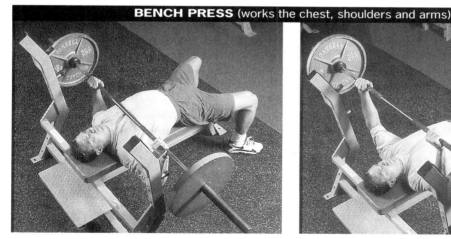
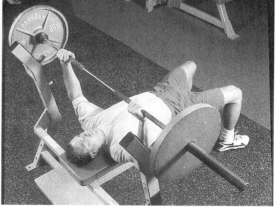

BENCH PRESS (works the chest, shoulders and arms)

Chest. Lower the bar until it touches your chest just above your nipples. Bringing it down too far below or above this point puts more stress on the shoulders and robs you of strength needed for the lift. Remember to let your muscles, not gravity, lower the bar to your chest. "There's as much muscle building going on in lowering the bar as there is in pushing it up," says Sprague. To achieve the best results, concentrate on controlling the weight throughout the exercise.

Elbows. Keep your elbows out as far as possible from your sides. Bringing them closer to the body takes the effort off the chest and puts it on the shoulders and triceps.

Feet. Your feet should be flat on the floor, pointing away from the body. If you raise or shift them during the exercise, you might lose your balance.

Hips. Keep hips flat on the bench at all times during the exercise.

Eyes. To help you concentrate on the weight as you lift, focus on the center of the bar. Also, position the bench away from any distracting overhead lighting.

Head. Avoid turning your head from side to side or pressing it into the bench as you push up the weight. This can strain your neck and trapezius muscles. Instead, rest your head flat on the bench and don't move it.

Arms. At the top of the movement, straighten your arms but don't lock the elbows. This keeps constant tension on the chest muscles.

Legs. Straddle the bench so that your knees are 1½ to 2 feet from each other.

Lower Back. An arch in the lower back is natural when you lift, but don't overarch to help push up the weight. There should be just enough space to slide a hand between your back and the bench. "Overarching places your body on an angle similar to a decline bench press, a movement you're naturally stronger with," says Sprague. You may be able to press more, but because you're working primarily the lower chest, you're cheating yourself out of two-thirds of the benefits and risking back injury.

Hands. Your hands should be slightly more than shoulder-width apart on the bar in an overhand grip. The bar should rest comfortably across the palms. This displaces the weight of the bar in a straight line through the wrists to the elbows and down to the shoulder joints to prevent injury. The surest way to avoid a big hurt is to have a spotter assist you.

Build Powerful Legs

In just 30 minutes a week, you can craft yourself a nice set of wheels.

We know that when you're in the gym, you want to concentrate on the muscles that show. But the next time you spend 40 minutes in the weight room buffing your biceps and chiseling your chest muscles, consider what you're missing by not working your lower half.

First, well-developed legs keep your physique in proportion. Unless you're a bartender or a TV anchorman, you need a lower half that measures up to your torso. Second, in almost every sport, power is generated from the legs, especially the hips and quadriceps. "Keeping them strong can improve your overall performance in whatever sport you play," says Brett Brungardt, former strength coach for the University of Houston and co-author of *The Complete Book of Butt and Legs.* And third, a set of well-built legs comes in handy during everyday chores, whether you're lifting a box or pushing a lawn mower. More power in your legs means less stress on your back when you're doing these mundane tasks of manhood.

Now the best part: You can reap all these benefits in just one 30-minute routine, and you can do it as little as once a week. Honest. "Your legs can respond and grow even if all you use is a once-a-week workout plan," says Brungardt.

Try two sets of each of these exercises, resting 45 to 60 seconds between each set. You'll get a complete leg workout in the time it takes to watch an average sitcom.

LEG PRESS (works the quadriceps, hamstrings and gluteal muscles)

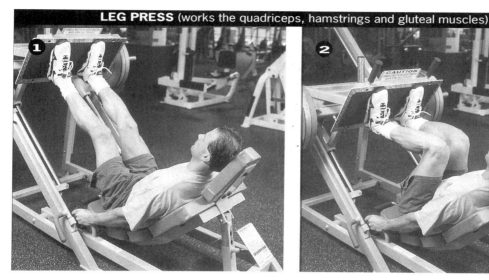

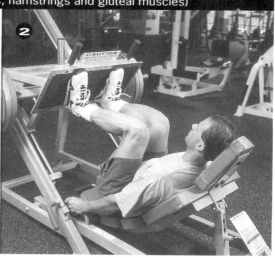

1. Sit in a leg-press machine with your back against the pad and your feet on the platform above you. Your feet should be slightly less than shoulder-width apart.

2. Slowly lower the weight until your legs are bent a little less than 90 degrees. Push the weight back up until your legs are straight, making sure not to lock your knees. Do 12 to 15 repetitions.

LEG EXTENSION (works the quadriceps)

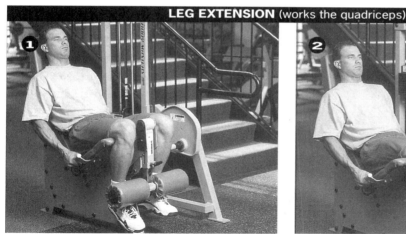

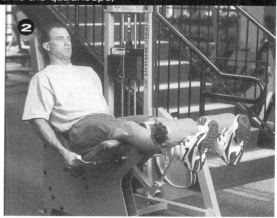

1. Sit in a leg-extension machine, with your ankles behind the leg pads. Grab the handles at the sides of the seat. Make sure you keep your back against the pad throughout the exercise.

2. Slowly extend your legs until they are straight. Hold for a second, then slowly lower your legs, making sure not to let the weights touch the stack. (This will keep tension on the muscles.) Do 8 to 12 repetitions.

TWO-UP, ONE-DOWN LEG CURL (works the hamstrings)

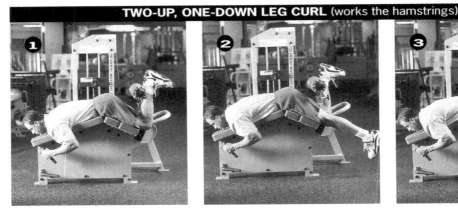

1. Lie facedown on a leg-curl machine, with both feet under the pads. Your knees should be hanging slightly over the edge of the bench. Slowly curl your lower legs until your feet almost touch your buttocks.

2. Lower your left leg so that your right leg supports the weight.

3. Lower your right leg, resisting the pull of the weight as you go. Use both legs to curl the pad to your buttocks. This time, use your left leg. Do ten repetitions (five for each leg).

STIFF-LEG DEAD LIFT (works the gluteal and hamstring muscles)

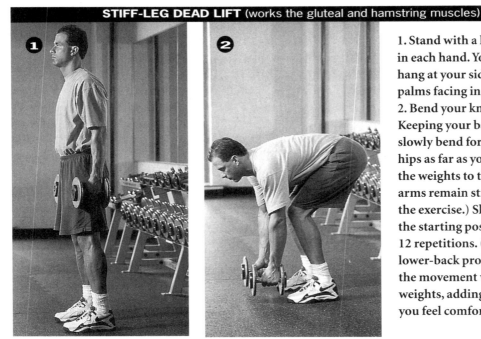

1. Stand with a light dumbbell in each hand. Your arms should hang at your sides, with your palms facing in.

2. Bend your knees slightly. Keeping your back straight, slowly bend forward from the hips as far as you can, lowering the weights to the floor. (Your arms remain straight during the exercise.) Slowly rise into the starting position. Do 10 to 12 repetitions. (If you have lower-back problems, perform the movement without any weights, adding weight when you feel comfortable.)

STEP-UP (works the hip extensors, knee extensors and quadriceps)

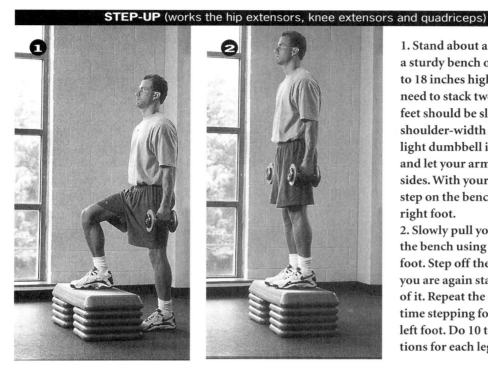

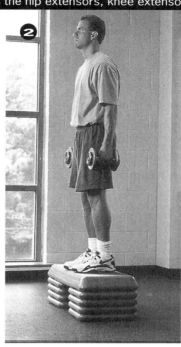

1. Stand about a foot in front of a sturdy bench or step that's 12 to 18 inches high. (You may need to stack two steps.) Your feet should be slightly less than shoulder-width apart. Grab a light dumbbell in each hand and let your arms hang at your sides. With your back straight, step on the bench with your right foot.

2. Slowly pull yourself up onto the bench using only your right foot. Step off the bench until you are again standing in front of it. Repeat the exercise, this time stepping forward with the left foot. Do 10 to 12 repetitions for each leg.

CALF RAISE WITH DUMBBELLS ON KNEES (works the calf muscles)

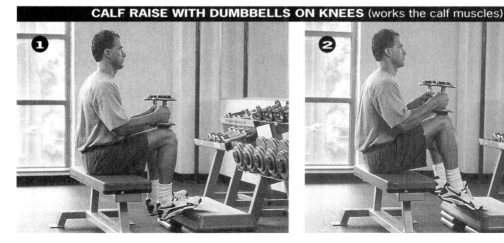

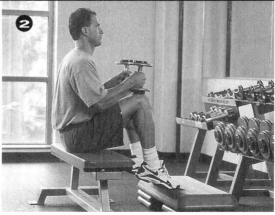

1. Sit on a weight bench with a small step (8 to 12 inches high) in front of you. Put the balls of your feet on the step so that your heels hang off the edge, your legs bent at an angle. Place a light dumbbell on top of each leg, right above the knee.

2. Slowly push up as high as you can on your toes, raising both heels. Hold a second, then slowly lower your heels as far as you can. (This will help stretch the calf muscles.) Do as many repetitions as possible.

STANDING TOE RAISE (works the front of the lower legs)

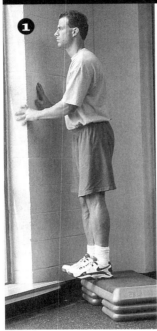
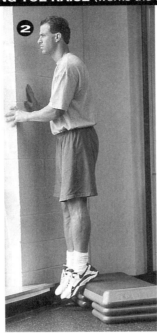

1. Place a step (at least eight inches high) next to, but not touching, a wall. Step onto the platform facing the wall, and move forward until only your heels are on the platform. (Use a stable platform, since you'll be putting your weight on the edge of the platform.) Your feet, from your arches to your toes, should be hanging off the platform. You'll need to use the wall for support throughout the exercise. Slowly raise your toes as high as you can and hold for a second.

2. Lower your toes as far as you can and repeat. Do as many repetitions as possible. (If this becomes easy, do the exercise one foot at a time, with the other foot wrapped behind the calf you want to work.)

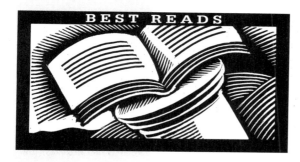

Strength-Training Myths

Ellington Darden, Ph.D., knows fitness. For 20 years, he was director of research at Nautilus Sports/ Medical Industries. He has written more than three dozen books on exercise, diet and healthy living. Living Longer Stronger: The 6-Week Plan to Enhance and Extend Your Years over 40 *(Perigree Books, 1995) is among his best. In it, he details the attitudes, exercise programs and eating habits that not only can trim your body but also can extend your life. This excerpt, from the "Reworking Strength-Training Basics" section, debunks several widely held myths about resistance training.*

Old myths, even after science proves them wrong, often continue to thrive.

Such is the case with the muscle-bound myth. A common belief still equates muscular development with being stiff, tight and inflexible. It is true that some men with large muscles lack a normal degree of mobility. Large muscles can be developed through training regimens that do little to improve flexibility. In rare cases, the activity that made the muscles larger concurrently produced a loss of movement. But in the vast majority of cases, muscle size has a positive correlation to extensibility. When strength training is conducted properly, and especially when certain exercises and machines are used, the full-range movements that improve muscular size and strength simultaneously increase flexibility.

Besides the fear of becoming muscle-bound,

there are many other myths that may discourage men in their second middle age from getting involved with strength training. Let's examine some of the most prevalent of these false beliefs.

Myth: Strength Training Will Slow You Down

If everything else is equal, the stronger, larger-muscled man will move faster because he will have a greater muscle-mass-to-body-weight ratio. Put a larger engine with more horsepower in an automobile, and it will travel faster even though it weighs more.

Suppose you want to curl an 80-pound barbell as fast as possible. If your biceps muscles are capable of curling exactly 81 pounds, then your speed of movement with 80 pounds will be very slow. Perhaps five seconds will be needed to move from the extended to the flexed position. On the other hand, if your biceps are capable of curling 100 pounds, you'll curl the 80-pound barbell in half a second or less. If your curling capacity is 110 pounds, your speed of movement will be even more rapid. Since skill is not significantly involved in curling a barbell, increases in speed must be accomplished by strengthening the involved muscles.

The same holds true with movements not related to strength training. Any type of muscle-powered movement is met by some kind of resistance: air, water, gravity or friction. Given equal resistance, the stronger man will invariably be faster.

Myth: Strength Training Takes Too Much Time

Contrary to popular belief, properly performed strength training takes only 20 minutes per workout. Performed three times per week, that's one hour of training time for every seven days. Investing one hour per week in exercise yields the best returns attainable in such a small amount of time.

Myth: If Something Hurts during an Exercise, Stop Doing It

There's productive pain during exercise, and there's destructive pain. The productive pain is a burning sensation in the muscle that usually occurs during the last repetition or two of an exercise. High-intensity exercise works a maximum percentage of the involved muscle's fibers, increasing demand for nutrient importation and waste exportation. This is accomplished by elevated blood volume to and from the muscle. The muscle swells and becomes engorged with intercellular fluid.

Engorgement of the involved muscles impinges on various nerves and creates the burning sensation. Within minutes after termination of the exercise, the pain and burning dissipate as the engorgement diminishes. Such burning in the muscle should not cause concern. It merely indicates a highly effective exercise.

On the other hand, if you ever feel a sharp pain in a joint, stop the exercise immediately. Sharp joint pain can indicate injury to the joint and/or connective tissues. If the condition does not improve or worsens, see your physician.

Myth: Whatever Muscle You Gain from Strength Training Will Turn to Fat Once You Stop Exercising

Muscle is muscle, fat is fat, and there is no way to turn one into the other.

Muscle is 71 percent water, 22 percent proteins and 7 percent lipids. Fat is 22 percent water, 6 percent proteins and 72 percent lipids. Like apples and oranges, muscle and fat are genetically and chemically different.

But why is it that people fall for this myth?

When you stop training, you seldom decrease your caloric intake. The result is a gradual decrease in the size and strength of your muscles and an increase in body fat stores. Since muscle and fat are so close to each other that they can intermingle, it appears that your muscles have turned to fat. Fortunately, muscle and fat levels don't change immediately when you stop exercising. You can work back to your previous level in a fraction of the time it took you to get there.

Myth: Strength Training Increases Your Risk of Coronary Artery Disease

Strength training can reduce certain risk factors for coronary artery disease. Dr. Linn Goldberg of the University of Oregon Health Sciences Center in Eugene studied the effect of strength training on fat buildup in the blood vessels. His participants trained three times per week for 16 weeks. Results included a significant lowering of low-density lipoproteins (the "bad" cholesterol) and a reduction in total cholesterol levels.

Other studies also indicate that strength training, especially when combined with low-calorie dieting, can significantly reduce triglycerides, increase high-density lipoproteins (the "good" cholesterol) and lower the important risk factor of total cholesterol divided by high-density lipoproteins.

Myth: Strength Training Is Dangerous for People with High Blood Pressure

Many earlier studies determined that isometric contractions elevated blood pressure to very high levels. Some people, including physicians, incorrectly assumed that weight training did the same. This is not the case.

Dr. Wayne Westcott, strength consultant to the YMCA of the USA, studied the blood pressure responses of over 100 subjects as they completed an 11-exercise Nautilus circuit. He noted a small increase in systolic blood pressure and a small decrease in diastolic blood pressure, a perfectly normal response to rigorous exercise. He concluded that sensible strength training does not have an adverse effect on blood pressure in healthy adults. Dr. Westcott warned, however, that maximum lifts, breath holding, isometric contractions and hand gripping can produce excessive blood pressure responses. Such activities should be avoided.

Researchers at Johns Hopkins University in Baltimore found that strength training can be a valuable method of lowering high blood pressure. They concluded that appropriate strength training is a very safe—but often neglected—mode of exercise for heart patients.

Myth: Strength Training Will Make You Look Like Arnold Schwarzenegger

This is a double-edged myth. Many younger men involved with bodybuilding desperately want to look like Schwarzenegger. They read his articles and books, adhere to his routines and eat his recommended foods and supplements. On the other hand, many older men do not want to look like Schwarzenegger. They find his muscularity unappealing, and they fear that strength training will overdevelop their muscles.

Both of these concepts are incorrect, and much of the reason centers around genetics. Genetics is an important factor in excelling in particular sports. For example, being tall improves your chance of being successful in professional basketball. For horse-racing jockeys, just the opposite is true. Your height can help or hurt you depending on the sport, but it's obvious that bouncing a basketball won't make you taller, nor will riding a horse make you shorter. Your height is primarily determined by genetics.

Champion bodybuilders are born with the genetic potential to develop excessively large muscles. Muscular potential, like height, can be judged quickly if you know what to look for. The length of your muscles—from the tendon attachment at one end to the tendon attachment at the other—is the most important factor in determining their potential size. The longer your muscles, the greater the cross-sectional area, and

thus the greater the volume your muscles can reach.

A long muscle presumes above-average size in that muscle. A short muscle implies that the muscle will be below average in size. Both extremes are rare. Having extremely long or short muscles exclusively throughout your entire body is seldom seen. Approximately one person in a million has such genes.

Schwarzenegger is one of those men. He has very long muscles throughout his entire body. Woody Allen, on the other hand, is an example of someone born with short muscles. Frame size is less important than muscle length in determining your ultimate muscular mass.

The majority of people have muscles that are neither long nor short, but average. Average-length muscles produce average-size muscles, even after years of training.

If you have long muscles, you're probably already stronger than other men your age—even if you've never trained. With properly applied strength training, your results will be significant and rapid. Gains in muscular size and strength will be several times faster for you than for the average trainee, whose gains will always be more difficult to produce.

How to Get Fit Fast

Ever wonder which exercise gives you the most bang for the buck? In a chapter from Covert Bailey's Smart Exercise *(Houghton Mifflin, 1994), he offers some interesting facts about how quickly certain exercises start providing benefits to your body.*

If you look at the following list of exercises and the number of minutes I suggest for each, you can see that you have to walk a long time to get the same benefits as you'd get from a short session of cross-country skiing. Why is that? Some people think that the difference comes from the amount of effort required. Not so. Even if walking is done with lots of effort and cross-country skiing is done with little effort, the difference is still seen. It's the amount of muscle involved in the exercise that matters.

How Long Should You Exercise?

Exercise	Minimum Time Required for Systemic Response (min.)
Walking	40
Bicycling, indoor	25
Bicycling, outdoor	20
Swimming	20
Jogging	15
Rowing	15
Cross-country skiing	12

When we walk on the level, our legs are almost straight, so little muscle is required to swing them. Walking is a good exercise, but you have to do it for a long time before your body feels the need to adapt to it. Biking, on the other hand, involves more muscle even though you're sitting. It requires the quadriceps, hamstrings and sometimes the abdominal muscles as you pull on the handlebar. Because it uses more muscle, more deeply, biking brings about a systemic response more quickly. After 20 to 25 minutes your body knows you've been exercising and responds with chemical changes in the heart, blood, bone and a host of other areas.

Jogging uses even more muscle. I laugh when I hear claims that walking and jogging are the same exercise. That's ridiculous. You need much more muscle to jog—for the added speed, for vertical movement (up-and-down bouncing), for deeper breathing, even for unconscious balance adjustment. There's no comparison between the effort needed to jog 15 minutes and the effort to walk 15 minutes. Don't let anyone tell you that they are the same. Jogging uses so much muscle that you don't have to do it long

to get a whole-body response from it.

Of course, you can make walking a harder exercise than jogging, can't you? Put a 50-pound pack on your back, then hike up Pikes Peak. Now you're using much more muscle. When people have joint problems from jogging, they can switch to backpack walking, hill walking, even to using ski pole–type walking sticks so that they're using enough extra musculature to get the same systemic improvement as in jogging, but with reduced trauma.

Cross-country skiing uses practically every muscle you have—arms, legs, back, thighs, buttocks, everything. In just 12 minutes your body says, "Wow! He's really exercising. I'd better make my muscles and organs healthier as fast as I can."

Swimming appears to be a multi-muscle activity, but, in fact, it is mostly an upper-body exercise. It uses the arms with their small muscles much more than the legs with their big muscles. In doing the crawl, you swing your legs much as you do when walking. There is little of the pumping you must do in running or cross-country skiing. Swimming is an excellent exercise, but you need to swim for at least 20 minutes to get systemic changes.

I've only touched on the common exercises. You may be wondering about inline skating, trampolining, stair climbing, step aerobics or something else. I could devote pages to each exercise, but it all boils down to this: How much muscle are you using? You can use a lot or a little muscle with something like a stair-climber. I've seen people on stair machines who look like they've invented a new tiptoe dance and others who really go at it. And the minutes listed for each form of exercise are only guidelines. If you have a way of walking that uses a lot of muscle—race walking, for instance—then you don't need to spend as much time doing it. Just remember my rule: "The more muscle you use, the less long you gotta do it!"

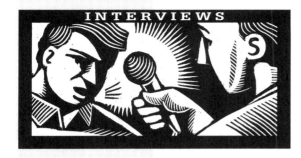

Louis Garcia on
Freestyle Jump Roping

If, during your daily channel surfing, you've noticed some agile young guy jumping rope like no-body's business, chances are that the man you saw was Louis Garcia. Considered by many to be the pre-eminent jump roper in the country, Garcia has been a jumping bean on everything from Coca-Cola commercials to Sports Channel fitness specials, demonstrating enviable deftness, speed and energy.

Garcia's more than a performer, though. He's a professional jump-roping athlete. He's also the creator and promoter of "FreeStyle Roping," a dynamic aerobic fitness program that anyone can do. Even you. So put down that remote and grab some rope. In this interview, Garcia tells you how to hop to it.

When most guys think of exercising, they're thinking heavy weights, big machines. What's so great about a jump rope?

You can use a jump rope for so many different things. It's a lot more versatile than any weights or machines. You can use it to warm up before weight training, you can use it as an aerobic exercise or you can use it as a drill to improve your hand-eye coordination or your performance in a specific sport.

For instance . . .

Well, basketball is a great example. Jumping rope improves the explosive power that you need in your legs for basketball. Spend some time with a jump rope, and pretty soon you'll notice that you're getting some altitude when you go up for those rebounds.

Is there any science to jumping rope, or is it pretty much like we remember from gym class?

First you have to have the right length of rope. Before you even start jumping, check the length. Put one foot on the middle of the rope and pull up on it. Both ends should be chest-high—right about where your armpits are. Once your skill level increases, you'll want to shorten your rope a few inches. A shorter rope will give you more speed and control. I recommend getting a rope that's adjustable, because you can shorten it without having to buy a new rope.

Once you have a rope that's the right length, hold the handles like you're shaking someone's hand. The emphasis should be on your thumb and index finger. You want to grab the handle where the rope and handle meet—not toward the end. Then keep your elbows in, not away from body.

Keep your shoulders down and relaxed. You don't want to lean too far forward or back. Keep your weight over the balls of your feet, knees slightly bent. This way, your legs are acting like shock absorbers. Don't land flat-footed. And don't jump too high—just a few inches off the ground, enough to clear the rope. A good visualization technique I tell people is to pretend they're jumping on a glass floor—that way you'll try to be lighter on your feet.

Finally, when you start jumping, you want to rotate the rope from your wrist, rather than swinging it. You're making a small, tight circle with your wrists using a slight amount of arm movement.

When you teach FreeStyle Roping, what do you focus on?

I use two techniques when I'm teaching. One is what I call neutral or resting moves. The other is a three-step breakdown. Neutral and resting moves are based on the idea that when you're a beginning jump roper, you can't jump over the rope continuously without getting tired and tripping up. You'll probably have to stop after a couple minutes. That's okay. That point in time is when you build in a neutral or resting move.

Basically, you turn the rope to the side of your body, either holding both handles in one hand or crossing one arm over your chest. So now you're not jumping inside the rope, you're turning it to the side of the body. This gives you a moment of less intense exercise, plus you don't have to concentrate on jumping over the rope. But the main advantage to these moves is that you're still jumping, you're still turning the rope, so you're keeping your heart rate up, which is important if you're jumping rope for aerobic training.

So FreeStyle Roping incorporates as much time doing neutral resting moves as it does jumping over the rope?

Well, it depends. But it's true that with FreeStyle Roping, we try to make it so that the time that you aren't jumping rope can be as much a benefit to your fitness as when you are.

We saw your exercise video _FreeStyle Roping: The Ultimate Jump-Rope Workout_ (available by calling 1-800-ROPE-132). In it, you go through an entire roping routine from the basics to advanced routines. Once you've picked out a rope for yourself, what's the best way to ease into a roping routine?

For a start, when you're learning any new jump—or you're just getting back into the practice of jump roping—use what I call the three-step breakdown. First, practice the foot and arm movements of whatever jump you're doing—only don't use the rope. This will help you build basic coordination without having to worry

about tripping on the rope. Step two, do the same jump, only this time turn the rope at your side—it's like the neutral or resting moves I was talking about. Finally, when you're used to the motions, the third step is to do the jump over the rope.

Give us some basic jumps to work with.

Well, the simplest one is the basic two-foot jump, which we all know. From there, you can do classic jumps like a boxer shuffle: You jump, land on the ball of the back foot and extend your front foot out so your heel touches the floor. Then switch legs. There's also a basic run—it's just like jogging in place, only now you're using a jump rope. From there you can go to more elaborate moves, where you cross your feet, cross the rope in mid-turn, step out to the side and back—there are hundreds of variations.

Does it matter in what order you do these?

Not at all. Do them in any order. Throw in new ones or make some up. Switch to resting moves when you get tired or think you're going to miss. The important thing is to take your time and have fun.

Carlos DeJesus on
Faster, Better Workouts

Carlos DeJesus doesn't believe in doing things twice—especially when he exercises. The champion bodybuilder turned personal trainer imparts this philosophy to his clients—many of them busy guys like you who don't have a lot of time for a workout.

You don't need a lot of time, he says. All you need is a plan. His plan. He outlined it for us, along with some other pet fitness theories of his—including how failure can be a good thing.

A lot of trainers adhere to a very strict recipe for building muscle—the old three-set, 12-rep formula. But you don't, do you?

Not really, no. I'm a bit different from many of my fellow trainers. I advocate doing one set for each exercise. Not three sets, just one set. But what a set. It seems to really work for my clients.

We're not surprised. In a study at the University of Florida's Center for Exercise Science in Gainesville, volunteers who did only one set of leg extensions showed strength gains similar to those who did a full three sets.

I'm not saying kill yourself, of course. That one set should be 8 to 12 slow reps of a heavy weight, somewhere at the upper end of your max.

How did you come to advocate this format of exercise?

My clients, my own observations. You hear guys all the time saying, "I just don't have enough time during the week to do all those exercises." Think about it—three sets of 12 reps of 10 to 12 exercises. That takes up a lot of time. On the other hand, doing a single set will cut your time by more than half. You could be out of the gym in a half-hour.

But you don't consider this a corner-cutting routine?

Not at all. Cutting corners can be dangerous. There are some things you don't want to cut out of your workout. One thing is a proper five- to ten-minute warm-up. Here's the scenario. You walk into the gym, do a warm-up that's going to get your arms and legs moving. I like the ergometer—that's the device that you pedal like a bike, and it has rowing arms that you push and pull. So pedal with your feet and move your arms for five minutes. You can use the stair-climbing machine, but don't hold onto the rails—swing your arms as you step.

The idea here is that you want to warm up the larger muscles—back, arms, chest and legs. Those are the largest muscles, so warming those up will warm your body up faster than anything else.

What's next?

Next is a few minutes of stretching and limbering up. Avoid bouncing stretches. Do this once your muscles are warmed up—you don't want to stretch a cold muscle. Do some leg stretches and some forward bends (toe touching). Then, since you're going to be doing lifts like bench presses, do elbow circles. Put your hands on your shoulders and rotate your elbows in each direction ten times.

Once again, these are things you don't want to cut out of your workout for the sake of time. Don't—I repeat—do not cut these out of your workout. That's how you get hurt. Where you make up the time is in the weight training.

How do we start? Just go in there and start lifting the heaviest weight we can?

No. Starting out, you want to err on the side of caution. For the first week or so, I say do a much lighter weight than you know you can handle—it's better to start light.

Give us an idea of the program you put your clients through.

Actually, I have two programs—A and B. In both programs, you do legs first. Legs have the largest muscles, and you want to progress from largest to smallest. Here's what you do for program A.

Leg extensions, 8 to 12 reps, one set. That's with a moderate weight. Now do leg curls, because you want to work the hamstrings. This gives your upper leg a balanced workout. Now we focus on the lower leg. Do standing calf raises. And that's it for legs.

Now we move on to the bench press. We do 8 to 12 reps, one set. Now that we've done a pushing exercise, we do a pulling exercise. So do lat pulldowns. Then the overhead press or the seated press. For these, you should do as many reps as you can to failure.

You do it until you fail?

For the general public, let's define what failure means. Failure doesn't mean that you're not a success at exercise. It means that your muscles won't move anymore and you've done all that you can do. That's why I'm saying—and I've seen the scientific evidence to back it up—that one set is as good as three sets, if you work the muscles to exhaustion on that one set. Once you get past the first week—where you're learning your limits and learning your way around the gym—you will always be working your muscles to failure on that one set.

Okay. Give us the rest of the workout.

Now you're doing the arms. Do standard barbell curls for your biceps. After biceps, do triceps extensions. Then shoulder shrugs—that way you work all the major muscle groups.

Finally, do your abs last. If you don't, you rob your torso of what we call a girdle of strength, which your abs provide. A lot of people like to warm up by doing a lot of sit-ups first. If you do that, then you've weakened your middle. So if you should then do, say, an overhead press, you might not have the strength to stabilize your body. It can lead to an injury.

You've mentioned that the way to work the muscles to total failure is to make sure that you do slow reps. How do you know how slow to go?

Use a rep protocol. I have a metronome in my studio, like piano players use. I set it on 60 beats per minute. I have people lift in rhythm to the metronome. You can do it, too, and you don't necessarily need a metronome. The trick is to do the lift through a count of six. You do a count of four on the positive movement—the part of the exercise where you're pushing or exerting. You do a count of two seconds on the negative phase of the lift, when the weight's coming back to you. And breathe on demand. Don't breathe in time to the metronome or hold your breath—this is a six-second lift. You need to breathe through it.

What's the benefit of lifting slowly?

You may be lifting slowly, but you make fast strength gains. You'll gain more strength because you're contracting slowly throughout the entire movement, fully working all the muscle fibers. You'll notice the difference between a slow lift and a fast one where your momentum and speed are helping you do the lift. The slow ones are more intense. With a slow lift, you'll really feel the burn. Try it, you'll see.

Okay, that's program A. What's program B?

It's the same principle, but you vary the exercises. You want your body to be doing all different kinds of exercises. It makes for a more well-rounded workout, and you won't be as bored. Here's all you do.

Squats

Dead lifts

Seated calf raises

Dips

Barbell rows or seated rows

Upright rows

Dumbbell curls, seated, arms at sides

Triceps, overhead extension—holding one dumbbell with two hands

Wide-grip shoulder shrug, reversed

Leg raise for abs

Can you alternate these programs during the week?

Absolutely. Do program A Monday, some aerobic circuit work on Wednesday—whatever you like. Then do program B on Friday.

Sounds simple. Any other strategies you can suggest?

Well, once you've been working out for a while, chances are that you're going to hit a plateau, where your strength gains just seem to level out. This is a problem for a lot of men. How I suggest getting past it is by doing rep inroads.

Here's how you do it. When you start your workout, start it at 50 percent of max. Do three to five reps, then go up ten pounds and do one rep; go up ten pounds, do another rep. Keep doing this, ten pounds and one rep at a time, increasing the weight with each rep. Do this until you're lifting as much weight as you can lift for one good rep with good form. Do that with each exercise you do.

Another example of a rep inroad is a little more complex. Let's say that the exercise you're doing is the leg extension and your max is 150 pounds. With this inroad you take 80 percent of that weight—120 pounds—and do as many reps as you can with 80 percent. Plus or minus 1 rep on either side of that number is your rep range. If you can do 10 reps, your rep range is 9 to 11.

So now when you work out, you lift 120 pounds and do 9 reps. When that becomes easy, do 10 reps. When that becomes easy, do 11. When you get to 11 reps and you can lift comfortably, you increase the weight you're lifting by 5 percent or 5 pounds—whichever is less. A lot of people use a variation of this rep inroad. Keep track of your progress on a chart, because each muscle group is going to have a different weight, different rep range and different rate of improvement. It can be hard to keep track of without a chart. Write it down.

Any final words of motivation?

Keep a positive mind-set. So much of your success in weight training depends on getting yourself in the frame of mind that you can do this. I have a saying: Whether you think you can or whether you think you can't, you're always right. So you might as well think that you can.

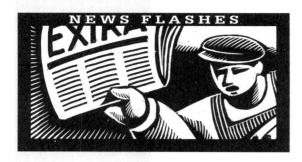

Treadmills Rate Well against Other Exercise Machines

MILWAUKEE—Treadmills burned more calories than five other popular exercise machines tested by researchers at the Medical College of Wisconsin and the Clement J. Zablocki Veterans Affairs Medical Center, both in Milwaukee.

The study of the equipment involved 13 healthy young-adult volunteers and compared six commonly used indoor aerobic exercise machines. The goal was to determine which machines burned the most calories at different exercise intensity levels, from "fairly light" to "hard." The machines included a stationary exercise bicycle with handlebars that are pulled and pushed, a cross-country ski machine, a regular stationary exercise bicycle, a rowing machine, a stair-climber and a treadmill.

Of these machines, the researchers found that, when it comes to burning calories and raising the heart rate, the treadmill provided the most effective workout.

On average, the researchers determined that when the participants were working on a treadmill at a "somewhat hard" exercise level, they burned approximately 700 calories per hour. In contrast, the average participant working at the same level of exertion on the regular stationary bicycle burned less than 500 calories per hour. Put differently, 40 percent more calories can be burned by walking/running on a treadmill than by cycling on a regular exercise bike.

Exercise Order Does Make a Difference

LOS ANGELES—Aerobic workouts may be less effective if done after—rather than before—a weight-training session, according to a study conducted at California State University, Los Angeles.

Researchers at the school studied 11 men in their twenties to determine what effect a 50-minute weight-training workout might have on subsequent aerobic exercise. Each man was tested during aerobic workouts that were performed both fresh and following a weight-training session.

The results: When subjects lifted weights prior to aerobic exercise, some physiological parameters such as heart rate, perceived rate of exertion and blood pressure were all significantly affected at some point during the aerobic portion of the workout. What these results mean in practical terms is that when you want to do both resistance and aerobic exercise, but the aerobic portion is more important to you, it is probably better to do the aerobic workout first and then follow it with the weight training. Or alternate the days you do your aerobic exercise and your weight training.

Exercise Blood Pressure Readings More Accurately Predict Heart Trouble

OSLO, Norway—Blood pressure readings taken during exercise more accurately predict heart attacks than resting blood pressure, Norwegian researchers at Oslo's Ullevaal University Hospital have concluded.

Nearly 2,000 apparently healthy men ages 40 to 59 were studied to determine whether a rise in systolic blood pressure (the top number) during a period of stationary exercise cycling could predict nonfatal and fatal heart attacks more accurately than a blood pressure reading taken after five minutes of rest. Tests demonstrated that while 520 of the participants had mildly elevated resting systolic blood pressures of 140, 304 of these men showed increased systolic readings of 200 or higher during six minutes of strenuous cycling.

Ultimately, the 304 participants who demonstrated the sharp increase in systolic blood pressure during exercise had twice the rate of heart attacks (18.8 percent versus 9.5 percent) compared to the 1,294 subjects with resting pressures below 140 and exercise pressures below 200. This group also had a much higher cardiovascular death rate than the rest of the subjects. As many as 58 percent of those who had a heart attack in this group died, compared to 33 percent for all of the other subjects.

So for apparently healthy men, an early rise in systolic blood pressure during exercise is a danger signal for future heart trouble.

Leisure-Time Activities May Postpone Death

TAMPERE, Finland—Middle-age men who are active during leisure time have a much lower risk of premature death than men who are sedentary during their free time, Finnish researchers announced.

After following more than 1,000 middle-age men for almost 11 years, researchers found that the men who burned less than 800 calories per week in leisure-time physical activities had an increased risk of 2.74 times for all-cause premature death and an increased risk of 3.58 times for cardiovascular death, compared to those men who burned at least 2,100 calories per week during their leisure time.

One of the purposes of the study was to determine the type and intensity of physical activity necessary to reduce the chances of dying prema-

turely. The study included 16 types of activities, along with some specified daily chores, in its definition of leisure-time physical activity. The results showed that while some of the most strenuous activities demonstrated the strongest decreased risk of death, many of the moderately intense activities such as gardening and repair work were also strongly associated with the decreased risk of death.

The study suggests that when it comes to maintaining cardiovascular health, it is more important to consider the total energy expended during leisure-time activity rather than the intensity of the activity.

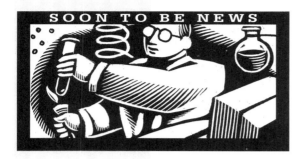

Will Wakeboarding Catch On?

Wakeboarding—best described as a cross between snowboarding and waterskiing—might be emerging as the next big water sport. Wakeboarders get pulled by a boat while standing on a board that is just a tad over four feet in length, made of molded fiberglass and fitted with rubber bindings on the top and a small fin under each tip. The board's fins give the wakeboarder the ability to accelerate. So even more than trick waterskiing, wakeboarding is known for its spectacular airborne acrobatics performed off the boat's wake.

More and more companies are manufacturing and selling the boards. The number of boards sold in 1996 greatly exceeded the 95,000 boards sold in 1995. Some attribute wakeboarding's notable initial success to its similarities with other more established "adrenaline" sports that push athletes to new and extreme levels of competition. *With an expanding pro tour and its inclusion in ESPN's Extreme Games in 1996, wakeboarding is moving from fad stage to being a firmly established sport.*

Is "Crew" Aerobics Coming to Your Gym?

For those who participate in aerobics classes because they let you exercise (and complain about exercising) as part of a group, here's a new alternative: aerobic crew classes.

The new style of aerobics class is similar to another recent trend—spinning classes. In these, a group of exercise cyclists pedal at various speeds and intensities as an instructor shouts commands and loud music urges you onward. Spinning classes were perhaps the first real group alternative to the traditional aerobics classes offered at health clubs.

The new crewing classes will look a lot like spinning classes, with the biggest difference being the substitution of rowing for cycling. The rowing machines would most likely be set in a circle, and an instructor would guide you through a high-energy workout. The program might start with a basic review of rowing techniques and a briefing on the rowing machine settings and then move on to include interval training, distance work, sprinting or power rowing. Since rowing gives both the lower and upper body a great workout, the new crewing classes may have an edge on the spinning workouts. *Crewing classes have begun showing up in big-city gyms and should be on their way soon to a health club near you.*

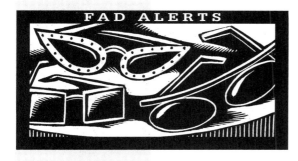

Sports Performance Bars

 If you think that sports performance bars are the best way to give your body the carbohydrates it craves for a workout, then chew on this: You can get just as many or more carbs from foods like fig bars, low-fat granola bars or bananas as you can from the average sports bar. But what a difference: The average granola bar costs about 30 cents, compared with the two- and three-dollar performance bars.

Does that mean that you should throw away your Powerbars and start foraging for Fig Newtons?

Not at all, says Nancy Clark, R.D., author of *Nancy Clark's Sports Nutrition Guidebook.* "Don't get me wrong. I'm not saying that sports bars are bad," says Clark. "The sports bars are a convenient and fashionable way to fuel up—but you pay a premium price for that convenience." Here's how the sports bars compare.

Bar	Calories	Carbs (g)	Protein (g)	Fat (g)
Powerbar	230	45	10	2.5
Clif Bar	250	52	5	2
PR Bar	190	19	14	6
Met-Rx	320	68	16	5
Granola bar	109	16	2.4	4.2
Fig bar	200	42	2.2	3
Banana	105	27	1	0.6
Bagel	163	31	6	1

Knee-Injury Repairs

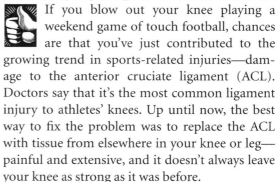 If you blow out your knee playing a weekend game of touch football, chances are that you've just contributed to the growing trend in sports-related injuries—damage to the anterior cruciate ligament (ACL). Doctors say that it's the most common ligament injury to athletes' knees. Up until now, the best way to fix the problem was to replace the ACL with tissue from elsewhere in your knee or leg— painful and extensive, and it doesn't always leave your knee as strong as it was before.

Now, researchers say that they've discovered a method that may help injured knees "grow" new ligaments. Instead of using your own tissue, doctors could do what's called a collagen allograft—rebuilding your ACL with raw material from the outer portion of bones. The collagen allograft would grow into a ligament-like structure that acts more like the ACL you blew out. If the procedure is approved, patients would stand a better chance of regaining almost full knee flexibility. This method of processing avoids the dangers of tissue rejection that can crop up using current methods, says Douglas W. Jackson, M.D., medical director of the Orthopaedic Research Institute in Long Beach, California.

Don't go asking for this collagen allograft just yet. Dr. Jackson stresses that the procedure is still in the experimental phase. But once the research is completed, Dr. Jackson expects that more men will be asking for his allograft.

For more on knee-injury trends, see our interview with Edward Laskowski, M.D., co-director of the Mayo Clinic Sports Medicine Center on page 195.

Chewing Tobacco

For years, baseball players have sworn that the nicotine hit from chewing tobacco and snuff gives them an extra edge in the game. Researchers at the University of Washington School of Dentistry in Seattle have given them something new to chew on. They found that using smokeless tobacco doesn't improve your game one bit.

After reviewing the batting and fielding averages of 158 professional baseball players, researchers saw that players who used smokeless tobacco didn't play any better than the guys who favored a nice, pink wad of bubble gum. The study found that players who chewed tobacco did have an edge in one dangerous respect—they had far more instances of precancerous oral lesions and receding gums.

Wet Suits for Swimmers

 If you've ever watched a triathlon or competed in one, you may have started to notice a few folks dressing like Navy SEALs. There's a scientific reason for that.

In a study of competitive swimmers, experts found that wearing a wet suit improved performance in less efficient swimmers. According to the study, the smooth surface of a neoprene wet suit can reduce drag by as much as 14 percent.

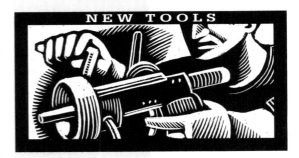

NEW TOOLS

Better Breathing

Breathe Right Nasal Strips

Do those late-season allergies have you more congested than a rush-hour expressway? Instead of medicating yourself with stupor-inducing decongestants, slap a Breathe Right on the bridge of your nose. Praised by pro athletes as a drug-free method of improving breathing and increasing oxygen flow, the Breathe Right strips have earned approval from the Food and Drug Administration as an effective treatment for nasal congestion. The strips, which come in three sizes, adhere to the bridge of the nose. When you bend the Breathe Right to fit your nose, a plastic strip inside the product springs back; the tension in the strip pulls your nasal passages open slightly, making breathing easier. $5 to $7 for a package of ten.

Safer Roughhousing

EZ Gard Shock Doctor

If you're planning a Saturday morning of high-impact football with the guys, make sure that the doctor is in. The Shock Doctor, that is. Touted as the most protective mouth guard on the market, it's also one of the comfiest. In tests, the Shock Doctor scored an 8 out of 10 on the energy absorption scale—the measure of how much punishment a mouth guard will soak up when you get hit. High-impact plastic cushions not only feel better than the old boil-'n'-bite mouthpieces from our younger days but also protect better against jaw fractures, chipped teeth and other head and mouth injuries. Plus, the manufacturer puts its money where your mouth is—Shock Doctor comes with a $7,500 dental warranty. Available at most sporting goods stores, the Shock Doctor can be purchased with or without a convenient strap so that you can let it hang around your neck while you're on the sidelines. $20.

Better Aerobic Workouts

Reebok Sky Walker

The Force will be with you in the Reebok Sky Walker, one of a number of all-body aerobic machines hitting clubs and gyms across the country. Unlike other aerobic machines, such as stair-climbers and stationary cycles, the Sky Walker works both upper and lower body at the same time. Four rods—two for the arms, two for the legs—swing in pendulum fashion on a platform. Adjust the hand grips and foot pads and step in. It feels—a bit awkwardly at first—like you're walking on air. That can be an advantage if you're prone to lower-leg troubles: The smooth arc of the rods takes unwanted pressure off knees and ankles. A console control allows you to set positive and negative resistance. $3,995.

Higher-Accuracy Free-Throw Shooting

Advanced Sports Concepts Big Ball

Improving your free-throw average just got a lot easier, thanks to the Big Ball. As the name suggests, this ball is big—approximately two inches larger than the average basketball, although it weighs about the same.

Practicing with the Big Ball forces you to shoot for the center of the basket, otherwise you'll hit the rim. Spend enough time shooting with this ball, then switch to a smaller regulation ball, and you'll notice a serious improvement in your accuracy. Evidently, college and professional players are noticing it, too—NBA and National Collegiate Athletic Association teams have started training with it. It's available at most sporting goods stores. $60.

Easier Weight Lifting

Manta Ray

We all know that barbell squats are a great muscle-building exercise, especially for legs. The problem is that squats are also especially hard on the neck, shoulders and upper back. That unyielding steel bar digging into your flesh can be an inconvenience—even an injury-causing problem.

Unless you're using the Manta Ray, a molded plastic device that snaps onto the barbell and fits over your shoulders and back. The smooth plastic spreads the weight evenly across your shoulders, and keeps pressure from building up on any one spot, such as the back of your neck. More comfortable than a rolled-up towel and safer than a foam pad (the Manta Ray has a raised lip that keeps the barbell from rolling off your back), the Manta Ray is great for any exercise where you're holding the bar across your shoulders. Call 1-800-258-8516 to order. $45.

Smoother Skiing

K2 Four Super-Sidecut Skis

It had to happen. In an age where onboard computers guide our cars and smart bombs are the terror of foreign despots, it was only a matter of time before electronic brains made their way into our sporting equipment. Case in point: the K2 Four, touted as the world's first "smart" skis.

The brain in these skis is a piezoelectric device that detects unwanted vibrations in the skis and then converts it into electrical energy, which is used to smooth out the vibrations so that the skier can maintain a smoother ride and greater control over his run. Because of these control features, the Four is slightly shorter than most skis, which also improves maneuverability. $650.

Safer Biking

Trek Lunar

You know you're supposed to wear protective headgear when you go bicycling. But most bike helmets make you look like the Human Cannonball. You want something that says you're fast, sleek and cool. Not something that makes you look like a guy who has to wear a goofy bowl on his head.

In which case, you need to check out bicycle helmets like the Trek Lunar. A new sleek visor and flashy colors make you look like a superhero, not a mild-mannered cyclist. Vents in the top and sides keep your head cool, while super-tough construction keeps your bean safe. $39.

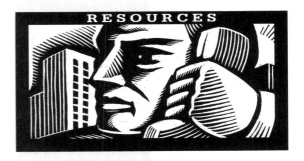

RESOURCES

Sports

Do It Sports
http://www.doitsports.com

A fitness fanatic was sitting at his kitchen table after a long bike ride, bemoaning to his friend about how hard it is to register for 10-K races and other competitions. The idea emerged: create a Web site where you could register for any public sporting event anywhere in the country, straight from your computer. And so was another Web site born. The site offers particulars on sporting events, races and tours, and lets you apply to many. The site also provides the average weekend warrior with information on any of a number of outdoor sports, including running, bike touring, mountain biking, in-line skating, rock climbing and various paddle sports.

Running

Runner's World Online
http://www.runnersworld.com

Run, don't walk, to this site if you are at all interested in running. Whether you run for fun, fitness or competition, *Runner's World* Online, which is brought to you by the world's leading running magazine, *Runner's World*, will provide you with the latest running information available. Here you can check out the Shoe Buyer's Guide to learn about which shoes might fit your running needs best. You can also get nutrition and training advice from experts and find out about the latest top-notch running products. If you are just starting a running program, the site has a spot devoted to beginning runners that gives you tips on how to get started.

Adventure Hiking

Merrell Hiking Center

http://www.merrellboot.com

No matter what your experience level is, this is a great site for anyone interested in hiking. The Merrell Hiking Center's Web site provides information on regional routes, hiking tours and self-guided adventure trails. The site, operated by Merrell Footwear, also gives briefs on about a dozen Merrell Hiking Centers, where you can rent or buy boots and other gear for day hikes.

Golfing

United States Golf Association

Home Page

http://www.usga.org

Golfers can have a field day visiting this site. The United States Golf Association's (USGA) Home Page offers answers to questions about its official rules and regulations, provides information on how to use the USGA Handicap System and gives golfing tips. You can also check out a catalog of golfing clothing and gear. On top of all that, go ahead and order tickets to the U.S. Open, start a USGA membership or just visit the site to view its elaborate graphics.

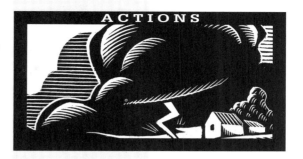

Looking for some new strategies for getting or staying fit? Here are 20 easy options, based on recent research and new findings by doctors and exercise specialists.

1. **Drink more water.** Yes, health experts have drowned you with their entreaties to drink more water, so just consider this another drop in the bucket. In its latest statement on the benefits of exercise and drinking fluids, the American College of Sports Medicine in Indianapolis says that drinking fluids before, during and after exercise will vastly improve your performance in that activity. Prehydrating—with either water or a sports beverage—helps maintain your normal body temperature, while keeping your heart rate low. The college suggests that athletes drink at least two eight-ounce cups of fluid about two hours before exercising. If you're participating in an endurance event—something that lasts longer than an hour—the college recommends drinking two to four eight-ounce cups of a sports beverage with carbohydrates in it for every hour of activity.

2. **Stay away from smokers.** Never mind that hanging around smokers will increase your risk of getting heart disease and cancer. Now some doctors are saying that exposure to secondhand smoke can severely limit your ability to exercise. According to Stan Glantz, Ph.D., a physiologist at the University of California, San Francisco, men exposed to secondhand smoke got exhausted faster during a run on a treadmill.

After the exercise, their heart rates took longer to get back to normal, too.

3. **Work out with your wife.** Can't seem to stick to that fitness routine? Next time you go to the gym, invite your wife along. Researchers at Indiana University in Bloomington concluded that married couples who exercised together are much more likely to stick to a regular exercise regimen than married people who exercised without a spouse. In the study, the couples had a higher regular attendance rate at the club. Moreover, only 6 percent of the couples dropped out of their routine. Married people working out alone had a 43 percent dropout rate.

4. **Get a tennis lesson.** Michael Dake, M.D., chief of cardiovascular and interventional radiology at Stanford University, says that snapping your arms or wrists during a throw or swing can cause a blood clot in your shoulder. The injury is more common in athletes who use snapping motions routinely, such as pitchers or martial artists. But the condition also crops up in amateur athletes who may not have learned the proper technique for handling the racket or bat in their favorite sports. The clot isn't life-threatening, but it can cause finger numbness and lead to more serious circulatory problems in the arm. Dr. Dake says that a simple surgical procedure can remove the clot, but you're better off learning how to swing right in the first place.

5. **Walk it off.** Injuries to the Achilles tendon of your heel are one of the most common sports injuries around—and also one of the hardest to heal. First, a surgeon has to repair the tendon, which connects your heel to your calf muscles. Then, typically, sufferers have to spend three months in a cast until their heel heals. Now researchers in this study are saying that you may be better off without the cast. In a study presented at the American Orthopaedic Foot and Ankle Society, researchers found that Achilles tendon injuries heal faster if they aren't immobilized for extended periods of time. By subjecting the ankle to rehabilitation exercises shortly after surgery, patients will develop a stronger tendon and greater mobility than if they leave the cast on.

6. **Sink that putt.** It's the eighteenth hole, it's a 12-foot putt, it's a round of drinks and your self-esteem on the line as you set up for your putt. Suddenly, your muscles seize up and you whack the ball past the hole and into the sand trap. Yes, it's the "yips," golf's very own version of performance anxiety. What is the best way to sink the yips? Focus on another part of your game, says Randy Myers, fitness director of the Professional Golf Association National Resort and Spa in Palm Beach, Florida. "Focus on improving another aspect of your game—driving more consistently, for example. Not only will this take your mind off the problem, but you may also find that you'll start getting the ball closer to the hole, and you won't have to putt as far anyway," says Myers.

7. **Try it on for size.** Many home gyms don't follow what champion bodybuilder and fitness trainer Carlos DeJesus defines as a natural range of motion. "There's one model I'm thinking of with this design—a bar coming outward, then a bar going across, forming a T. You face the machine, grab the bar and do a curl," says DeJesus. The problem is that you're arcing toward you and the bar is arcing away, toward the machine. That's not a natural motion. If it were a real barbell, it would arc in the same direction as you're curling, he adds. As it is, some of these machines can injure the joints in your arms, shoulders or back. Before you order or buy, make sure that the home gym has a no-questions-asked refund policy.

8. **Go easy on the leg machines.** Leg extension and leg curl machines—they're standards of circuit training and the mainstays of many gyms. Don't make them the mainstay of your leg-exercise routine, though.

"We'd like to see people do other leg exercises," says Tom Jackson, physical therapist with ARC Physical Therapy in Anaheim, California. "They don't really follow any motion that you would do in real life." Plus, given the amount of knee problems people have reported in conjunction with these exercises—especially leg extensions—Jackson says that they're just not worth the trouble. "To work those muscles, you're far better off with squats and lunges," he says.

9. **Make your arms stronger.** If you really want to build the arms—biceps and triceps—the best exercises are isolation exercises, says Jeffrey Stout, Ph.D., assistant professor of exercise physiology at Creighton University in Omaha, Nebraska.

"The idea is to do an exercise with one arm—say, a dumbbell curl—until the arm completely fatigues," says Dr. Stout. "Once that happens, you can use your other arm to assist and do three to five more reps. If you want your arms to grow, you have to push them to total exhaustion." Dr. Stout says that since he started doing more isolation exercises, he's gained an average of one inch on his arms each year.

10. **Exercise in the late afternoon.** If you can manage to hit the gym between 4:00 and 5:00 P.M., you'll be delightfully surprised to find that you have energy and power you didn't know you possessed. Why? A simple matter of biological rhythms, says Phyllis Zee, M.D., Ph.D., director of the sleep disorders program at Northwestern University Medical School in Chicago and an expert on biological rhythms.

"We call this time of day the power hour," says Dr. Zee. Why isn't entirely clear, but Dr. Zee says that various functions in the body governing awareness and physical strength seem to converge at this time. Studies have shown that athletes perform better at this time of day than any other. Maybe you can, too.

11. **Sharpen your "sports vision."** To track a moving object better—such as the golf ball you just launched or the clay pigeon that's whirling toward the horizon—do exercises to improve your visual acuity. Paul Planer, a doctor of optometry, optometrist and author of *The Sports Vision Manual*, suggests writing numbers and letters on an old softball and playing catch with a pal. Each time the ball flies toward you, call out the last number or letter you see before you catch it. Doing such exercises helps you focus sharper, faster.

12. **Do push-ups on your knuckles.** Sure, it sounds hard, but it actually saves you from serious wear and tear. "Push-ups place enormous pressure on hands and wrists, since they're bearing most of your weight during the exercise," says James J. Pedicano, M.D., a wrist and hand surgeon in Ridgewood, New Jersey.

So knuckle under. "By making a fist, you're straightening out the line of your hand and arm—and the force won't get channeled into that delicate point on the wrist," says Dr. Pedicano. Of course, you should place those knuckles on an exercise mat, not bare floor. Even more effective: Put two dumbbells on the floor (the octagonal kind, which won't roll) and grip them like parallel bars. "You get a better range of motion and virtually eliminate joint problems that way," says Dr. Pedicano.

13. **Change your shoes.** Even if they look brand-spanking-new, once you've logged over 100 hours of use on those cross-trainers, consider buying a new pair. "No matter how good they look, after 100 hours of use, cushioning and various support material—things you can't see—are going to be broken down and compressed from all those hours of use," says Tom Brunick, director of the Athlete's Foot Wear Test Center at North Central College in Naperville, Illinois, and a technical editor for *Runner's World* magazine. Continue to use an old, flawed shoe and you could risk injuring the joints in your lower legs and feet. "Shoes weren't meant to last a lifetime," says Brunick.

14. **Skate like a hunchback.** So you want to give in-line skating a shot? Here's a tip to keep you from falling over every ten seconds or so, courtesy of Joel Rappelfeld, in-line skating instructor and author of *The Complete Blader.* "Whenever you start to feel off-balance, just go to your stable position," he says. When you're on skates, that means leaning forward with your hands on your knees. Any time you feel like you're about to keel over, Rappelfeld says that going immediately to this position restabilizes you. Best of all, you won't look stupid doing it. If you do take a tumble, fall on your plastic protective gear.

15. **Lift it nice and slow.** When you're pumping out those bench presses, pay attention to proper form. "Do the lift slowly—especially any presses," says Allen Kinley, assistant strength and training coach at Texas A&M University in College Station. Not only does this work the muscles more fully, but it will also likely prevent you from doing the barbell bounce. Kinley says a lot of men try to use the momentum of rapid reps to get through a set—what they end up doing is bouncing the barbell off their chests. "It's a good way to break your sternum—or at least get a heck of a bruise," he says.

16. **Use the granny gear.** When you're out on your bicycle and you're trying to crank up a hill, don't be afraid to shift up to that largest back gear, also known as the granny gear.

"I think the name makes guys shy away from it. But it's there for a reason—to make your life easier. Go ahead and use it," says Don Cuerdon, senior editor for *Mountain Bike* magazine. As you climb, lean forward, almost putting your chest to the handlebars. This will also make your climb easier.

17. **Watch your eats.** If you follow a regular fitness routine, it's okay to reward yourself once in a while with a beer or a burger after a workout. But try to keep your postexercise meals especially high in carbohydrates and low in fats. Carbohydrates are better for refueling for your next workout, says Cheryl Hartsough, R.D., a dietitian at the Professional Golf Association National Resort and Spa in Palm Beach, Florida. In one study of postworkout fueling, when given high-fat food choices, men ate so much fat that they canceled out the benefits of their workouts. When given high-carbohydrate food choices, the men ate their fill with calories to spare.

18. **Take shorter rests.** When you're weight training, it's not uncommon to rest two to three minutes between sets. Don't. If you want bigger muscles, shorten your rest to 1 to 1½ minutes. This strategy is more likely to completely fatigue your muscles and thus promote better muscle growth, according to strength-conditioning expert Tom Baechle, Ed.D., professor and chairman of the exercise science department at Creighton University in Omaha, Nebraska.

19. **Add a mile a year.** As you get older, no matter how much exercising you do, it's inevitable that you're going to gain a little weight. Or is it? According to the National Runners Health Study, increasing your weekly mileage by about 1½ miles each year should be enough to help you keep the waistline of your youth, says Paul Williams, Ph.D., principal investigator of the National Runners Health Study at Lawrence Berkeley National Laboratory in Berkeley, California.

20. **Protect your ankles.** If your favorite sports involve running and basketball, consider keeping your ankles under wraps. In a study of basketball players, researchers found that wearing canvas or leather ankle braces prevented sprains without hindering performance.

2

EATING

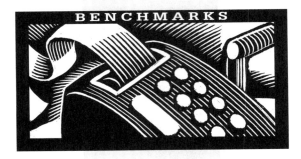

AVERAGES

■ Percentage of men who say they really enjoy cooking: 31

■ Amount of food a 160-pound man will eat during his lifetime: about 45 tons

■ Number of times men eat out per week: 4.3

■ Number of Americans who eat Spam regularly: 60 million

■ Percentage of American workers who eat lunch at their desks: 49

■ Amount of chips, pretzels, cheese puffs and other salty snacks that the average American eats annually: 22 pounds

■ Percentage of Americans who prefer milk chocolate over dark chocolate: 71

■ Amount of ice cream an American eats annually: 13 quarts

■ Number of Americans who died in 1994 of acute food poisoning: 9,100

■ Percentage of American adults under 35 who have eaten pizza for breakfast: 75

■ Percentage of Americans over 55 who have eaten pizza for breakfast: 25

■ Percentage of Americans who skip breakfast: 10

EXTREMES

■ Biggest burrito: 3,960 pounds of eggs, refried beans, cheese, tomatoes, lettuce and salsa wrapped in a 3,055.4-foot-long tortilla

■ Hottest spice: the red "Savina" habanero, belonging to the genus *Capsicum*; one dried gram of this spice is able to produce detectable "heat" in 719 pounds of bland sauce

■ Most expensive glass of wine: $1,447 for the first glass of Beaujolais Nouveau 1993

■ Number of Hostess Twinkies consumed in the United States every year: more than 500 million

Another Look at Salt

Long hailed as heart-helping, low-salt diets may actually decrease your energy, blur your thinking and leave you at increased risk for a heart attack.

Sure, you watch what you eat, avoid fast food and overly processed foods and reach for anything with "low sodium" on the label. Then why do you feel so tired all the time? It may be because you've been duped by the media and by members of the medical profession. Oh, the intentions have been good, but new research suggests that the information may have been seriously flawed. For nine out of ten men, a low-salt diet might actually leave you more vulnerable to a heart attack and create symptoms such as foggy thinking, fatigue, fainting spells and difficulty exercising.

According to a recent study, men who maintained a low-salt diet (less than 2,000 milligrams a day) had four times as many heart attacks as those who ate three times as much salt.

In an unrelated study, researchers found that low-salt diets may be at the root of extreme fatigue. In 96 percent of the chronic-fatigue sufferers studied, researchers noted a blood pressure control difficulty called neurally mediated hypotension (NMH), which is known to be exacerbated by a lack of dietary salt. In fact, 61 percent of those studied reported avoiding salt on a regular basis.

In light of this new evidence, which is undoubtedly the tip of a large iceberg, how did our culture go from one that valued salt highly (heck, it used to be used as money) to one that despises it? About 15 years ago, researchers found that in about one out of ten men (those known as salt-sensitive), cutting salt intake drastically could translate into a 2 mmHg (millimeters of mercury) drop in blood pressure.

When scientists who study whole populations plugged those numbers into equations linking blood pressure levels with overall mortality, the equations predicted that thousands of lives would be saved. Hence, the American Heart Association's recommendation that "it is prudent for most people to restrict their intake of salt in case they are salt-sensitive." Not only does it seem strange to issue a public health warning in case a person has a constitution similar to a small minority population; the recommendation is doubly odd considering that no study has directly shown that high blood pressure increases a man's risk of dying from heart disease.

"To ask Americans to turn their diets upside down in the hope that a low-salt diet will translate into health benefits strikes me as faith worthy of the church fathers. In God we trust—all others show data," says Michael Alderman, M.D., chair of the Department of Epidemiology and Social Medicine at the Albert Einstein College of Medicine of Yeshiva University in New York City, president-elect of the American Society of Hypertension and co-author of the recent heart attack study. He adds, "The essential problem with the low-salt argument is that it misses the reality of biology."

The Renin Factor

Salt is a central player in almost every bodily function, especially blood flow, so it's not surprising that your body has prepared an intricate emergency response to the lack of it. When your kidneys detect low blood levels of salt, they kick into action and increase the production of a hormone, renin, to compensate for the loss.

The trouble is that renin narrows blood vessels and reduces blood volume and flow. Sounds like a recipe for a blood clot, and it may well be: Relatively high levels of renin have been linked with an increase in heart attacks in several studies. "An increase in renin may just make that extra difference between having and avoiding a heart attack, especially in men with atherosclerosis," says Dr. Alderman.

Some antihypertensives, such as ACE (angiotensin-converting enzyme) inhibitors, lower blood pressure by restricting renin action. In men who aren't salt-sensitive, coupling a low-salt diet with a drug that suppresses renin can produce a blood pressure dive. "When your renin system is blocked and you're on a low-salt diet, you have no way of holding your blood pressure up and there's a danger that you might actually go into shock," explains John H. Laragh, M.D., professor of medicine and director of the Hypertension and Cardiovascular Center at New York Hospital in New York City.

To Each His Own

One of the reasons that the medical community's attempts to broadcast general recommendations have gone awry is a basic biological reality: We're all very different. "Everybody's salt factor is different, and everybody's renin factor is different," explains Dr. Laragh. In other words, you may need 3,000 milligrams of salt a day to perform at your best, and I may need 10,000. No one knows.

Researchers do know, however, what symptoms can arise if you're not at your particular optimum sodium level, if you're salt-depleted. "If you're salt-depleted, your blood is very thick and sluggish, you don't exercise well, you don't function overall as well," says Dr. Laragh. Runners

have long known this: It's why they chug salt solutions as they make their way around the track.

The Fatigue Link

From the description of salt depletion, it's clear that salt intake below your individual optimum will make you tired. For people with NMH, that tiredness can be agonizingly constant. When most of us stand for long periods of time, our bodies compensate. In people with NMH, a miscommunication occurs: Blood pools excessively in the legs, triggering the heart to pound faster. But the brain misinterprets the heart's exertion and, at the worst possible moment, sends a signal to lower blood pressure. After such a drop in pressure, symptoms may include fatigue, light-headedness and blurred vision—and they may last for days.

"Many people with chronic fatigue trigger this NMH reflex throughout the day, which makes them feel tired much of the time," says Peter C. Rowe, M.D., associate professor of pediatrics at the Johns Hopkins Children's Center in Baltimore. "For some, the fatigue seems to come out of the blue; but for many, it happens after they've reduced their salt intake."

Since the blood pressure drop can occur as long as 20 minutes after standing, traditional measurements can't catch NMH. It takes a tilt-table test, in which a person is tilted back slightly and blood pressure readings are taken at intervals. If you've been feeling tired for more than six months, check with your doctor. Treatment begins with an increased intake of salt and water.

The Bottom Line

All things in moderation. If you're not salt-sensitive and have no medical condition (such as kidney disease) in which low salt is especially advised, your best bet is to eat a diet high in fresh produce and low in fat and just let the salt fall where it may.

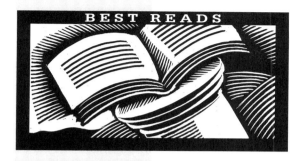

A Plateful of Miracles

Most men's picture of getting older includes the classic signs of age: wrinkled skin, fading memory, diminished physical capacity and increased susceptibility to infection. A growing body of research, however, views these "signs of age" as little more than deficiencies of critical chemicals called antioxidants.

"We can view aging as humankind's inevitable destiny and idly sit by as our bodies disintegrate. Or we can take action to hang onto and replenish our biochemical vitality that is slipping away," writes Jean Carper, a syndicated nutrition writer and author of the book Stop Aging Now! *(HarperCollins, 1995). She argues that by eating foods high in antioxidants—chemicals that disable harmful substances that attack cells and cause them to malfunction—we can turn back the clock. In this chapter from her book, she reveals the power of fruits and vegetables.*

While any fruit or vegetable you eat is bound to make known and unknown chemical contributions to your quest for youth, here are ten with so much known potential that you shouldn't ignore them.

1. Avocado. It's one of the super-guardians of cells because of its abundance of glutathione, the "master antioxidant" that, among other miracles, helps neutralize highly destructive fat in foods. True, avocado is high in fat, but much of it is good fat—monounsaturated, a type that resists oxidation. Eating avocados also lowers and improves blood cholesterol better than a low-fat diet does, according to research.

2. Berries. Blueberries, for example, have more antioxidants called anthocyanins than any other food—three times more than the second-richest sources, red wine and green tea. Both blueberries and cranberries help ward off urinary tract infections. In one study, the older people who ate the most strawberries had the lowest rate of all kinds of cancer.

3. Broccoli. Broccoli is blessed with an awesome array of antioxidants. Particularly strong is one called sulforaphane, discovered by Johns Hopkins University scientists. Fed to animals, the broccoli chemical revved up the activity of detoxification enzymes that slashed cancer rates by two-thirds. Broccoli is packed with free-radical fighter vitamin C, beta-carotene, indole, glutathione and lutein. Broccoli is one of the richest food sources of the trace metal chromium, a life extender and protector against the ravages of out-of-control insulin and blood sugar.

4. Cabbage. Like broccoli, cabbage is a cruciferous vegetable with potent antioxidant activity. Men who ate cabbage once a week compared with once a month had only 66 percent of the risk of colon cancer, one classic study found. Cabbage also seems to deter stomach cancer. Savoy cabbage (the crinkly type) is strongest— eat it raw or lightly cooked for best effect.

5. Carrots. Carrots are legendary in fighting off aging diseases. In a recent study, men eating a couple of carrots a day lowered blood cholesterol by 10 percent. Countless studies pinpoint beta-carotene, carrots' main antioxidant asset, as a powerhouse against aging and disease. People with low levels of beta-carotene in their blood are more apt to have heart attacks, strokes and various cancers.

6. Citrus fruit. The orange is so full of antioxidants that officials at the National Cancer Institute have called it a complete package of every

class of natural anti-cancer inhibitor known, including carotenoids, terpenes, flavonoids and vitamin C. Grapefruit, too, has a unique type of fiber, especially in the membranes and juice sacs, that reduces cholesterol dramatically and even may reverse the aging disease atherosclerosis.

7. Grapes. The anti-aging secret of grapes is simple and powerful: Grapes contain 20 known antioxidants that work together to fend off oxygen free-radical attacks that promote disease and aging, according to researchers at the University of California, Davis. The antioxidants are in the skin and seeds, and the more colorful the skin, the greater the antioxidant punch.

8. Onions. Full of antioxidants, onions help prevent cancer, thin the blood (discouraging clots) and raise the good-type HDL (high-density lipoprotein) cholesterol. Red and yellow (but not white) onions are the richest foods in quercetin, a celebrated antioxidant that inactivates cancer-causing agents, inhibits enzymes that spur cancer growth and has anti-inflammatory, antibacterial, antifungal and antiviral activity.

9. Spinach. One of the most striking antioxidants in spinach is lutein, thought to be as strong an anti-aging agent as the well-known beta-carotene. Spinach, however, has both, plus a good dose of folate, a brain and artery protector.

10. Tomatoes. Tomatoes are by far the richest source of the remarkable antioxidant lycopene. New research suggests that lycopene preserves mental and physical functioning among the elderly. High levels of lycopene also reduce your risk of pancreatic cancer.

A Man's Kitchen

Here's a topic that you probably haven't given much thought to: how to stock a kitchen with the right cooking equipment. Most guys—women, too, for that matter—own an oddball assortment of hand-me-down dishes and pots, gift woks and *toaster ovens, flea-market potato mashers and college beer mugs. But as Jeff Bredenberg and Alisa Bauman point out in* Food Smart: A Man's Plan to Fuel Up for Peak Performance *(Rodale Press, 1996), just like the workshop, it's essential to have the right gear in the kitchen to get the job done right. In this excerpt, they outline the essentials for a man's kitchen.*

Junu Kim grew up with his mother's admonition ringing in his ears: "If a man steps into the kitchen, his testicles will fall off."

Now in his thirties, Kim is married and does most of the cooking. And fortunately for Kim and millions of other modern men, it turns out his mom was wrong. "Both of those boys are still there," Kim says proudly.

It all leads us to wonder where this idea came from that a man's castle stops at the kitchen door. Kitchens are full of guy stuff. And we're not just talking about the beer and leftover pizza in the fridge. The kitchen is the place where lettuce gets slammed against the countertop, the place where huge, sharp knives dismember chickens and turkeys. And it's the place where slabs of meat are beaten with wooden hammers. Indeed, in many ways a man's kitchen is a tool-shop in disguise. Some comparisons:

Workshop	Kitchen
Saw	Chef's knife
X-Acto knife	Paring knife
Pliers	Tongs
T square	Measuring cup
Workbench	Cutting board
Table saw	Food processor

Just like the workshop, you need to choose your kitchen equipment carefully. Here's what you need to outfit a man's kitchen.

Going under the Knife

Enter the world of kitchen knives. You have your fillet knife, your butter knife, your boning knife and your bread knife. Then there's your ham knife. And the cook's knife. A carving knife. An oyster knife.

Seems like they make a different knife for every cutting job around. But you only need two: a big chef's knife for chopping and pulverizing and a smaller paring knife for whittling and dissecting. Here's what you need to look for.

Steel yourself for action. If you can find a carbon steel knife, you're in business. That's the best kind of knife around. But it also rusts easily and is hard to come by, says Annemarie Colbin, founder of the Natural Gourmet Cookery School in New York City and author of *Food and Healing* and *The Natural Gourmet*. To prevent rust, wash it and dry it immediately after each use.

Stainless steel is also a good buy. It will need more sharpening than a carbon steel knife, so you'll have to buy a sharpener as well. If you're the kind of guy who lets dishes and utensils pile up in the sink until you run out of clean ones, it might prove to be a wise investment.

Look for rivets. Rivets are those small, flat circles you see in the knife's handle. Think of them as screws that hold the blade to the handle. A good knife has at least two rivets on each side, Colbin says.

Better check your tang. If you look down at the handle, you can see where the blade runs through the middle of it. That's called the tang. The best knives are called full tang, which means the steel goes all the way to the end of the handle. A half-tang, where the steel goes halfway down the handle, is much better than no tang. If you buy a knife without rivets and without a tang, expect it to fall apart.

Make it resin-ate. The handle should be treated with resin so that it's smooth and waterproof.

Be ready to pay. You'll have to fork out a lot of dough to buy a good set of kitchen knives. They can run more than $200, but if you demand quality, they're the top of the line. *Consumer Reports* rated kitchen knives and chose J. A.

Henckels Four Star, J. A. Henckels Professional "S" and the Cuisine de France Sabatier as the top three lines. Just a chef's knife from any of those companies might cost close to $100. If you just want a good, inexpensive knife, *Consumer Reports* rates Ekco Best Results Professional as tops. A four-piece set will run you only about $30.

Stay sharp. Once you get your knives, you'll want to keep them sharp. "Knives that are dull will slide and therefore can hurt you more easily," Colbin says. "Most people think it's the other way around."

Your knife is dull when:

- It slides a lot when cutting.
- It makes cracking sounds when cutting. Knifes should be quiet.
- You run it lightly across a tomato and it doesn't break the skin.

If your knives are really dull—we're talking about going back and forth over the tomato four or five times with no result—you should get them sharpened professionally, Colbin says. Look under "Sharpening Service" in the phone book.

You could try to do the job yourself with an oilstone or diamond-impregnated block, both of which are sharpening tools that can be found where you buy knives or in some hardware stores. The process requires lots of patience. There are also electric sharpeners that will fix super dull knives.

The idea, though, is to keep your knives from getting that dull, and that means sharpening them every time you use them. So when you buy your knives, you should also get a sharpening steel from the same company. Hold the blade at a 20-degree angle against the steel and draw the blade across the steel from handle to tip. Do that three or four times on each side of the blade before each use.

Some knives come with holders that will sharpen them for you. Every time you pull out or put back the knife, the blade drags across a sharpening mechanism. But be wary. *Consumer Reports* warns that many of the samples they tested did not function properly.

Be an Iron Man

You'll need pots (deep containers you can boil water in) and pans (shallow containers you can make pancakes in) of at least four different sizes, says Colbin.

- A one- to four-quart pot
- A huge six- to eight-quart stock pot
- A ten-inch skillet (with deep sides)
- A seven- to ten-inch sauté pan (with shallow sides)

If you have a big family or just tend to use every burner on the stove when you cook, you'll want some additional pots and pans in various other sizes. You're looking for stuff that's easy to clean and hard to break. Here's what to look for.

Get a good conductor. No, not the kind who comes in tails waving a baton. You need pots and pans that conduct heat evenly so that you won't burn as much food. The best heat conductor is silver, but unless your last name is Trump or Forbes, you can't afford that (more than $2,000 a pan). Copper also conducts heat well, but it's easily damaged, is a major-league pain to clean and can release copper into your food, says Colbin. What's left? Aluminum. Because aluminum can make food smell funky, you want the aluminum sandwiched between some other metal, preferably stainless steel—it's easy to clean.

Work out with iron. A cast-iron skillet should last a lifetime. It adds crunch to foods and blackens catfish extremely well. You don't have much sticking, and you'll boost your iron intake, says Colbin, because some of it gets in your food. It's also versatile, working equally well on the stove or in the oven, and it's easy to clean, too.

But cooking with cast iron is a workout. The typical cast-iron pan can weigh about three times as much as the typical stainless steel one.

Also, you'll need to season a new one and keep it seasoned to prevent rust. A completely seasoned cast-iron pan takes several months of continuous use and proper care. After that, the pan turns a dark color, possibly black. But you can get great results from a just-seasoned pan. Once you remove the label and the adhesive underneath the label, pour a half-cup of vegetable oil into a 12-inch skillet (use less for a smaller pan) and use a paper towel to spread it evenly over the surface (the sides, too), making sure to rub the oil in well. Pour off the excess oil, leaving a thin film on all the surfaces, and bake the pan at 300°F for an hour. Then turn the oven off but leave the skillet inside for a few more hours, preferably overnight, says Tom Ney, food editor for *Prevention* magazine. After that, put the pan on a stove burner and heat it for five minutes on medium high. Let it cool. It's now seasoned.

Don't be a stickler for cost. If cast iron seems like too much work, then go for either stainless steel or a pan with a nonstick coating. Fancy nonstick pans can run you close to $100, and they're not indestructible. If you're a freshman cook, Nancy D. Berkoff, R.D., a culinary instructor at the Los Angeles Trade Technical College, suggests buying the cheapest nonstick pan possible. After all, odds are that you're going to destroy it. Once you've learned to be gentle, then you can advance to the more expensive kinds. Just remember not to use metal spoons or metal spatulas with it.

Get a grip. Pots and pans come with wooden, plastic and metal handles, and each material has its strengths and weaknesses. Metal handles get really hot, but a pan with a metal handle can be used for baking as well as stove-top cooking. Wooden handles are sturdy and attractive, but you can't put them in the dishwasher if you want them to continue to look nice. *Consumer Reports* pushes plastic handles. Though they aren't as handsome, they are dishwasher-safe, rugged and can usually withstand oven temperatures up to 300°F.

Everything but the Kitchen Sink

You could spend your weekly paycheck on a lot of unnecessary kitchen stuff that you'll probably never use, or you could buy what you really need and use the money you save for a weekend getaway for two to a romantic bed-and-breakfast (breakfast optional). It's up to you. Here's what you need.

• Cutting board. Get a big, maple butcher block. "It looks better, it smells better and it lasts longer," Colbin says. How big of a block you buy depends on the size of your kitchen. It should be at least an inch thick and measure at least 12 inches by 24 inches. Which is safer, wood or plastic?

Despite some research that gives the safety edge to wood, the jury is still out at this point. Mona R. Sutnick, R.D., Ed.D., a nutrition consultant and spokesperson for the American Dietetic Association, says the real issue is keeping whichever material you use for a cutting board very clean.

• Food processor or blender. Look for a small, inexpensive one that's easy to clean. Use either appliance to puree or chop. A blender will also mix drinks and crush ice, and you can use the blender to make a cream soup without the cream. Any starchy vegetable or grain such as potatoes, carrots or oatmeal will create a creamy texture in the blender, says Colbin.

• Mixing bowls. Look for something easy to clean that can go from the fridge to the oven and back to the fridge without exploding. Stainless steel bowls are the best, in Colbin's opinion, because they are the lightest and most durable, but they can't go into the microwave like glass or plastic.

• Tongs. You want a pair that fits your hand comfortably and is sturdy enough to pick up an ear of corn without snapping in two.

• Ladle. Make sure it's man-size. It should be big enough to dish out chili a serving at a time.

• Mixing spoons. Think about what you look for in a paint stirrer. That's right: wood. You want wooden spoons for the same reason you want wooden cutting boards. They look better, and they are easy to clean. "Also, the wooden spoons last forever. The plastic ones react badly to heat," Colbin says.

• Peeler. The kind that works best, according to Colbin, has the blade sandwiched into the handle.

• Grater. Instead of nicking your knuckles on the rectangular kind, you can buy the circular kind with a hand crank.

• Spatula. For scraping goop out of bowls, buy rubber on a wooden stick. "All of the plastic ones disintegrate. They get really weird," Colbin says. "They get very sticky and disgusting after a short time. Rubber lasts the longest."

Some other things you'll want: garlic press, metal spatula for flipping pancakes, juicer, whisk, strainer, can opener and a hand beater.

Mapping Out Your Kitchen

She's coming for dinner tonight. The one you met in the grocery store olive oil aisle. You lured her to your place by boasting about your culinary skills. Now you're sautéing shrimp, mixing up chocolate mousse and slicing strawberries. She will arrive in less than half an hour, and where are the (expletive deleted) measuring cups? You tear the place apart. In your blind frustration you fling open the freezer door. It happens. Measuring cups are sometimes in the freezer. Wham. A pound of ground beef lands on your foot.

Miss Olive Oil arrives at your front door, and you have a broken toe. A little disorganized, are we?

Not to fear. Here's a seven-step program that any clutteraholic can follow.

Keeping It Cold

Refrigeration and freezing allow us to store food for a long time, but not forever. Assuming you have your refrigerator set at 40°F and your freezer at 0°F, here's how long you can keep some common items.

Food	Refrigerator	Freezer
Eggs, fresh, in shell	3 weeks	Do not freeze
Egg yolks and whites	2–4 days	1 year
Eggs, hard-boiled	1 week	Do not freeze
Liquid egg substitute, unopened	10 days	1 year
Liquid egg substitute, opened	3 days	Do not freeze
Mayonnaise	2 months	Do not freeze
TV dinner, unopened	Do not refrigerate	3–4 months
Soups and stews	3–4 days	2–3 months
Burger/stew meats	1–2 days	3–4 months
Ground turkey, veal, pork or lamb	1–2 days	3–4 months
Hot dogs, unopened	2 weeks	1–2 months, in freezer wrap
Hot dogs, opened	1 week	1–2 months, in freezer wrap
Lunchmeat (unopened)	2 weeks	1–2 months, in freezer wrap
Lunchmeat (opened)	3–5 days	1–2 months, in freezer wrap
Bacon	7 days	1 month
Raw sausage	1–2 days	1–2 months
Smoked breakfast links or patties	7 days	1–2 months
Canned ham	6–9 months	Do not freeze
Whole cooked ham	7 days	1–2 months
Sliced cooked ham	3–4 days	1–2 months
Beefsteaks	3–5 days	6–12 months
Pork chops	3–5 days	4–6 months
Lamb chops	3–5 days	6–9 months
Beef roasts	3–5 days	6–12 months
Lamb roasts	3–5 days	6–9 months
Meat leftovers	3–4 days	2–3 months
Whole chicken	1–2 days	1 year
Chicken pieces	1–2 days	9 months
Fried chicken	3–4 days	4 months

1. Organize around the stove. "You want to have things within easy reach," Colbin says. "Whatever you use the most should be closest to you." So keep your two knives, your cutting board, maybe a mixing bowl, your pan and your pot near the stove. Think about what else you usually need and put them in plain view. A few exceptions: oils and spices. Nix the wall spice racks. Spices should be stored in darkness. Ditto for oil.

2. Only buy as many appliances as will fit on the counter. Thanks to modern ingenuity, you can get creative about where you put them. Just about everything can be mounted to a cabinet. "If you don't have the space, you have to keep it underneath the counter. A lot of people don't want to take the time to get it out and plug it in," says Jennifer Anderson, nutrition consultant and spa dietitian at Bonaventure Spa and Fitness Resort in Fort Lauderdale, Florida. "It sounds silly, but you don't want to go past all of your other appliances, pots, pans and mixing bowls and drag it out."

3. Ask for help. Any department store carries an array of organizational helpers. One kitchen helper looks like a circular plastic or wooden rack. You can hang your measuring spoons and cups, a can opener and some other stuff on the sides and stick your mixing spoons, spatulas and other stuff in the center. "I find that to be pretty handy because when I'm cooking, the measuring spoons are right there and they are all together," Anderson says. "It's not like they're mixed up in the drawers and I can't find my quarter-teaspoon."

4. Get a drawer separator. It has slots for your forks, knives and so forth.

5. Keep like things together. Make a breakfast section, a starch section for lunch and dinner and a canned-food section. Putting your cereals, oatmeal, oat bran and other morning eats together allows you to go to one place to figure out what you want for breakfast. "Everything's right there, so you're not looking all over your kitchen and thinking, 'Oh, nothing looks good in this cabinet, let me try another cabinet,'" Anderson says.

6. In the freezer, keep meat, poultry and fish on the bottom. That way, if some juices accidentally escape, they won't contaminate anything else that's not going to be cooked at a high temperature. Keep the frozen vegetables on top.

7. In the freezer and refrigerator, use the door shelves to stack small items that will easily get lost in the depths.

Quality Counts

You'd think that something called refined would be better than the original version. But those who follow the world of nutrition know that refining often strips much of what's good out of food. But how, exactly? Ann Louise Gittleman, a certified nutrition specialist, answers the question with fascinating clarity in her book Super Nutrition for Men and the Women Who Love Them *(M. Evans and Company, 1996). Here is an excerpt.*

The refining of grain was made possible by the invention in 1862 of machinery that removes and disposes of the outer husks of the grains. It is in these outer husks that most of the nutrients are concentrated. Typically, in the production of flour, the bran and germ are removed, resulting in extensive losses of nutrients.

During World War I, the milling of grains was forbidden in Denmark because of economic cutbacks. The death rate fell 34 percent, and the incidence of cancer, kidney disease and diabetes dropped significantly. During World War II, when grains were only partially milled in England, much the same thing happened. The less we refine food, the more it supports our health.

Among the nutrients lost in the refining process are the B vitamins, a family or "complex" of vitamins that plays an important role in nourishing the nervous system. We need extra amounts of the entire B family when we're under stress, but refined products, even though "enriched" with a few of the Bs put back, can't meet this need. A continuous diet of refined food cripples the body's ability to deal with stress, a prominent feature in the life of today's man.

Also lost in the refining process are many of the important "antioxidant" nutrients—vitamins A, C and E and the minerals selenium and zinc—so necessary for their role as "free-radical" scavengers in the body. Free radicals are renegade chemical fragments caused by such stresses as pollution, oxidation, exposure to ultraviolet radiation, ingestion of rancid oils and surgery. They are believed to play a key role in aging and in the degenerative disease processes, particularly cancer. Men need antioxidant nutrients to protect their bodies against damage from free radicals. Consuming a diet of refined foods creates deficiencies in these important protective nutrients and therefore increases vulnerability to degenerative diseases.

Also lost in the refining process is fiber, needed to move food residue through the intestines and prevent constipation. Many of the vitally important trace minerals are lost as well. According to Henry A. Schroeder, M.D., who did extensive research on the trace minerals over 20 years ago, "most of the energy in the average American diet which comes from white flour, white sugar and fat, is not supplied with the trace substances needed to utilize that energy efficiently and properly." The refining of sugar removes 93 percent of the ash and, with it, the trace minerals needed to metabolize the sugar. The milling of wheat into refined white flour and the refining of raw cane sugar into white sugar remove minerals in the following percentages, according to Dr. Schroeder:

Mineral	White Sugar (%)	White Flour (%)
Cobalt	98	89
Magnesium	98	85
Zinc	98	78
Chromium	93	40
Manganese	89	86
Copper	68	83

Additionally, white flour has lost the following minerals originally present in whole wheat: 60 percent of the calcium, 71 percent of the phosphorus, 77 percent of the potassium, 78 percent of the sodium, 76 percent of the iron, 48 percent of the molybdenum and 75 percent of the selenium.

Iron is the only mineral that is later added back to food when it is enriched. It is put back in an inorganic form, iron sulphate. Inorganic iron taken into the body stays out of solution. The body is unable to absorb it properly. The absorption problem is compounded by the lack of other minerals in refined foods. As a consequence, this iron often ends up being deposited in the arteries and joints, leading to degenerative disorders like heart disease and arthritis. Enriching foods with iron can cause more problems than it solves. In Sweden, liver cancer rates tripled when the bread makers began fortifying their flour with iron.

While inorganic forms of iron are not well-absorbed, natural iron supplements, such as iron peptonate, are—especially when electrolytes are balanced. The "heme" form of iron found in animal products is also well-used, making liquid liver extract a good supplemental source of iron for those who need it.

Iron deficiencies among men are rare, however, except possibly among those who have low thyroid function, have lost blood, have been ill or have engaged in endurance exercise. If in doubt about iron levels, have laboratory tests performed, but as a general rule, men should avoid taking supplemental iron and consuming foods enriched with it, for iron overload can create serious problems, including heart disease, arthritis, diabetes and impotence. Also, excess iron is stored in the central nervous system and is found in many psychiatric patients. High levels of the free form of the mineral are found in the brains of those suffering with Parkinson's disease.

Following the refining process, which removes most of the eight vitamins present in whole wheat, only three are replaced in the enriching process. Altogether, refining removes over two dozen nutrients and replaces only four.

White "polished" rice is also a refined product. After processing, it retains only the following percentages of trace minerals present in the whole grain: 17 percent of the magnesium, 25 percent of the chromium, 73 percent of the manganese, 62 percent of the cobalt, 75 percent of the copper and 25 percent of the zinc. Choose brown rice over white for a more nutritious meal.

When we remove bran and germ from whole wheat, nothing is left but the starch. It is in the starchy portion of the grain that the heavy metal cadmium is concentrated. Cadmium toxicity is strongly associated with hypertension. If enough zinc is present in the body, it can defend against the cadmium. Unfortunately, zinc is found in the bran and germ portions of the grain and is discarded in processing. This means that when we eat refined grains, we are vulnerable to the ill effects of cadmium, particularly if our body stores of zinc are low. This is not a problem with the whole grains. In the absence of chromium and fiber, also removed in the refining process, the body has trouble processing the starch that remains. Pure starch stresses the pancreas and throws the blood sugar into turmoil.

Most of the oils consumed in the standard American diet are highly refined. According to Dr. Schroeder, separating oil from corn results in a refined product with less than 1 percent of the magnesium and only 25 percent of the original zinc. Vitamin E, needed to help retard spoilage, is also removed, as is lecithin, a fat emulsifier. The fat-digesting enzyme lipase is destroyed by the heat used in processing, making the oil undigestible. Beta-carotene is also virtually destroyed by processing methods. And, perhaps worst of all, refining destroys much of the valuable omega-3 and omega-6 essential fatty acids.

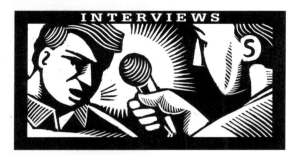

Mary Friesz on
Eating Strategies for Men

As a nutrition consultant and spa dietitian at Bonaventure resort and spa in Fort Lauderdale, Florida, Mary Friesz, R.D., has heard just about every excuse there is when it comes to why we don't eat as healthy as we would like. But eating healthy doesn't have to be hard, Friesz says. You just need to be creative. During an interview she explains how to overcome some of the pitfalls of unhealthy eating.

How much nutritional knowledge do men have?

Sometimes they don't even know what fat is. For instance, some don't even know that potato chips are fattening. I had a weight lifter who didn't realize that eating a couple of crackers is better than eating potato chips.

For men who want to lose weight, calorie counting can be a real drag. Do you have to do it?

Some people really love to count calories and fat grams. But other people would really rather not worry about it—especially men. They don't want to sit there and write down everything they ate. They don't want to be precise and figure out exactly how many cups of rice they ate. That's why many times I have them work on portion size instead. That means knowing that three ounces of meat is the size of a deck of cards. That means maybe using a smaller plate if you are the type of person who has to cover it with food.

Is there any one easy rule men can follow that will pretty much keep them in the clear when it comes to eating healthy?

Make 50 to 65 percent of what you eat carbohydrate. That's baked potato, rice, bread, cereals and grains.

What do you think is the easiest change men can make that will help them eliminate fat from their diets?

Eating smaller portions of animal protein, such as cutting down on the size of that steak.

Could you list some easy cooking strategies men could use that would quickly cut some fat from their diets?

• Use chicken or vegetable stock instead of oil when stir-frying. You don't need to make it yourself. You can buy a low-sodium broth in the canned-food section of the grocery store. Another option is the low-sodium bouillon powder that comes in packets. You can mix it up as you need it.
• When you have to use oil, use a spray such as Pam. But don't drench the pan. A light coating is fine. Or you could lightly spray the surface of the food. People often think the spray is low fat but it's still vegetable oil. If you hold the button down for long, you'll get a lot of fat.
• When a recipe calls for oil, try cutting the amount of oil you use in half.
• Take the skin off your chicken or turkey after you bake it. If you bake poultry without the skin, it will dry out.

You make it sound easy. But I'm no whiz in the kitchen. I think if I started fooling around with recipes, I might create something really foul-tasting. Any suggestions?

There is a lot of frustration because sometimes men think that cooking healthy is over-

whelming. There's just too much to do, too much to prepare. That's why I always tell them they have to take it one step at a time. The idea is to use food substitutions. You can replace oil with an equal amount of applesauce when baking cookies or muffins. Just remember to cut down on the sugar a bit when you do this. Try some of the new fat-free products that are available, like mayonnaise. If you want to break yourself in slowly, mix some of the new fat-free product with your old favorite. When you are cooking healthy, you really need to be creative. And that's where some people really don't enjoy it. They feel like they don't have time to be creative—to make things taste good.

So it sounds like you need to make time for trial and error. And you need to be prepared. You need to be able to find things when you are looking for them so that you don't burn your vegetables while searching for the vinegar. Can you offer some wisdom to people like me whose kitchens are probably the most cluttered places in our home? How can we get organized?

The easiest thing is to keep all of your breakfast stuff together, your starches and pastas together and other food groups together. That way when you are in a hurry in the morning, you only have one place to look. You don't have to look all over your kitchen in search for something to eat. Also, you'll notice when something is low. For instance, when you use up that box of pasta, you know there isn't any more left. You don't have to wonder whether there really isn't a box in some other cabinet. You know to put it on your grocery list. It also helps to keep the grocery list on the refrigerator door.

In the freezer, you want to keep individually portioned and wrapped meats and a couple bags of frozen vegetables. Individually wrapped portions make defrosting in the refrigerator easier and help you control the portion size. Frozen veggies are easy to toss into a soup or casserole.

Too many gadgets can be a problem when it comes to finding somewhere to put them all. But is there one gadget that can go a long way to helping you eat healthier?

One big, good cast-iron pan about eight inches in diameter with a lid can do almost anything you would want. You can use it to sauté, steam, stir-fry and make sauces. Make sure that you use a plastic spatula so that the surface doesn't get nicked.

You talked about how steaming and stir-frying can be healthy ways to cook. What are some others?

Grilling is good, because it allows the grease to drip somewhere else. Roasting at 475° is also healthy. And baking is good as long as you take the skin off the chicken and turkey before you eat it. Broiling is healthy, and it's also easy. You can throw in a chicken fillet, broil it for 20 minutes and you're set for dinner.

What do you do when the cooking is really out of your control, like when you are on the road eating out each meal?

I work with one man who travels a lot. I told him that it's harder because he is eating out. When you are eating out, you can always count on bigger portions (sometimes twice the amount of food you need) and more fat.

But there are always better alternatives. Ask to go light on the sauce or, even better, for sauces to be served on the side. Choose wine- and tomato-based sauces over cream and cheese sauces. Ask for steamed vegetables. You can have that baked potato instead of the french fries. You can have a salad with the dressing on the side, and while you are at it, ask them to hold the croutons and cheese also. Even if you are eating fast food, you can try to stay away from the cheeses and special sauces. You can always make what you have a little bit better.

Doreen Virtue on
Having a Romantic Dinner

Relationship expert and psychologist Doreen Virtue, Ph.D., is an expert on food and sex. Her recent book In the Mood *details not only what to eat for a more potent sex life, but also how to eat. And it's the how that we were interested in. So we gave her a call and asked her to talk with us about just what is needed to create a romantic dining atmosphere.*

What is the most common misconception couples have about romantic eating?

They think that it has to be reserved for a romantic restaurant. Couples can make ordinary dinners at home into warm, romantic meals that help them to reconnect. Most people realize this but need to be reminded.

You have said before in one of your books that having a romantic dinner shouldn't be a special occasion. It's something families should do every day. Why is it so important to eat together?

Dinner is one of the few opportunities for those of us with dual careers to sit down and spend a few moments getting to know one another, reconnecting and having fun. Based on my own childhood, my parents were very adamant about no television during dinner. They would have candlelight or dim lights. It wasn't like we had to dress up for dinner. But it was an occasion where we shared what went on during the day. And that ritual was very important for my family to be healthy.

You said no television. Why?

There's a number of reasons. First, the news tends to cause indigestion and upset people. Stress adversely affects the metabolism. It slows it down, triggering the production of cortisol in the brain, which increases our appetite for carbohydrates. Having the news off reduces your appetite and gives you the opportunity to have a soothing discussion.

What else should you do to make a meal romantic?

I recommend playfulness. I think it's a really good idea for couples to feed each other with a bite or two. It's loving. Look for opportunities to help one another. If you can see that your mate needs the butter, go for it and give her the butter. Those little acts of kindness at the dinner table really create feelings of warmth and unity. It also enhances the feelings of sexuality later in the evening. You don't want to sleep with someone you don't like or who you feel doesn't care for you. Everything is a prelude to a sexual encounter. We need not separate sex as the minute we take off our clothes and are in bed.

How should couples prepare the meal?

Men and women can have very different kitchen personalities. The man might stand there and order the woman around, telling her exactly how he wants her to chop the onions. She's going to feel offended and criticized. When that happens, couples need to talk about their feelings. They need to create definite duties. If he's really into how the onions should be chopped, then onion chopping should be his job.

In your book, you talked about why it's important to keep stress to a minimum if you want to enjoy a healthy sex life. Can you go into that more?

There are a whole bunch of studies that were done on animals—rats, monkeys and cats—looking at sexuality and serotonin, a chemical released in the brain. The sperm count was lower, virility was lower and ejaculation was less impactful when serotonin was low. So physiologically, serotonin is linked especially to men's sexuality. Stress is a big factor. When you are stressed out, your serotonin is depleted, so you feel tired. When you are tired, who is in the mood? It's like, "Uch. It's too much work." Also, when you are stressed, the central nervous system goes into a sympathetic mode. When you are sympathetic, you can't get aroused. It's only when you are relaxed and in the parasympathetic nervous system that you can get sexually aroused. You would probably think that it's the other way around, because sex seems like such an intense physical reaction. It seems like sex involves being stressed. But sex is actually a result of being relaxed. As a clinician, I see this all the time. And I also see people feeling guilty about that.

Is there any food that helps put us in the mood?

Meals like pizza, pasta with cheese, Mexican food or any menu that combines carbohydrates with dairy products. Let me explain why. You want the amino acid tryptophan to get to your brain to stimulate serotonin production. Usually, amino acids are always competing to get into the brain. And tryptophan usually gets blown away by all the other amino acids. But when you eat carbohydrate, it acts like a magic carpet that helps the tryptophan get into the brain.

What is a common eating habit that can sabotage your sex life?

Some people drink Pepsi, Coke or coffee all day at work. Because they are feeling tired, they keep pushing themselves with sodas and chocolate. When they come home, they are buzzing. They are so stimulated from all the caffeine they have ingested that they try to turn it off with too much alcohol. Then their systems are just overwhelmed with the up-and-down effects. You end up blown out. How can you enjoy your sexuality if you feel like a washrag?

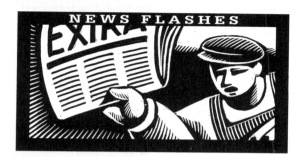

Tea, Beer Might Help Heart

MADISON, Wis.—Black tea and dark-colored beer can be added to a growing list of beverages that might help keep the heart's arteries from forming clots, according to research out of the University of Wisconsin Medical School in Madison.

The same cardiac researcher who first discovered that red wine and grape juice might help in the preventive battle against heart disease believes that black tea and dark-colored beer may have the same protective effect. The reason: These beverages contain large amounts of vitamin-like compounds called flavonoids.

Flavonoids are believed to offer protection against heart disease because they are antioxidants that "soak up" hazardous oxygen molecules called free radicals. Researchers also suggest that flavonoids prevent sticky cells called platelets from forming dangerous clots on arterial walls, which can eventually lead to heart attacks or strokes.

In the study, researchers created a scientific model that duplicates how blood clots when it flows through narrowed arteries with damaged walls. Dark-colored beer, with its high flavonoid content, did a better job of inhibiting platelet activity than did light-colored beer, which contains fewer flavonoids. Black tea, which contains many flavonoids as well, was also found to be better at lowering platelet activity levels than coffee.

Fast Food Can Be Part of a Low-Fat Diet

CHICAGO—People who want to reduce the fat in their diets do not have to eliminate fast-food meals to achieve results, according to researchers at the Chicago Center for Clinical Research.

In a recent study, researchers gathered 113 people who ate higher-fat foods on a regular basis and split them into two groups. One group was put on a diet that followed the healthy-eating guidelines of the National Cholesterol Education Program, while the other group was placed on a diet that balanced fast-food fare with lower-fat meals.

After about eight weeks, researchers found that both groups had been able to reduce the total percentage of fat, percentage of saturated fat and cholesterol in their diets in a similar manner. Those participants who eliminated fast foods completely from their diets demonstrated significantly greater drops in total serum cholesterol than those who included some fast food in their diets. The results, however, indicate that with proper education, people can make fast foods part of their healthier low-fat diets.

Salt–High Blood Pressure Link Broken

TORONTO—In a finding that contradicts widely held notions about the benefits of reducing salt intake, researchers at the University of Toronto have concluded that reducing the amount of salt in a diet does not lower blood pressure for most individuals.

The researchers looked at the results of 56 separate sodium-restriction trials (28 involving people with high blood pressure, 28 involving people with normal blood pressure). The studies involved more than 3,500 participants.

Researchers found that the largest blood

pressure response to sodium restriction involved hypertensive people 45 years or older. In trials involving younger hypertensives, there was only a slight decrease in systolic blood pressure (the top number) and a negligible change in the diastolic pressure (the bottom number).

In the trials that included subjects with normal blood pressures, the researchers saw no evidence of a systematic change in blood pressure as a result of sodium restriction.

Sodium restriction might be beneficial to older hypertensive individuals, the researchers concluded. But the wisdom of universal dietary sodium restriction has been called into question with the results of this study.

Pork Measures Up to Chicken in Fight against Cholesterol

DURHAM, N.C.—Eating lean pork is just as beneficial as eating chicken for those needing to cut their cholesterol levels, according to a study performed by researchers at Duke University Medical Center in Durham, North Carolina.

The study examined 51 men and women with high cholesterol levels for a period of 28 days. The participants ate two large servings per day of either skinless chicken breast or lean pork as part of an overall diet that included 25 percent of its calories from fat.

The researchers discovered that pork and chicken were equally effective in helping the subjects lower their cholesterol levels by as much as 8 percent. So for those who need to keep their cholesterol levels in check, pork can serve as a healthy dietary addition, offering both variety and cholesterol-lowering benefits.

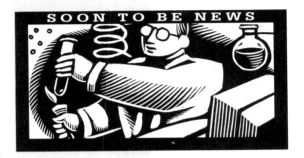

SOON TO BE NEWS

Can Eating Less Keep You Young?

There is mounting evidence that eating fewer calories throughout adult life may lead to a reduction in the diseases of aging.

Over the past 50 years, studies with rodents have demonstrated that much longer life spans can be attained when the animals were kept on a diet consisting of 50 to 65 percent of their preferred calorie consumption.

In a recent study of pigs, researchers fed the animals anywhere from one-third to one-half fewer calories than they would have normally eaten on their own. By the study's end, the pigs that were kept on the low-calorie diet well into their old age did not have the same deterioration in glucose and lipid metabolism that usually occurs in humans and laboratory animals as they age.

Currently, studies involving monkeys are testing this same theory and appear to be showing the same slowing of the aging process that the rodents and pigs showed.

Since pigs and monkeys are both good models for humans because of their similarities in physiology and biochemistry, the studies offer convincing evidence as to one possible method of slowing the aging process in humans. *Research in the area continues. If the premise holds true, look for more specific diet recommendations for humans, with the goal of improving longevity and reducing diseases linked to old age.*

A Healthier Carrot?

Eating lots of carrots has always been a good way to get beta-carotene into your diet. Now a new kind of carrot called a Beta Sweet promises to provide even more beta-carotene—about twice the amount in an average carrot.

Researchers at the Vegetable Improvement Center of Texas A&M University in College Station have cultivated a new vegetable that looks like a carrot that is deep maroon on the outside and dark orange at the center. They named it the Beta Sweet because of its high beta-carotene content and its sweet taste.

Since its cultivation at the center, the researchers have sold the new vegetable to local restaurants and Texas A&M fans because the new carrots happen to be the school's color (maroon). The Beta Sweet has received rave reviews in taste tests mostly because of its crisp texture and sweetness. In particular, the restaurant industry is excited about the vegetable's prospects because its two-tone color makes it so visually appealing. The first small-scale commercial production of the maroon carrots will be in early 1997. *Initially, the carrots will be available for retail purchase only in a few test markets. If the public response is favorable, expect to see the vegetable's availability expand rapidly.*

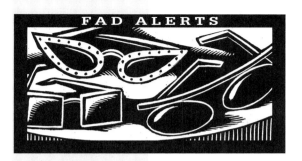

Tasty Low-Fat Foods

 Low-fat food seems to have pasted itself to supermarket shelves much the same way diet soda glued itself to weight-conscious women during the 1980s. In 1995, more than 1,900 new low-fat products hit the shelves in just about every food category, from ice cream to potato chips to granola bars. "That's a record," says Lynn Dornblaser, editor/publisher of *New Product News.* "That's a lot of products finding their way onto store shelves."

And those products are not just new. They are new and improved. While you could rightfully cringe at the thought of stomaching a low-fat cookie or chip a few years ago, you don't have much of a case today. Manufacturers have found numerous innovative ways to make up for the fat deprivation of their products.

Some use benign ingredients such as fruit juice. One company, though, is experimenting with a fat substitute called olestra, under the brand name Olean, in potato chips and tortilla chips. The fat-free versions of Lay's, Ruffles, Doritos and Tostitos are being tested in three American cities.

Though some patrons have complained of intestinal problems after eating fat-free chips, olestra has opened the door for other foods to be made in more creative ways, says Dornblaser.

(For more on olestra, see Weight Loss Fad Alert on page119.)

Specialty Foods

 In tough economic times, we might not buy the biggest house we want. We might settle for a Honda Civic instead of an Accord. And we might decide to spend our vacation close to home instead of in the Bahamas.

But somewhere, somehow we will treat ourselves to something. We will throw all financial prudence out the window.

And usually, we throw it out the window of a specialty food store. "Consumers are more willing to experiment and try unusual things. We've seen a real growth in the number of products that are sold predominantly in specialty stores or health food stores. It's in those stores that you find $30 bottles of balsamic vinegar. Consumers may not be willing to buy a new house, but they will spend a few extra dollars on a specialty cheese or a hot fudge sauce where the first ingredient on the label is chocolate instead of corn syrup," says Dornblaser.

Though they have no health claims to make, such products have grown at close to the same pace as low-fat products, says Dornblaser. "For every trend, there's an opposite trend. So for every low-fat product you see, there are at least as many interesting, significant and unique products that are not low-fat and that don't make any health claims at all. We see a lot of those products in specialty food stores," says Dornblaser.

Convenience Foods

 On average, a 1990s family spends about 15 minutes less than a 1980s family did in front of the stove each day and uses two fewer ingredients to whip up a meal. But that doesn't mean that 1990s families don't take dinner seriously. American families ate dinner as a family an average of 4.8 times a week, according to a 1995 survey. The families say that eating together strengthens family unity, though time and scheduling problems create barriers.

To make dinner more convenient, 1990s families are using speed-scratch kits that come with all the basic ingredients needed to make meals like pizza, fajitas, tacos and salads. They are also buying fully cooked, ready-to-eat meals at grocery stores. In response to that demand, convenience products continue to proliferate, says Dornblaser.

"It runs the gamut from fully prepared meals to partially prepared to easy-to-prepare. It can be marinades and sauces to use to make a meal or a frozen package of vegetables and pasta in sauce that you put in a skillet and add meat," says Dornblaser. "Consumers have less and less time. They want to do things quicker than ever, but they want food to taste really good."

Along with the convenience-food trend has come convenience cookbooks. Cookbooks started with 30-minute dishes, then moved to 20-minute dishes. Then they began with meals that needed only five ingredients. And now cookbooks are coming out with meals that need only three ingredients, says Dornblaser.

Coffee and Tea Products

 America is deep into a coffee craze, with cappuccino bars opening most everywhere you look (we particularly like the ones inside bookstores). Tea is pretty hot, too, with exotic flavors filling grocery store shelves and tea houses also popping up in big cities. What's next? Coffee- and tea-flavored products, of course.

Pepsi has come out with a coffee-flavored soda, Pepsi Kona.

Olive Oil

 Olive oil is as popular as ever. U.S. consumption has quadrupled since the early 1980s, perhaps in part spurred by medical reports of its heart-friendly nature. Or perhaps more Americans are realizing that olive oil has the same coolness factor as dark beer. Whatever the reason, the result is rising olive oil prices. And those prices are expected to increase as much as 30 percent more in the coming months because of droughts in olive oil–producing countries in the Mediterranean.

Girl Scout Thin Mint Cookies

 Thin Mints are the most popular selling Girl Scout cookie, selling 1.6 billion in 1995. The problem is that the mints are a bit of a misnomer. One measly serving contains 8 grams of fat. But Girl Scouts are now selling more heart-healthy cookies: Strawberries 'n' Creme and Chalet Creme, which have only 2.5 and 4.5 grams of fat per serving, respectively. But it seems that cookie buyers would rather have the old standby. During their first year on the market, the low-fat brands didn't come close to outselling Thin Mints.

Salsas

 Hundreds of new salsas hit the market each year. And that will continue with salsas containing many new ingredients, possibly including sweet potatoes, squash, beets, pickles and cauliflower, according to *Prepared Foods* magazine. Prognosticators expect salsas even to make it into the dessert category, with dried-fruit chunks in a chocolate sauce made for cookie dipping.

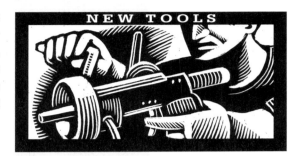

Healthier Pasta Toppers

Mail-Order Olive Oil

Label a product by its degree of virginity and guys are sure to go crazy about it. Enter olive oil. The Etruscan variety is the best you can find this side of Genoa, and you can get it with a phone call. Zingerman's delicatessen in Ann Arbor, Michigan, boasts an array of extra-virgin olive oils fresh from Spain, Italy, France, Greece and Israel. Besides being low in saturated fat (the artery-clogging stuff) and high in monounsaturated fat (which can lower cholesterol), the imported oils are made from handpicked, stone-crushed, cold-pressed olives. You can choose from exotic oils pressed with Sicilian lemons and oranges to rare buttery juices ripened on French hillsides. Call Zingerman's at (313) 769-1625 to get a free catalog of oils with complementing cheeses, teas, breads and meats of equal caliber. $24 to $45 per bottle.

Zestier Drinking

Blenheim Ginger Ale

Just south of the border, they produce an elixir that'll curl your tongue and make your nose hairs do the jitterbug. And the liquid does not have a lick of booze in it. It's Blenheim (pronounced BLEN-um) Ginger Ale, an old-fashioned, spicy-hot soda pop that packs a wallop four times stronger than the wimpy ginger ale you buy down at 7-Eleven. It's made on the grounds of that tourist attraction known as South of the Border on Interstate 95 in South Carolina, 27 miles from where the original plant cranked out cases for 90 years. The spicy ginger ale is made from mineral-spring water, Jamaican ginger, sugar cane and something secret for extra kick. It comes in three grades: Old #3 Hot, #5 Not as Hot and #9 Diet. They have recently added a nonalcoholic #11 Ginger Beer to the lineup. And they'll mix cases if you want them to. To order, call 1-800-270-9344. But take our advice and let Old #3 get nice and cold in the fridge before you sip it. At room temperature, it's just too damn hot. $24 per case, including shipping, or just $20 per case if you order three or more.

Easier Cooking

Gourmet in a Box

Although taking a date out to dinner and a movie is nice, you'll earn more points if you tie on an apron and cook her a meal yourself. Unfortunately, Chef Boyardee ravioli is out of the question. Never fear, Gourmet in a Box comes to the rescue. It helps you make such exotic fare as herbed pasta with sun-dried tomatoes, porcini mushrooms and chicken, Caesar salad, and stuffed mushrooms and rosemary garlic bread with relative ease. You receive a kit containing premeasured spices, dry foods, baking tins and instructions for making a four-course meal. You buy the other ingredients—chicken, lettuce and so forth—along with a nice bottle of wine. Call 1-800-224-4404. $19.95 plus $6.95 shipping and handling.

Tastier Ribs

Barbecue Sauce

There's a hole-in-the-wall in Dallas called Sony Bryan's Smokehouse that serves up some of the most delicious ribs and sides of beef barbe-cue on either side of the Mississippi. The secret is the sauce, a sweet tangy concoction that's been staining the ties of presidents, entertainers, sports legends and Dallas faithful since 1910. Now you don't have to live in Texas to get yourself a jug to slather over your own smoked ribs. A mail-order company called Specialty Sauces will ship off a supply of Sony Bryan's sauce. You can also order the sauces of other famous barbecue pits such as Charlie Robinson's #1 Rib Restaurant in Chicago; Arthur Bryant's Barbecue in Kansas City; McClard's Bar-B-Q in Hot Springs, Arkansas; and King Street Blues in Alexandria, Virginia. Call 1-800-728-2371 for a free catalog. $29.95 for a sample set containing one of each plus $5.95 for shipping.

Heartier Sandwiches

Fresh Bread

Men cannot live without bread. What would we use to sop up our marinara sauce? What would hold the turkey against the Swiss cheese? We need gutsy bread that you have to chew, like those big round loaves that sustain a French farmer for days. Now you can get the best bread in Paris without leaving home. Deborah's Country French Bread in Chicago will ship luscious breads anywhere in the United States. The breads come from the famous bakery Poilane on the Rue du Cherche-Midi in Paris. The breads are frozen right out of the bakery's wood-burning ovens and are flown to the United States, where they are shipped within two days to your door. Call 1-800-952-1400. $27.95 plus shipping for the 4.2-pound, 13-inch-diameter, sourdough loaf.

More Adventurous Eating

Jody Maroni's Sausages

For 13 years, the musclehead-and-Roller-blade set on California's Venice Beach boardwalk has savored Jody Maroni's Sausage Kingdom sausages. The place is famous for "haut dogs"—that is, sausages filled with all sorts of unusual ingredients, such as tangerines, wine, cheeses, pine nuts and raisins. Most of the sausages get only 25 percent of their calories from fat. Now you can sample the West Coast phenomenon even if you live in Hoboken, New Jersey. Maroni's ships 24 frozen varieties of its sausages by next-day air. We tried the Yucatan chicken and duck sausage with cilantro and beer mostly because it has one-third the fat of traditional sausages. It had a good spicy and garlicky flavor. Call 1-800-428-8364 for a free brochure. $65 for a five-pound box of any-flavored sausages, including shipping.

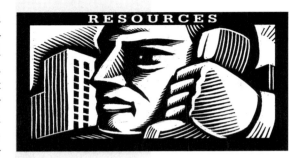

RESOURCES

Healthy Snacking

American Institute for Cancer Research

Department HS

Washington, DC 20069

The American Institute for Cancer Research offers a booklet titled "Sneak Health into Your Snacks" for those interested in healthy snacks and healthful snacking habits. The booklet includes lists of healthy snacks broken down by taste. Send a stamped (55 cents), self-addressed, business-size envelope to the above address for your free copy. The institute is an independent, nonprofit research and education organization that gets its support from individual gifts, foundations and industry.

Food Safety

International Food Information Council

Web Site

http://ificinfo.health.org

Do you have questions about how to cook your favorite foods safely? If you do, head on over to the International Food Information Council (IFIC) Web site. This site can provide you with the latest information on nutrition, food allergies and food safety. It also offers simple suggestions for healthy eating. The IFIC is a nonprofit organization based in Washington,

D.C., that receives funding from several leading food and beverage companies.

Nutrition

Nutrition Hot Line of the American

Dietetic Association

1-800-366-1655

Call up the nutrition hot line offered by the American Dietetic Association to hear an assortment of messages on a variety of subjects associated with healthy eating and food preparation. You can also order fact sheets on food-related topics, speak to a registered dietitian or get help to locate a registered dietitian in your area. The message line operates from 8:00 A.M. to 8:00 P.M. Central Standard Time, Monday through Friday. The registered dietitians are available from 9:00 A.M. to 4:00 P.M. Central Standard Time on those days.

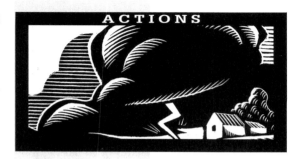

Sick of hearing about all the foods whose synonym is death wish? We agree. Fearing food is no way to get through life. Food should be your friend. Here are 17 actions to take, based on new findings about the power of food.

1. **Press here for wellness.** The fact that your beef is brown doesn't necessarily mean it's safe. Meat that's old or has been exposed to too much air can brown prematurely, making it appear properly cooked when, in fact, it may only be a half-step past raw and possibly laden with killer germs. But you can eat burgers without fear if you perform this easy safety test. Press down on the burger and look at the color of the liquid that oozes out. If the juice is almost yellow, with no trace of red, the burger is safe to eat, says Cheryl Hartsough, R.D., a dietitian at the Professional Golf Association National Resort and Spa in Palm Beach, Florida.

2. **Swab that tongue.** To find out how sensitive you are to the hotness of chili peppers, take a cotton swab dipped in blue food coloring and run it over your tongue. Then look at your papillae, the little bumps on your tongue where your taste buds are located. If they are as big as a pinhead, you're capable of eating the hottest of the hot. If they are much smaller, you might want to stick to more mild peppers, says Melissa Stock, former managing editor of *Chili Pepper* magazine. Jalapeño peppers are good starter peppers, Stock says. But if you have really small papillae, you may want to remove the seeds and white fleshy stuff to cool them down a bit.

3. **Have some wine with that water.** In the eighteenth century, a wine-and-garlic concoction seemed to protect grave diggers against the plague. While garlic is known as a bacterial fighter, researchers at the Tripler Army Medical Center in Honolulu are finding out that wine also played a role. When scientists pitted wine and the active ingredient in Pepto-Bismol against bacteria known to cause traveler's diarrhea, they found that wine was ten times more effective in killing the bugs. Tequila and pure alcohol had little protective effect. The two wines tested—California white and Spanish red—proved equally effective in killing off bacteria.

4. **Eat your tomatoes.** Harvard researchers who surveyed the eating habits of more than 47,000 men for six years say that a diet high in tomato-based foods may protect men from prostate cancer. The diets rich in tomatoes, tomato sauce and juice, and pizza seemed to have a dramatic protective effect against this most common cancer in men. Those who ate more than ten servings a week had a 35 percent reduction in the rate of prostate cancer. Researchers theorize that lycopene, an antioxidant nutrient found in large amounts in tomatoes, may be responsible. But this doesn't mean that you can live on pizza. A high-fat diet has been linked to prostate cancer. Your best bet is to indulge in the red sauce and go easy on the cheese.

5. **Test your vitamins.** Make sure that your vitamin will deliver what it promises by dropping one in a glass of white vinegar. If the pill doesn't break down in a half-hour, switch brands. Most nutrients are absorbed in the first part of your small intestine—where food and supplements linger only for 20 to 30 minutes, says Hartsough.

6. **Put some tea on that clogged artery.** Doctors have long known that eating a lot of vegetables can help ward off heart problems. But it wasn't until recently that they found that vegetables could also ward off stroke. And even more surprising was this discovery: Drinking a lot of black tea has the same effect. According to researchers at the National Institute of Public Health and Environmental Protection in the Netherlands, men who drank 4.7 cups of tea a day had a 69 percent lower risk of stroke than men who drank less than 2.6 cups per day. The researchers suspect that it's the antioxidative compounds in tea that keep cholesterol from binding to artery walls, thus keeping the passageways clear for blood to run.

7. **Eat a big meal? Exercise harder.** After overeating, older men burn fewer calories than younger ones. So as you age, if you want to stay the same weight, you'll need to compensate by doing a little more exercise, say researchers at the Jean Mayer U.S. Department of Agriculture Human Nutrition Research Center on Aging at Tufts University in Medford, Massachusetts. The theory is that aging slows down the metabolism, which means that the body burns fewer calories. Researchers tested out that theory by feeding a group of men in their sixties and seventies and a group of men in their twenties an extra 1,000 calories a day for three weeks. The older group ended up storing 87 calories a day as fat, which amounts to 2.2 pounds of fat a year, while the younger men's metabolisms increased to burn off the extra calories. This increase was not as significant in the older men, so they gained weight. The solution may be to take a walk after eating, the researchers suggest.

8. **Trim fat.** You can eat the food you like and still eat less fat. Here are a few strategies.

• Blot pizza grease with a napkin to eliminate up to a teaspoon of fat per slice.

• At McDonald's, order two small regular burgers instead of one quarter-pound cheese-burger to save ten grams of fat.

• Wipe half of the special sauce from your fast food sandwich to save six grams of fat.

• Use small-curd, low-fat cottage cheese instead of high-fat ricotta in lasagna, manicotti and other cheese-filled Italian dishes.

• Heat the oil in a skillet before cooking so that the meat absorbs less fat.

9. **Eat before you drink.** The more a man drinks, the more he eats, say researchers at Laval University in Quebec and Wageningen Agricultural University in the Netherlands. When the researchers had eight men eat lunch and dinner, sometimes drinking Molson, sometimes an alcohol-free beer at each meal, they found that the men ate more when drinking an alcoholic beer, especially when they were eating a high-fat meal. In a larger, related study, investigators found that people seem to eat more protein and less carbohydrate as well as take in more calories when drinking alcoholic beverages.

10. **Eat another fruit a day.** When British researchers studied the records of 96 men and women over 65 years of age, they found that those consuming 65 milligrams of vitamin C (roughly the equivalent of one orange a day) had reduced immune functioning, more respiratory illnesses and a higher risk of heart disease than those taking in 125 milligrams (about two oranges). The researchers caution that supplements may not fit the bill. Other chemicals present in fruit may enhance vitamin C absorption. If you are not in the mood for an orange, try guavas, kiwifruit, papaya, cantaloupe, grapefruit or a handful of berries.

11. **Take five-minute sun breaks.** The farther north you live, the more likely you need some extra vitamin D during the winter. Sunlight is the only cue the body uses to make the vitamin, which has been shown to strengthen bones and ward off prostate cancer. "But if you're living in a low-sunlight area during the winter, you could stand outside naked all day and still not make any vitamin D," says Michael F. Holick, M.D., Ph.D., director of the Vitamin D, Skin and Bone Research Laboratory at Boston University Medical Center. What to do? Make a point to get sun on your arms, face and neck three times a week for five minutes (before putting on sunscreen).

12. **Don't catch this buzz.** Someone at some point may have told you to start eating honey for various and sundry reasons, all of which were linked to the notion that honey is made from bee pollen. Myths would have you believe that bee pollen is good for you. It's all hornet wash. Bee pollen offers no health benefits. Plus it doesn't even come from bees. It's flower pollen and is useful only to other flowers. "It has been purported to cure impotence, allergies, immune problems, arthritis, you name it," says John H. Renner, M.D., president of the Consumer Health Information Research Institute in Independence, Missouri. "Because it came from nature, it was mystical enough to be alluring. But the fact is, there is no evidence that it has any benefit."

13. **Know your cuts.** The fish you buy over the counter at the fish store come in particular cuts. Read and learn from Aliza Green, a food and restaurant consultant in Philadelphia.

• Whole-dressed: It's a whole fish that's been gutted, scaled and possibly deboned.

• Pan-dressed: It's been gutted, scaled, beheaded, definned and detailed, the same as whole-dressed without the head.

• Steaked: It's a cross-section of a fish, usually about an inch thick. Rib steaks are cut from the front half of the fish, tail steaks from the back. When buying steaks, make sure that they are consistent in thickness so that they cook evenly.

• Filleted: It's a slab of fish removed from the bone from head to tail. It may come with or without skin. Be sure to remove the tiny pin bones from each layer of flesh.

• Surimi: It's imitation crabmeat, probably made from Alaskan pollack that has been ground into fish paste, supplemented with starches, flavorings and stabilizers, then molded to look like crab or lobster.

• Scrod: It's an old New England term for a small, white fish—which could be cod, haddock or pollack.

14. **Eat fish on thyme.** When buying fresh fish, keep it on ice. Ask the shop for a bag of ice or bring your own cooler. At home, keep fish in the refrigerator on ice, with wax paper between the fish and ice, and eat it the same day. To bring out the unique flavor of the sea creature, spice it with thyme.

15. **See red.** Sweet red peppers often cost twice as much as green ones, but they might be worth it. Red bell peppers contain nine times as much vitamin A as green peppers do. Vitamin A is a disease fighter known to speed the healing of wounds. Also, red peppers have more than double the amount of vitamin C.

16. **Follow the 30-second rule.** If you want to lose weight, eat slower. Put down your fork and wait 30 seconds between bites, says Art Ulene, M.D., medical correspondent for NBC's *Today*.

17. **Drop that beer belly.** There's a reason we refer to big tummies as beer bellies. Researchers measured the waists and drinking habits of men and found that you can drink as much wine as beer, but the wine won't saddle you with nearly as much of a belly as the beer will. In fact, wine may even reduce your waistline. Researchers speculate that it might contain substances that counterbalance the ill effects of its own alcohol.

3

SEX

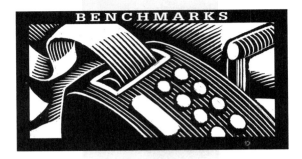

BENCHMARKS

AVERAGES

- Percentage of American men who say that they would marry the same woman if they had to do it all over again: 80

- Percentage of women who say that they would marry the same man: 50

- Percentage of adults who say that they were first told the facts of life by their mothers: 17

- Percentage who say that they were first told the facts of life by their fathers: 2

- Number of minutes a man makes love: 10

- Number of sexual partners a man has during his lifetime: 5 to 10

- Number of times a month a man has sex: 7

- Age at which men marry: 26

- Age at which men lose their virginity: 17

- Length of a penis at rest: 3.75 inches

- Length of a penis when erect: 6 to 7 inches

- Age at which a boy first ejaculates: 13 years, 2 months

- Percentage of American men who say that they would allow their spouse to have sex with a stranger in exchange for $1 million: 10

- Percentage of women who cite vulgar language as the biggest turnoff in a man: 81

- Percentage of women who've agreed to a date because they like the car a man drives: 7.5

EXTREMES

- Price of a wedding ceremony at the coin-operated 24-hour Church of Elvis in Portland, Oregon: $1

- Cost to replace a missing penis, à la John Bobbitt: $50,000

- Cost per minute to hear the Bill of Rights read over the phone "in a provocative manner" by a woman named Bambi: $1.98

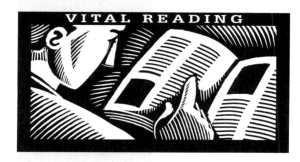

VITAL READING

Herbs for Better Erections

If your erections aren't as strong or as long-lasting as they used to be, check out these herbal products uncovered by new research.

Maybe you don't get as hard as you did ten years ago. Maybe you can't last as long. Maybe your erections switch on and off during a sexual encounter. Whatever the manifestation, more than 40 percent of men between the ages of 40 and 70 suffer from moderate-to-minimal erection problems. Not so bad that they'd seek major medical help, but not exactly a quality-of-life plus either.

That's where herbal remedies and simple devices come in. Recent research has shown that a myriad of products as close as your local drugstore or mail-order vendor can significantly boost erections. Here's the pick of the litter.

Ginkgo biloba. In a recent study out of Germany, investigators studied 20 men who could have erections only when injecting special drugs into their penises. After nine months of taking an 80-milligram capsule of ginkgo biloba three times a day, all 20 were able to have spontaneous erections (without drugs), and experienced measurable increases in the hardness of the penis throughout its length.

"This research has definitely made believers out of skeptics," says Steven Margolis, M.D., a family physician practicing in Sterling Heights, Michigan, who has long recommended ginkgo biloba to his patients with erectile problems.

To understand how ginkgo biloba, an herb that increases blood flow, could make a soft man hard, you have to understand a little about erections. When you're aroused, your brain sends a message to your penis to accept as much as ten times more blood into two long tubes. The body then traps the blood (via the tubes themselves and valves on veins) into the hard, full erection.

As men age and plaque builds up on arteries, blood flow throughout the body is impaired. This reduced blood flow can result in leg pain, memory problems, heart disease—and erection softening. By revving up the travel of blood throughout the body, ginkgo biloba hardens erections, perks up the mind and strengthens the heart in some men.

Your best bet: If you're an otherwise healthy older man suffering from minor-to-moderate erection problems, it might make sense to give ginkgo biloba a try. "First, see your doctor to make sure that your blood pressure and cholesterol levels are normal and that you have no possible complicating medical issues," says Dr. Margolis. You'll probably want to start with 60 milligrams twice a day (research has found that's all it takes to help 50 percent of men with mild erectile problems).

If you don't see a result in four weeks, move up to 80 milligrams three times a day. Before buying ginkgo biloba, check the label to be sure that it's a standardized formula, that it contains 24 percent flavonoids and that it meets the German standards ("listed in the German Kommission E").

Chinese ginseng. For centuries, Chinese healers have valued ginseng as a male virility tonic. Now, modern-day Chinese research suggests that ingredients in ginseng, steroidlike chemicals called ginsenosides, play a key role in erection. After studying rabbit erectile tissues, the investigators found that ginsenosides encourage tiny penile muscles responsible for the inflow of blood to relax. This relaxation has long been known to be the central event in erection hardening.

Your best bet: Since the key to Chinese ginseng's effect is the ginsenosides, you should aim to get between 15 and 45 milligrams of ginsenosides a day, advises Michael T. Murray, a doctor of naturopathy in Seattle and author of *Male Sexual Vitality*.

Yohimbine. Derived from the bark of an African tree, yohimbine (in one form or another) has been used to boost male virility for centuries. While yohimbine may increase libido, its main action is to drive more blood to erectile tissues. Indeed, 34 to 43 percent of men with moderate erectile problems have been shown to benefit greatly from taking yohimbine daily.

The catch? Many possibly dangerous side effects, including elevations in heart rate and blood pressure, anxiety and hallucinations. "You should take yohimbine under a doctor's supervision," advises Dr. Margolis.

Your best bet: Talk to your doctor about taking 125 milligrams of a generic yohimbine formulation (the brand names are as much as three times more expensive).

Penis rings. Who says that you have to ingest something to boost an erection? For as long as man has had a penis, he's devised ways of maintaining an erection centered on the concept of trapping blood in the penis using something that circles the organ's base.

Most of these devices have a dual-ring structure: You drop one testicle at a time through the lower ring and then tuck your flaccid penis through the upper ring. As you become erect, the penis ring gets tighter, trapping blood in the penis and heightening penile sensation and erection du-

ration. Doctors caution never to keep a ring around a penis for more than 30 minutes—it's especially crucial not to fall asleep with the ring on.

Your best bet: Rings come in three varieties: latex, metal and leather. Forget the metal: If your erection won't subside for whatever reason, you'll have to go to the emergency room for removal. We prefer leather—simply because a man can unsnap a leather penis strap after 30 minutes whether his erection has subsided or not. The latex is a compromise—less expensive (and less appealing) than the leather, but easier to remove (by cutting) than the metal.

Slip Sliding Away

Using personal lubricants could revolutionize your sex life.

Something's changed. You're not sure what, but sex just isn't what it used to be. Maybe your partner seems distant and uninterested, maybe her remoteness just comes and goes, or maybe it's you who just can't seem to get things going. Although it may seem as though the relationship is on the rocks, you may have just literally hit dry ground.

"A common cause for both men and women to lose interest in sex is a simple lack of lubrication," says Bruce Bekkar, M.D., an obstetrician and gynecologist practicing with the Southern California Kaiser-Permanente Group in San Diego. Think of two pieces of sandpaper rubbing against each other and you'll start to get an idea of how unsatisfying "dry" intercourse can be. It's none too healthy either: Rubbing sensitive skin on the penis or vagina lining too vigorously can cause abrasions and infections.

Since arousal is the primary stimulant for lubrication, dry sex can set in motion a destructive cycle. "Less lubrication creates less pleasurable sexual sensations. The diminishment in pleasure then leads to less arousal, which in turn creates even lower levels of lubrication," explains Dr. Bekkar.

And that downward lack-of-slide cycle can have a big effect on the performance of the penis. When men have anything less than a rock-hard erection, lack of lubrication may make the situation worse by making intercourse more difficult. "If a man's attempting penetration and is not succeeding, he can get so frustrated and disappointed that he loses the erection altogether," says Laurence Levine, M.D., director of the Male Sexual Function and Fertility Program at Rush–Presbyterian–St. Luke's Medical Center in Chicago.

All of these side effects can take a real toll on your relationship. When a man starts to notice that his wife seems remote and sexually uninterested, he may start to wonder if she's having an affair or if he's simply not able to satisfy her anymore. "It's very threatening to men when they're used to having their partners respond in a certain way and suddenly, or gradually, she just seems to lose interest," says Dr. Bekkar.

Think back on a recent sexual encounter. Did you feel a lot of friction, or have trouble with initial penetration, or did things seem to slide together without much trouble? If you had several orgasms, did the later ones seem to generate more friction? Does the friction tend to increase the longer you keep going? Does your partner need more time before penetration than she used to? Do the lubrication levels seem to vary at different times of the month? If the answer to any of these questions is "yes," your sex life may be in need of a little lube fine-tuning.

Different Causes

First, it's important to understand that men don't make much of a contribution in the slippery realm of sexual lubrication. While some men produce a bit of lubrication from tiny glands that line the urethra (the tube that carries semen and urine through the penis), most release nothing more than a little early seminal fluid. "Lubrication falls almost entirely to the woman. Men don't really contribute in a noticeable way," says Dr. Levine.

It's critical then to throw off our studied ignorance of all things related to the female cycle. By understanding when lubrication might not be available, no matter how aroused your partner is, you can learn when it might be critical to have a little lube tube handy.

Menstrual cycle. If your partner seems very lubricated at some times and fairly dry at others, it may simply be because of her monthly cycle. Women in their childbearing years ride a veritable hormonal roller coaster, undergoing shifts in the quantity and quality of lubrication at different points of their cycles.

About two weeks after menstruation, certain hormones peak and the egg is released. It's during this time of the month, ovulation, that the opening to the uterus, the cervix, begins to release a watery mucus that forms a slick highway to facilitate the sperm's journey to the egg. "This increase in cervical mucus adds to a feeling of vaginal 'wetness,'" says Margaret Polaneczky, M.D., assistant professor of obstetrics and gynecology at New York Hospital–Cornell Medical Center in New York City. Some women also report heightened desire at this point in their cycles.

Postpartum. After the birth of a child, a woman's estrogen levels dive, and they stay fairly low as long as she's breastfeeding. "When estrogen levels are low for a prolonged period of time, the vaginal tissues just don't lubricate very well," explains Dr. Bekkar.

Menopause. Right around age 50, most women will undergo dramatic hormonal shifts that signal an end to their reproductive years— and a dramatic drop in their levels of lubrication. "Within a few months to a year after menopause occurs, a woman will notice a significant decrease in her amount of lubrication and the elasticity of her vaginal tissues," says Dr. Bekkar. Both of these effects are brought about by a reduction in the level of estrogen—and can often be reversed in the long term by taking estrogen supplements.

Choosing the Lubricant for You

So now that you know when and why you need a lubricant, the best thing to do is run out to your local drugstore and pick up whatever they have—right? Not exactly. "Widely available lubricants, like K-Y Jelly, were originally designed for medical use and aren't designed to stay slick as long as some of the products especially designed for sex," says Cathy Winks of Good Vibrations, an adult mail-order company based in San Francisco. In other words, you may want to buy your lubricant from a sex specialty store.

When it comes to selecting a particular lubricant, keep in mind your intended usage. If you're going to pair the lube with a condom, be sure to stick with water-based formulation: The oils in some brands can eat away at latex. If you'll be using lubricants in conjunction with oral sex, read the labels carefully: Glycerin and sucrose carry a sweet taste, and detergents such as nonoxynol-9, methylparaben and propylparaben are likely to impart a soapy, medicinal flavor. Some people have reported a slight numbing of the tongue with lubricants containing nonoxynol-9. "It's perfectly safe to use," assures Dr. Polaneczky.

The rules for using lubricants are simple: A little dab, lightly rubbed on the clitoris. penis or just inside the vagina, will do ya.

If you or your partner notices a problem with painful intercourse as a result of dryness, experts recommend that you get a physical to rule out any more serious problems such as a yeast infection or a sexually transmitted disease.

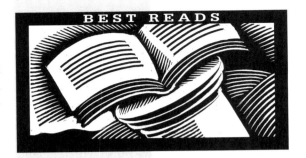

BEST READS

Peak Erotic Experiences

The most important sex organ of all is the brain, asserts Jack Morin, Ph.D., in his controversial book The Erotic Mind: Unlocking the Inner Sources of Sexual Passion and Fulfillment *(HarperCollins, 1995). It's intuitively true. Physical contact is pleasurable only if your mind is tuned in the right way. In this excerpt, Dr. Morin discusses what a man's turn-ons reveal about his sexuality.*

One of the most effective and enjoyable ways to unlock the mysteries of the eros is to reminisce about your most compelling turn-ons. During these moments of high arousal, the crucial elements—your partner, the setting, perhaps a tantalizing twist of luck—all mesh like instruments of an orchestra, producing a crescendo of passion. Look closely at a peak turn-on and you'll undoubtedly sense that something close to the core of your being has been touched. And because everything is accentuated during such moments, they reveal an enormous amount about how your eroticism works.

As a young psychology student in the 1960s, I was influenced by Abraham Maslow, who called for a "psychology of health" to counterbalance the overemphasis on problems that he believed was distorting our view of human beings. He broke new ground by studying people he called self-actualizers—those who are comfortable with themselves, relatively free of neurotic conflicts from the past and available to tackle the challenges of living with creativity and zest. Self-actualizers are still largely ignored by psychologists, even though they have much to teach us about emotional well-being.

Maslow was equally intrigued by a wide variety of peak experiences—such as being enraptured by a beautiful piece of music or a painting, a special communion with nature or the joy of bodily expression in dance or athletics, to name just a few. During these moments of ecstasy, we are fully present in the moment, unself-consciously expressing our truest selves with ease and grace, grateful to be alive. Even though peak experiences aren't productive in the usual sense, participants invariably describe them as profoundly positive and sometimes even life-changing.

According to Maslow, self-actualizers have peak experiences more frequently than the rest of us, but nearly everyone has them occasionally. Among his most provocative observations was that during and following peak experiences we temporarily take on many of the characteristics of self-actualizers. In other words, peaks offer us glimpses of our most authentic, healthiest selves and thus can serve us as guides to growth. Maslow saw peak experiences as crucial sources of "clean and uncontaminated data" about who we are and might become.

When I began my formal studies of eroticism as a practicing psychotherapist, I approached the challenge with Maslow's insights in mind. I was convinced that if I devoted as much attention to peak sexual experiences as I did to problems, I could eventually discern truths about eroticism that would otherwise elude me. My first discovery was rather discouraging: Even in the nonjudgmental atmosphere of therapy, people rarely bring up their peak turn-ons spontaneously. And when I started asking, I quickly learned that most clients required a high comfort level and a significant amount of courage before they were willing to disclose de-tails about this extremely intimate material.

I began encouraging clients who were grappling with sexual problems to explore their peak turn-ons, hoping the potential benefits of doing so would be obvious to them. In most cases I was wrong. The majority had trouble grasping the value of discussing their peak experiences; they just wanted to fix their problems. A prevalent comment was, "Sure, I've had good sex in the past, but what can that do for me now?" Out of necessity I became adept at gently challenging clients to set aside their preoccupation with problems for a while so that they might learn more about their eroticism.

I quickly saw that those who accepted my challenge typically made more rapid and long-lasting progress than those who insisted on focusing exclusively on their troubles. Some improvements came about when they used their peak turn-ons to help clarify their conditions for satisfying sex—an extremely important ingredient for successful sex therapy.

Fred: Centerfold Syndrome?

Fred consulted me because his sexual desire for Janette, his wife of six years, had been declining for more than a year. Although he assumed that she must have noticed the reduction in both the frequency of sex and his enthusiasm, Fred had no idea how to discuss his predicament with Janette without hurting her. Besides, he felt ashamed of himself and was convinced that she couldn't possibly understand what he was going through.

"I think I have the centerfold syndrome," he announced about halfway through our first meeting. He explained that as a young adolescent he had masturbated to photos in his dad's *Playboy* magazines. More than 20 years later, the majority of his fantasies were still populated by young women with picture-perfect bodies. "My wife still looks great," he added, "but she's no centerfold. I know it sounds horrible to say, but I can't help noticing her body changing. I love her too much to tell her the truth."

Clients, especially introspective ones like Fred, often enter therapy with theories about the origins of their problems. Fred was the first, however, to have invented and named a new diagnosis. Yet many other men—and more than a few women, too—had hinted that constant images of sexual perfection in the mass media sometimes reduced the allure of their actual partners. Obviously, Fred had named a very real problem.

However, as Fred talked about his sex history and his relationship with Janette, I sensed that his declining desire had less to do with flawless centerfolds than he believed. To help him find out for himself, I suggested that he think about his peak turn-ons. After overcoming his initial hesitation, he told me about a series of memorable encounters with a young waitress and aspiring model with whom he had had an affair when he was in the military. His obvious pleasure in telling these stories soon turned to discouragement because they seemed to confirm his theory. I suggested that before jumping to conclusions he consider other factors that also might have turned him on besides her gorgeous body.

As he revealed the details of these remarkably passionate encounters, it became clear that in each instance his excitement reached its zenith when the waitress unambiguously demonstrated her attraction for him by "losing control" and "going after what she wanted." Certainly, her appearance stimulated his desire, but it was her escalating enthusiasm that transformed simple desire into fiery passion. Fred discovered that when he fantasized about a centerfold-like woman, the visual enjoyment of her perfect body was merely a starting point. As his arousal built, he imagined her casting caution to the wind and "going crazy with lust."

Then I asked about peak encounters with his wife, of which there had been many, even some during the previous year. Because he had already recognized how much he valued a highly responsive and eager partner, he quickly saw that in every peak encounter with Janette, she, too, had been unusually expressive and uninhibited. Fred also stumbled on another important fact: Whenever Janette exhibited the impassioned fervor that excited him, he automatically perceived her differently; he completely ignored her imperfections and focused instead on her most appealing attributes.

As it turned out, Fred's declining desire was influenced—but not caused—by his fascination with centerfolds. Much more important than Janette's changing body was the fact that she had become increasingly passive in recent years, to the point where Fred was no longer sure if she particularly enjoyed sex with him anymore. Luckily, the two of them had always talked openly about most things, although it had been years since they had discussed sex. Spurred on by a deeper understanding of his eroticism and a reduction of his guilt, Fred initiated an extremely productive dialogue with Janette.

Once she felt assured that his intention was not to criticize her but to improve their sex life, she acknowledged her increasing passivity in bed. She explained how Fred's tendency to be sexually aggressive had led her to conclude that he preferred her to be submissive. She was just trying to give him what she assumed he wanted. She also divulged that her passivity was making sex less interesting for her, too. As she grasped how much Fred missed feeling her unbridled desire, she gradually felt freer to let her excitement show. And in response, Fred's passions once again began to stir.

Fred might have found a solution to his problem without examining his peak turn-ons. And, of course, this couple's ability to communicate so productively and become sexually experimental—skills that many sex therapy clients lack—were essential to their success. But by freeing him from the discouraging and mistaken belief that only physical perfection could excite him, Fred's memories of peak sex greatly accelerated his progress.

Breasts

One thing that men universally agree on is the beauty of a woman's breast. Stefan Bechtel and Laurence Roy Stains eloquently explain why this is true and reveal some intriguing characteristics of the female breast in an excerpt from their book Sex: A Man's Guide *(Rodale Press, 1996).*

It's hard to imagine anything more entrancing than a woman's breast, especially a breast swollen with sexual excitement, firmly pendulous as a sun-ripened mango, a succulent melon raised to your hungry lips, nipple erect, pert and uplifted, aflame with . . .

Oh—sorry.

But, hey, maybe we can be forgiven, since that's one of men's absolute favorite sexual daydreams. In fact, in one University of Missouri study of male sex fantasies, kissing a pair of monumental breasts was the second most frequently mentioned fantasy (outranked only by the thought of getting turned on by a pair of terrific legs).

The really interesting news is that when women in the same study were asked their favorite fantasies, the one they mentioned most often was . . . having a man kiss their breasts.

A "Distinctively Human" Act

The late Alfred C. Kinsey, a former zoology professor, pointed out that while the desire to kiss and fondle a woman's breasts may seem about as natural to you as anything can possibly be, it's actually fairly uncommon among other animals. "Mouth-breast contact," he reported, "constitutes the one technique in human petting behavior that is most distinctively human."

We must all be pretty human: Various sex surveys have shown that over 90 percent of men enjoy stimulating their lover's breasts during sex, whether by mouth, hand or otherwise. Oddly, women don't enjoy it quite as much as men do, some evidence suggests. In fact, if you think of female masturbation techniques as the key to understanding what actually turns women on most, it's interesting to note that only 11 percent of the nearly 8,000 women Dr. Kinsey studied said they liked to stroke their own breasts during masturbation (compared to 84 percent who stroked their clitoris or labia minora, the soft inner lips that surround it). Only a very small percentage of women can reach orgasm purely through stimulation of their breasts, other sex surveys have shown.

It seems a contradiction: Lots of women fantasize about having their breasts kissed, but when it really happens, many don't seem to enjoy it that much. "Women do report taking pleasure in watching their partners having pleasure," says Shirley Zussman, Ed.D., a certified sex therapist and co-director of the Association for Male Sexual Dysfunction in New York City. "She may be aroused, indirectly, by watching him kissing her breasts. That's what excites her."

The Pleasure of Breasts

American males are often accused of being obsessed with big breasts, and it's probably true. The French, by contrast, maintain that the ideal breast should fit inside a champagne glass. Don't forget, though, that the size of a woman's breasts has no more to do with a woman's sex drive than the size of your penis has to do with your sex drive, says Judith Seifer, R.N., Ph.D., president of the American Association of Sex Educators, Counselors and Therapists. A flat-chested woman is as likely to be sexually charged as a woman who is very well endowed.

And breast size has nothing to do with breast sensitivity either. Jolan Chang, writing in *The Tao of Love and Sex*, a book about ancient Chinese sexual techniques, observes that "strange as it may seem, the size or beauty of a woman's breasts is irrelevant to whether she enjoys them being kissed, sucked or licked." But he goes on to say: "With many women there is a direct connection between nipples and vulva. Stimulating these two delicate buttons either by kissing, sucking or caressing will... quickly result in the vagina overflowing with lubricant."

You may have discovered on your adventures that a woman's breasts may occasionally exude a few dewdrops of sweet-tasting liquid that isn't milk. This exotic exudate has been described in erotic literature as witches' milk, white snow or sometimes even the peach juice of immortality.

"The mammary glands can express sweet-tasting, plasmalike fluids when a woman is not lactating (producing milk)," Dr. Seifer explains. "We don't know why, but we've recently noticed that some women using Norplant (an implantable contraceptive) will drip from the breast. This also occurs when women have elevated blood levels of prolactin (a hormone that induces milk production), which is sometimes caused by a lesion on the anterior pituitary gland."

Interestingly, women with pituitary lesions also have difficulty reaching orgasm until the lesion is surgically removed, Dr. Seifer says. So if your woman is having trouble reaching orgasm and she has the peach juice of immortality on her blouse, consider suggesting that she see a doctor.

What Happens during Arousal

The sex researchers William H. Masters, M.D., and Virginia E. Johnson, of the former Masters and Johnson Institute in St. Louis, spent a lot of time carefully observing what happens to people's bodies when they get sexually aroused. (You've probably noticed a few things yourself, but you probably didn't take notes.)

One of the key things Dr. Masters and Johnson noticed about the female breast was that the "virgin" breasts of a young woman who has never suckled a baby undergo quite different changes than the breasts of a woman who has breastfed.

The first visible evidence of sexual excitement in an "unsuckled" breast, they found, is nipple erection. This usually occurs very shortly after any sort of stimulation. Often, her nipples don't become erect simultaneously—one may get erect very rapidly while the other lags behind. This is especially true if her breasts are markedly different sizes or one of the nipples is slightly inverted (nipples can be "innies," too, just like belly buttons).

At the same time, the areola (that beautiful dark disk around the nipple) also begins to swell. In fact, because the areola tends to swell faster than the nipple, there's often a momentary impression that the nipple has disappeared, or that she's lost her nipple erection. Well, that's not so; it's just that everything is swelling with the "vasocongestion" (damming up of blood) that's one of the essential elements of arousal. Her whole breast may swell as much as 20 to 25 percent; at the same time a fine tracery of veins appears on her breast, sometimes standing out in bold relief. You'll also probably notice a pink mottling of her skin called the sex flush, spreading like an ocean sunset from her upper belly to the top, sides and then undersides of her breasts.

After she's reached orgasm (or after she begins cooling off—the "resolution phase" of the sexual response cycle), the sex flush rapidly fades away. Her swollen areolae quickly return to their pre-aroused state. Because they shrink more rapidly than her nipples do, you may have the momentary impression that she's having a new nipple erection (sometimes called a false erection), but that's just nature trying to fool you.

The "Suckled" Breast

In women who've suckled babies (especially more than one), this sexual swelling is much less dramatic. In fact, women who have breastfed "frequently show little or no increase in breast size" when they're aroused, Dr. Masters and Johnson reported (partly because milk production increases the venous drainage of the breast). Older women's breasts don't swell during arousal so much either. And, as a general thing, the more slack and pendulous the breasts of a woman of any age (otherwise known as the National Geographic effect), the less likely they are to swell during sexual stimulation.

You may not have noticed it, but your own nipples probably also got erect the last time you were aroused. In fact, Dr. Masters and Johnson reported, "few men under 60 years of age ejaculate without an obvious turgidity (swelling), if not full erection, of the nipples." This other, tinier erection, which tends to fade away as a guy gets older—just like your other one—often persists for a long time, sometimes even hours, after ejaculation.

A Word about Technique

One of the most important things to remember about ravishing a woman's breasts is that you need to get feedback from her about what she likes and doesn't like, Dr. Zussman says. Breast sensitivity varies greatly from woman to woman, and at different times in the same woman. Especially during the few days before her period and during the first few months of pregnancy, her nipples and breasts may be so sensitive that she doesn't want to be touched at all. Be gentle, go slow. Don't knead them like bread. Adore them.

If She's Had Breast Implants

What about women who've had breast implants—do they have any less feeling in there?

"Well, some do, some don't—the more surgery involved, the less feeling they have," Dr. Seifer says. "Actually, there's usually a more profound loss of feeling in breast-reduction surgery than implant surgery because sometimes they move the nipple around and really reconstruct it."

Women who've had breast reconstruction surgery after a mastectomy for breast cancer often are struggling with their sexual self-esteem as well. In fact, "women with breast cancer are often more afraid of losing their husbands or lovers...than they are about the possibility of facing a cruel and untimely death," observes Helen Singer Kaplan, M.D., Ph.D., director of the human sexuality program at New York Hospital–Cornell Medical Center in New York City. The great majority of husbands and lovers don't lose sexual interest in their mates after mastectomy—provided they were turned on by her before the surgery, Dr. Kaplan says. But latent marital and sexual problems are likely to be stirred up by the mastectomy, and therapy may be useful. The most important thing is to keep the lines of communication open.

"The man may be grieving also, especially if he's a 'breast man,'" says Dr. Seifer. "It's important to be able to say, 'Damn right I'm gonna miss those things!' and not pretend that you don't."

Occasionally, a man who has ravished his wife's breasts for years will be filled with dread and guilt when she develops breast cancer—especially if the breast he tends to favor is the one that develops a tumor, observes Jude Cotter, Ph.D., a psychologist and sex therapist in private practice in Farmington Hills, Michigan. He'll harbor the terrible fear that it was he who caused the cancer. But there's no known connection between breast stimulation and breast cancer, so this is not really anything to worry about.

So enjoy yourself.

Welcome to the human race.

Aphrodisiacs

In an excerpt from Sex: A Man's Guide *(Rodale Press, 1996), Stefan Bechtel and Laurence Roy Stains tackle the age-old question of whether aphrodisiacs are for real. And, yes, they talk about Spanish fly.*

Take a tip from all those fancy hotels. Leave a piece of fine chocolate on your lover's pillow.

That first kiss afterward will be especially delicious. Then you can say, "Did you know that chocolate contains an amino acid that stimulates the brain to make phenylethylamine, a chemical released when we fall in love?" If she responds with, "That has to be the geekiest thing you've ever said," maybe you should soften your approach. Try something more romantic, like: "You know, Casanova always drank chocolate before entering the boudoir." Tell her that chocolate has been regarded as an aphrodisiac ever since the Aztecs handed a box to Cortés.

The sudden appearance of chocolate can even become your own little bedtime ritual. Whenever either of you wants to invite the other for a walk in the garden of earthly delights, you can reveal your intent, wordlessly. It will be your own private sex signal. Perhaps there will be nights when both of you find chocolate on your pillows. Those nights we live for.

But all that aphrodisiac stuff. Is there really anything to it? Well, maybe there isn't, and maybe there is. Stop being such a little inspector about it, will you? It's all in the suggestion. You see, when researchers have tried to prove the claims about aphrodisiacs, they often get a big placebo effect. For example: In one Canadian trial of the drug yohimbine, 42 percent of a group of impotent men responded to treatment—but so did 28 percent of the "control" group, who were slipped a simple sugar pill! Santa Monica family practitioner Cynthia Mervis Watson, M.D., writes in her book *Love Potions: The Doctor's Guide to Aphrodisia,* "it is entirely possible that as long as your brain *thinks* that any given substance or ritual will work, it will trigger the appropriate chemical responses and your body will experience all the physical signs of arousal."

An old Cole Porter love song said it: "Do, do that voodoo!"

Coming Soon to Your Local Pharmacy

If you insist, we'll tell you about some real, actual, bona fide, scientifically tested aphrodisiacs. They are drugs with names like L-dopa, apomorphine, trazodone, bupropion and fenfluramine. Unfortunately, you wouldn't take these drugs unless you were suffering from clinical depression, bulimia or Parkinson's disease. Patients who've been put on these drugs have experienced a quite unintended zing in the libido department. But when subsequently administered to healthy groups, the drugs produced only mixed results, and their side effects ranged from uncontrollable yawning to irregular heartbeats.

Nonetheless, the medical research community's experiences with these drugs have led to a greater understanding of arousal and the brain chemistry behind it. In the last few decades we've seen some drugs dampen sexual arousal—notably, drugs commonly prescribed for high blood pressure, depression and high cholesterol. Other drugs—those mentioned above, plus a couple others—awaken the libido. Most of them do it by mimicking a brain chemical called dopamine, one of the neurotransmitters that brain cells use to communicate with each other. Raymond C. Rosen, Ph.D., professor at the Robert Wood

Johnson Medical School in Piscataway, New Jersey, and a leading researcher in the field, has coined a term for these medications: "prosexual drugs."

The perfect aphrodisiac, says Dr. Rosen, would heighten sexual desire, pleasure and performance. That magic substance "is still eluding us," he says. But drugs that match part of that job description are in the pipeline. Specifically, new drugs to treat erection problems are now in clinical trials—oral medications, not the currently available drugs that you must, alas, inject into your penis before each use. "There's great interest and enthusiasm" about these drugs among researchers, he says. Also coming soon: a drug treatment for premature ejaculation. "We're understanding more and more about the neuropharmacology," Dr. Rosen says. "The future of prosexual drugs looks very good."

Well, that's nice for guys with performance problems. But what about desire? What about pleasure? What about people who can summon neither? The major pharmaceutical companies seem not to be so interested in that. "A few efforts to increase libido have not worked out," Dr. Rosen says. "We don't have a good libido drug that's free of side effects at this point." A few years ago, researchers had high hopes for the drug quinelorane. It went as far as clinical trials; once nausea appeared as a side effect, its maker, Eli Lilly, suddenly stopped the research.

So. We're back to using . . . what? Spanish fly?

Eating Wild Yams?

Once upon a time, when the authors were callow youths, we couldn't spell "aphrodisiac," but we'd heard about Spanish fly. It was supposed to make a woman beg you for sex. As pimply 14-year-olds, we figured that was the only way we would ever enjoy a liaison with the opposite sex. The whole notion of aphrodisiacs appealed to the era's playboy philosophy, magnified by early adolescence—the ultimate way to trick a young woman into having sex. Big fun.

Dr. Watson, in *Love Potions*, debunks our dweeby dreams of Spanish fly. She says that it isn't an aphrodisiac at all. The extract from a Spanish "blister beetle" (real name: cantharides), it does cause extreme irritation of the urogenital tract, among other horrid symptoms, although an indiscriminate roll in the hay is not the sort of relief that will leap to the poor sufferer's mind.

Forget Spanish fly. There are thousands of traditional aphrodisiacs, devised by every major culture, and most of them are listed in Dr. Watson's book. She argues that many traditional aphrodisiacs contain the vitamins, amino acids and enzymes that nourish our brain chemistry, creating the chemistry for love—"which is why they really do work," or so she claims. You should know that the Food and Drug Administration claims they really *don't* work.

Among her foods for love are avocados, carrots, figs, peaches, asparagus, garlic, onions, potatoes, artichokes, cucumbers, oysters, pomegranates, tomatoes, honey, royal jelly and "prairie oysters," the testicles of bulls and rams. Much less appetizing, and a lot harder to find in your local grocer's aisle: tiger penises, the index finger of a gallows corpse, the right lobe of a vulture's lung, edible nests made from the spittle of Malaysian sea swallows.

The plant world is where the pharmaceutical industry finds its compounds, so if you have any interest in herbs, you can eliminate the middleman. Among the venerable herbs of love: damiana (a shrub that grows in the desert of Mexico and Texas), saw palmetto berries (the saw palmetto is the palm tree that grows in the American Southeast), wild yams (native to Mexico), licorice root, kola nuts, ginkgo, sarsaparilla, red clover and bee pollen.

The strength of Dr. Watson's book is that she gets down to recipes. A recipe for damiana, for instance, involves soaking an ounce of the dried herb's leaves in a pint of vodka for five days, straining and then soaking them in three-fourths of a pint of water for another five days, heating the water, adding some honey, and recombining with the vodka. Dr. Watson says she has "personally observed its amatory effects."

For love potion ingredients try the Health Center for Better Living, 6189 Taylor Road, Naples, FL 33942; 1-800-544-4225. Health Center for Better Living sells blends containing most of the aforementioned aphrodisiacs. Just look for the labels "Love Formula," "Male Power" and "Man's Rejuvenator" in the catalog.

If you've always intended to become a junior herbalist, you're all set.

As for the rest of you . . . looking for something a little more conventional? There's always alcohol, America's favorite aphrodisiac. Only one problem: Alcohol is technically a depressant. It does remove inhibitions—hence the bit of bathroom-wall wisdom, "Candy is dandy, but liquor is quicker." But in anything more than moderation it can render you temporarily impotent. Numerous studies show that, at best, it reduces arousal and the intensity of orgasm in both men and women. Likewise its modern counterparts, the "recreational drugs" such as amphetamines, barbiturates, cocaine and marijuana. Perhaps you already know that, based on unfortunate personal experience.

Based on fortunate experiences, here's what does work: A great meal. A crackling fire. Candlelight. Soft music. Fragrances. Lingerie. Sweet nothings whispered in the ear. And chocolate.

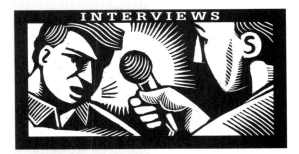

Richard A. Carroll on
Making Love through the Ages

Richard A. Carroll, Ph.D., is director of the Northwestern Medical Center, Sex and Marital Therapy Program in Chicago. As a veteran counselor, Dr. Carroll has seen it all when it comes to sexual issues. But one that continues to draw his attention is the relationship between age and sex.

Dr. Carroll says that a wealth of evidence, both societal, cultural and learned, seems to imply that sex and aging are mutually exclusive concepts. That's a serious shortcoming in a society as sexual as America—a society where a tremendous chunk of our population will be considered elderly in the next few decades.

"There's this archetypal picture of the elderly being asexual," Dr. Carroll says. "Aside from the pejorative dirty-old-man stereotype, there isn't a healthy, positive image in our society of older people as sexual beings."

We asked Dr. Carroll about the relationship between age and sex and, more important, to detail ways that you can remain sexually untarnished in the golden years. Here's what he said.

Do older people have sexual desires, and what exactly is sexual desire?

Sexual desire is best defined as "the urge to engage in sexual behavior," and older people have it as well as younger people. But desire as we know it really comes from several sources in our bodies. There's clearly a physical impetus to it. For example, much of our desire is biological, particularly hormonal. Sexual desire in both men and women is dependent on a certain level of testosterone. There's a critical level of testosterone that both sexes need. Below that threshold, you experience a decrease in desire. Beyond the critical level, it really doesn't matter how much you have. There's also a mental component to desire, based on emotion and your feelings for the other person. These, too, affect and influence sexual desire.

Is sexual desire the same in older men as it is in younger men?

Not really. Nothing in our bodies remains the same as it used to be, including our sexual urges. As a man gets older, it's likely that his level of testosterone will decrease. The key, of course, isn't the gross amount of testosterone coursing through his body. It's what's called bioavailable testosterone. That's the testosterone available in the bloodstream. The older you get, the less bioavailable testosterone you have.

In younger men, there tends to be more free-floating testosterone, which means there's a greater chance for desire, chemically speaking. As a man gets older, there tends to be less desire because of his fluctuating amounts of available testosterone. Most men find that their sexual desire peaks around the age of 18, 19 or 20. It begins to decrease thereafter slowly but probably won't be recognizable until later in life. Around 50, the changes are pronounced for most men, and they get more noticeable as time passes.

Does all this mean that men in their fifties won't be virile?

First of all, try to avoid using the word *virile*. I personally try to clean up our language whenever I can about these things, because our language is packed with so many loaded terms. The

implication of virility is that if a man isn't as sexually driven as he was in his twenties, he isn't as manly. *Virile* is such a loaded term, because if you're not virile, you're wimpy, as the thinking goes. And that's just not so.

If you don't use the word "virile," how do you describe it?

We describe more or less sex drive as normal fluctuating changes. It's normal for a man's body to react differently to sexual desires and impulses as he gets older. The travesty is that people think sex ends in retirement. We certainly don't want to foster an image of a man being an asexual being after age 60. There are plenty of men who are in their sixties who have strong sex drives, and plenty of men in their seventies who are still sexually active. You don't necessarily have to burn out as you age.

Speaking of those "normal changes," how do most men react to these fluctuations?

Because our language and society and culture are so permeated with sex, many men think that if they're not as sexually active as they used to be, there's something wrong with them. There's so much pressure and expectation for a man to be able to perform on demand or to be able to perform constantly that it's hard for him to accept the changes in his body. It's a shame, because these changes are purely natural and biological. What's important is that we try to get over the image of a man's masculinity being intricately tied to his sexuality. If a man can't get an erection or doesn't feel like having sex, he's still a man. Sex doesn't make the man.

This all sounds like a great attitude adjustment to make, but are there some specific things individuals can do to increase the chances that they'll be making love after 60?

Certainly, and perhaps the most important thing you can do is accept that change is normal.

Just because you don't have the same sexual response in your sixties as you did in your thirties doesn't mean it's the end of the line and that you can't have a normal, happy sex life. Feeling otherwise will only make you feel inadequate.

These changes you'll encounter somewhere along the road include a drop in desire, the occasional inability to get an erection, the necessity of more stimulation and more direct stimulation to get an erection, taking longer to achieve orgasm, orgasms that aren't as intense or forceful as they used to be and longer refractory periods, or recovery periods between orgasms.

What else? What physical steps can we take?

The best physical advice I can give you is this: Use it or lose it!

Are you serious? You mean have more sex? That sounds like advice every man wants to hear.

Yes. The more sex you have, the more sex you'll be able to have. This happens because there's a feedback cycle here. Orgasm and ejaculation stimulate the production of testosterone, so when this happens, you've got an insurance policy, so to speak, ensuring an increased sexual desire. If you stay sexually active, you'll keep producing testosterone, which helps keep you sexually active.

Another thing you can do—must do—if you want a healthy and full sex life is stay in shape. There's a direct correlation between your physical health and your sexual activity. The healthier and more energetic you are, the better sex you're going to have. If you're happy and enjoying yourself, you'll keep it up, so to speak.

Do we need to look like weight lifters or marathon runners?

Of course not. But erections are based, in part, on how healthy your vascular system is. If your arteries are clogged with plaque from not exercising enough and eating poorly for years, then chances are that the arteries in your penis won't be in good shape either. This means that you may not be getting enough blood to your penis to attain and maintain a good, solid erection.

Being in shape means raising your heart rate for 20 to 30 minutes at a clip, three or four times a week. It also means eating healthy, sticking to a low-fat diet and making sure that you're eating extra fruits, vegetables and whole-grain foods.

Your best bet to ensure sex in your later years is to live this kind of healthy lifestyle today. Don't wait until you're 50 and already having problems.

Anything else we can do? Is there a secret technique or maneuver that will boost our sex lives in the autumn years?

There aren't any secrets. But here's something that's often overlooked: Make your relationship with your partner as sound, intimate and comfortable as possible. Don't take her, her body, her support or her sexuality for granted. Continually work at your relationship, like you would a job. Continually work at pleasing your lover physically and nonphysically, and show her how to please you. Make sure that you're communicating well and aren't internalizing your emotions and thoughts. Make sure that you've built and are building intimacy and a deeper love and respect with each passing day.

These things, although they sound like common sense, are going to improve any relationship. And when it comes to the bedroom, they'll make making love much more satisfying and successful.

We men are not very well trained to be comfortable with emotion, intimacy and communication. But the irony is that these things can improve your love life at any time, especially in the golden years.

Marilyn K. Volker on
Foreplay: The Big Buildup

Marilyn K. Volker, Ed.D., is a sexologist in private practice in Coral Gables, Florida. She's a long-time counselor and a popular speaker on sex education and related topics. She also spent six years as a sex surrogate in the 1970s. Yes, that means she had sex with patients as part of their counseling therapy, though it rarely involved intercourse.

In her practice, Dr. Volker finds that many couples have sexual problems that can be avoided. Sometimes, it's just knowing that you don't have to do it every day to be happy. Other times, it's knowing that variety is the spice of life, and that can mean changing the pace or getting out of a rut.

"Some people think that couples must have intercourse every time they have sex and that if they don't, the sex will be boring," Dr. Volker says. "That's simply not true. I call sex without intercourse outercourse instead of foreplay because the term foreplay implies that something should always come afterward. It doesn't have to always be that way. Outercourse can be hot, pleasurable and sensuous and runs the gamut from kissing and hugging to licking and touching."

We asked Dr. Volker to name one thing that can keep the embers of lust glowing, and she said outercourse. Outercourse is something that can spice up even the blandest of sex lives, she says, as well as build intimacy and fulfillment. According to Dr. Volker, outercourse is the essential ingredient in a happy, healthy—and long-lived—sex life. Here's what she said.

Outercourse seems like one of those mythical times in sex that should be emphasized so much but, in reality, tends to be overlooked. Is this right?

Oftentimes, for couples who have been having sex for a while, outercourse can be dangerously de-emphasized. But you can't emphasize it so much that it becomes dogmatic. I like to ask, who made the rules? The myth that specific events, like outercourse, have to happen in a specific order or last a certain amount of time is simply not true. It's hogwash.

Any type of activity that raises the sexual response—outercourse or intercourse—is foreplay. Sex doesn't have to mean intercourse, and outercourse doesn't have to be done 15 minutes before penetration. Outercourse, as an art form, so to speak, can continue all day.

Daylong outercourse? Sounds exhausting.

That's because you're thinking with your body. Outercourse doesn't necessarily have to be physical. Touching or arousing your partner can be done emotionally and mentally as well. Just calling your partner at work and talking playfully, sensuously or sexy to her on the phone, or leaving a note on the car windshield telling her that you can't wait to see her tonight, is outercourse. Outercourse is nothing more than building sexual anticipation, arousal and excitement. There's an infinite variety of ways to do that, and they don't all include your body. They don't all take place immediately prior to sex.

So in other words, outercourse is almost as much a state of mind as it is something physical?

Exactly. And any man can learn basic skills for extending his time in outercourse, whether it's physical or nonphysical actions. It all leads to the same thing: a satisfying buildup of sexual energy that builds intimacy and makes your encounters more mutually pleasurable.

Will what works well today work well in the future? In other words, will outercourse change?

Definitely. Everyone's sex response changes. From a purely biological point of view, men may produce less testosterone as they age, so their sex drives may wane. Erections might require more stimulation and more time to form, and once they do, they may not be as firm as they used to be. Women, in the same vein, are unable to produce as much lubrication in their vaginas as they age, so they require more direct stimulation and some different approaches. But just because you and your partner are changing doesn't mean you need to scrimp on outercourse. You just have to adapt. In a loving, caring relationship, that's part of the fun: keeping things interesting and satisfying, even if it means doing them differently.

What's the worst thing you can do in outercourse? What should a man avoid?

One of the worst things you can do is make your lover feel neglected, and this can happen in lots of ways. You could skip outercourse and rush right into intercourse, not worrying whether she's lubricated or otherwise prepared. You could mechanically go through the motions without making sure that she's really enjoying herself. Or you can make negative comments about her body, particularly her breasts. Breasts are how women are measured in society, and making a negative comment about them for her is like her making a negative comment about your penis size.

What about the things we should do—is massage a good place to start?

Before you even touch her, build up the outercourse nonphysically, like I said before, by leaving notes on her window, flirting with her or complimenting her outfit on her way to work. It doesn't have to be that exactly—you probably already know what works for her, so concentrate there. Then, when you're together, set the mood. Too many couples forgo these important details, but it's the details that set the romantic scene. It's the details that made your sex lives so exciting when you first started seeing each other.

By details, do you mean planning a romantic evening, candles, music and all?

If that's what you both enjoy, sure. Whatever you do, start first with making sure that you're both relaxed and won't be disturbed for a while. Maybe you can get a sitter and escape to a nearby motel for an evening. Then it's up to you.

If you're at home, you can light a few candles, play soft music and burn some incense, if you both enjoy these things. Then make an erotic dinner together, something that includes lots of luscious fruit and finger food that you can feed each other. After dinner, leave the dishes and dance. It's probably been a while.

Other ideas are taking a comfy camping trip for two, if you're the outdoorsy type. Pamper yourself in a spa for a weekend. Or just sneak off like two teenagers to neck in your car on a desolate street. The key to this outercourse is to build up your excitement with whatever it is that you both enjoy.

Then massage?

I'd start with touching in a nurturing way first. Remember, you're moving into areas that unlock your arousal, so there's no need to rush the "hot spots" right away. Start by touching her in a nurturing way. Be playful. Be sensuous. And, finally, sexual. Massage is an excellent way to relax your partner and yourself, and it's a nice prelude to more intimate touching.

The important thing is not whether you have the hands of a professional masseur but that you're touching with love and pleasure in mind. You'll find that most women have what's called erogenous zones, or areas of their bodies that they find particularly arousing to be touched.

These erogenous zones don't necessarily include the genitals, right?

Right. Most women prefer to be touched first somewhere else other than the genitals.

That's one difference between the male and female sexual response: Men usually don't mind direct genital stimulation, while women like to warm up to it first. For a woman, the back, shoulders, lower hips, buttocks, anus and thighs are all good areas to be stroked. And don't neglect the face and neck. The head, face and neck are really up there on many women's lists of body parts to be gently touched and kissed. Most women really enjoy attention to these areas.

Anything to keep in mind as far as touching goes?

Yes. The skin is your biggest sex organ, and hers, too. Women are often more responsive to touch than men tend to be. Men are more visually excited; women are more turned on by touch. Try varying your touches. In sex therapy, we have what's called sensate-focus exercises that train you to touch for the sake of enjoying the touching, not to consciously try to please your mate. In other words, make your touching sessions in outercourse as much for your pleasure as for hers. And remember to vary the pacing and the type of touch to fit the mood. An invigorating massage might pep her up or relax her into falling asleep without necessarily arousing her. Make sure that you know what works for her and what doesn't so that you're not at odds during your touching. Touch can enhance what could get to be a pretty boring ritual if you don't try different things.

What other techniques can a man experiment with during outercourse?

Feel free to experiment with different things. You can both work on oral sex techniques, try sex toys, dress up, buy her lingerie, do stripteases for each other. The sky's the limit. Some couples once a month will try something different as a rule of thumb. They make a promise to routinely try something new, so they always have something to look forward to. To this end, you can make the sex equivalent of a "job jar" by writing down your ideas and putting them in a jar. Then pick an idea out of the jar once a month, once a week or once a session.

For example, say you want an invigorating foot massage but have been too shy to ask. Write it on a slip of paper and put it in a job jar. When both of you write down a number of ideas, you'll have a jar of sexual adventures waiting to supplement your lovemaking. These ideas can be an erotic boost to your outercourse.

Should outercourse end with orgasm?

There doesn't have to be orgasm. Some people want to climax after an invigorating outercourse session, others don't. I'm thinking of men and women who have said to me that they don't want to experience orgasm sometimes. Some men enhance their sex response by holding back; it helps them learn better ejaculatory control for the next time. Other times, it can be hard work for a woman to have intercourse, because she may have a medical problem that makes intercourse painful or because it would just take too much energy. As long as you're both happy, your outstanding outercourse can occasionally be a bonding experience instead of a prelude to sizzling sex.

Any parting thoughts?

One of the most important things you can do to improve yourself in the art of outercourse is to approach it like a businessman approaches work: How do you find out what your customer wants? You ask! And if you want to please customers, you deliver what you can. This type of communication and interaction works well in outercourse, too. Good, clear, honest communication is crucial to a continued happy sex life. Remember that the feeling you have when you walk away from a sexual encounter is the imprint that you're walking into your next encounter with.

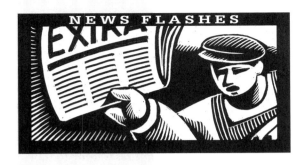

Sex–Heart Attack Link Proven False

CHICAGO—Putting to rest a long-held myth, a new study shows that sex is highly un-likely to trigger a heart attack, even among those with heart disease.

The study involved 1,774 patients who had suffered heart attacks, including 858 who were sexually active in the year prior to the attack. Among them, 27 reported sexual activity in the two hours preceding the attacks. Based on those numbers, researchers calculated that by having sex, patients temporarily increased their chances of suffering a heart attack from 10 in a million to 20 in a million. But the starting risk is so low that doubling it isn't dangerous, researchers say.

Researchers also found that heart patients who participated regularly in moderately strenuous exercise faced little or no added risk from sexual activity. Just walking briskly slightly uphill for 30 minutes a day can make sex as safe as non-strenuous activities for heart patients.

Sexual intercourse in familiar surroundings with one's spouse puts no more stress on the heart than climbing a flight of stairs or walking briskly for two blocks, researchers concluded.

Rigorous Sex Can Induce Vision Loss

PITTSBURGH—It's one of the oldest sex myths on record: Masturbation can make you go blind. The truth, it turns out, is even odder: Sex, either with a partner or alone, can indeed cause sight loss in extreme cases.

Researchers recently have documented six cases in which rigorous sex caused temporary blindness. Five men, ages 30 to 53, suffered bleeding of varying degrees in at least one of their eyes while having sex or masturbating. One woman, the only female documented, complained of losing vision in her left eye while being stimulated with a vibrator.

These surprising findings were published in the American Medical Association's *Archives of Ophthalmology*, which stressed that Valsalva retinopathy, as the condition's technically called, is indeed rare. Experts believe that bleeding occurs when pressure builds behind the eye, causing blood vessels to break and delicate tissue lining to tear. It can take five weeks to ten months for normal sight to return.

Although unusual, similar situations have been documented in athletes, who strained themselves, for example, while lifting weights. To avoid temporarily blinding yourself next time, avoid straining. Don't hold your breath during sex, as some people in the publicized cases did, and especially avoid overexerting yourself if you lead an otherwise sedentary life.

Pumpkin, Doughnut Smells Top Turn-Ons for Men

CHICAGO—Forget that bottle of Chanel. A study to determine which scents cause men to become most sexually aroused reveals that foods have far more impact than perfume. Topping the list as the most arousing food was pumpkin pie.

To get the readings, Alan Hirsch, M.D., neurologic director of the Smell and Taste Treatment and Research Foundation in Chicago, had men wear masks of varying scents and then measured blood flow to the penis. Unscented masks didn't increase blood flow at all, while different food scents had a range of results. The aroma of pumpkin pie increased penile blood flow by 40 percent. In comparison, a woman's perfume boosted blood flow by only 3 percent. Other winners for the men were a mixture of doughnut and black licorice, followed by combination pumpkin pie and doughnut, then orange alone. Scents you might as well not consider in the seduction scene include chocolate, cranberry, floral and Oriental spice—none scored highly.

Dr. Hirsch got the idea to test food smells in a study that was originally to measure the "turn-on" effect of perfume. Food scents were given to the control group, thinking it really wouldn't have an effect. The result? Baked cinnamon buns had a greater effect than all the perfumes put together.

Dr. Hirsch speculated that the smells evoked a nostalgic memory that relaxes the men, making them more aware of sexual cues around them. Further scent studies may lead to home-baked treatments for impotence, Dr. Hirsch suggests.

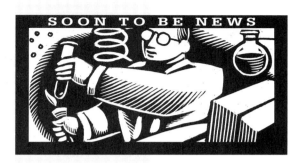

SOON TO BE NEWS

Cures for Impotence?

An estimated 18 million men suffer from some form of impotence. Given the diversity of causes, treatments for impotence have been all over the map, ranging from unwieldy pump devices to the psychiatrist's couch. But one key weapon was missing: a pharmaceutical solution.

Until recently. Two new medications—one in pill form, the other injected at the base of the penis—show considerable promise in remedying some forms of impotence.

One of the drugs, alprostadil (Caverject), has already been approved by the Food and Drug Administration (FDA) to treat erectile dysfunction. To use it, a patient injects the drug into the base of his penis via a pen-shaped tool that shoots a tiny needle into the skin. In 5 to 10 minutes, the drug stimulates blood flow to the penis. When the penis is full—and the erection is firm—the drug stimulates penile vessels to close off, giving the user from 20 minutes to an hour of hard labor. Caverject is up to 85 percent effective in treating most forms of impotence, whether its cause is physical or mental. Caverject is available by prescription, and its maker, Upjohn, continues research on related uses of prostaglandins, a naturally occurring chemical (Caverject is a synthetic version).

Separately, researchers from pharmaceutical manufacturer Pfizer are studying whether a drug named sildenafil (Viagra) can work as a remedy for impotence. The company already has completed three short-term European trials that included a total of 400 men whose impotence didn't have a clear biological cause. Nearly 80 percent of the men said that their sexual performance improved within an hour of taking the pill.

Sildenafil's effect on impotence was discovered by accident. While testing the drug's ability to help open blood vessels, researchers also found that participants reported added zip in their sex lives. Researchers have detected few side effects from sildenafil, although a handful of men complained that the medicine gave them headaches. Men whose impotence has a clear physical cause, such as diabetes or high blood pressure, are currently being studied. *Pfizer expects sildenafil to come before the FDA for review by the end of 1997.*

Male Birth Control?

Although it may be a few years before you'll find them in drugstores, all-new forms of male birth control are being concocted.

Recently, the World Health Organization and the National Institutes of Health (NIH) completed a study of men who received regular injections of testosterone as a method of reducing the overall amount of sperm being produced. There were some distinct drawbacks to the method—for example, the shot has to be administered in the butt, every week. However, the shot proved to be 98.6 percent effective in the study.

The NIH has already moved beyond this preliminary work and says that it has developed a male shot that need only be administered every three months instead of every week.

In addition, researchers hope to design a male birth control pill that would specifically shut down areas of the body responsible for sperm production. *Although a male pill won't be ready until well into the next century, expect the three-month shot to be a new option in male birth control sometime in the next few years.*

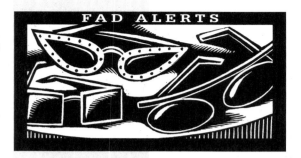

FAD ALERTS

Saw Palmetto

Seminoles are known for more than just being the team name for Florida State University. It turns out that the original 'Noles, the Indian tribe, caught on to the medicinal benefits of saw palmetto (*Serenoa repens*) early on—a plant that naturopathic doctors and herbalists say may help remedy enlarged prostates.

The Seminole Indians originally used the berries from the saw palmetto as an aphrodisiac. While there's no scientific proof that it'll lift your libido, it seems quite effective in treating benign prostatic hyperplasia, or enlarged prostate, according to Varro E. Tyler, Ph.D., professor of pharmacognosy in the School of Pharmacy at Purdue University in Lafayette, Indiana. The herb accounts for some 38 percent of all medications prescribed for the problem in Italy, a bigger market share than any other man-made drug can claim. One study of 500 men found that 88 percent of them experienced some relief of symptoms by taking the herb.

Drug experts in Germany think that saw palmetto works by preventing the conversion of testosterone into dihydrotestosterone, a more potent form of the male sex hormone that may trigger prostate growth. The dosage of many standardized extracts is 160 milligrams of saw palmetto twice a day. Don't run off to your health food store just yet. (Or worse, don't buy a saw palmetto from your local nursery.) Rather, ask your doctor to explore the opportunities with you.

No Sex before Sports

 It's an athletic tradition as old as athletics itself: Don't have sex the night before a big sporting event. And the tradition lives on—abstinence was a hot topic at the 1996 Summer Olympics. It turns out, exercise physiologists say, that the well-meaning counsel is a sham. In fact, abstaining from sex before any important event for fear of losing your competitive edge might be one of the longest-running illegitimate fads around.

Tommy Boone, Ph.D., professor of exercise physiology at the College of St. Scholastica in Duluth, Minnesota, who investigated this supposed phenomenon, tested eleven men on a treadmill twice, with and without their having sex the night before. Sex the night before maximal exercise did not work the heart any differently than when the same men abstained. Therefore, the study's authors concluded that having sex 12 hours before an athletic event won't adversely affect your performance.

Cybersex

 She's asleep in the next room. You're not tired—in fact, you're horny as hell. You fire up the computer, make your way to the "singles" chat room, and find yourself engaged in heated conversation with "Bunny44D" or "DonnaMatrix." In today's digital age, there's nothing quite so vogue as cyberchat, and electronic communication is apparently here to stay. But are adult-rated conversations online deleterious for you and your darling?

"It's a question of mind-set," says Phyllis Phlegar, author of *Love On-Line*. "If you're doing something that you are deliberately concealing from your partner, then you need to rethink what you're doing," she says.

Phlegar argues that an online affair can be just as damaging as flesh-and-blood infidelity. "What's most injurious about an affair is not that you're having computer sex with someone else. It's the deception. It's the understanding that you are carrying on something secret and illicit outside of the marriage or relationship," she says.

If you're single, of course, you're a free digital agent; go forth and sow your electronic oats, according to Nancy Tamosaitis, author of *net.sex*. But if you're in a relationship and want to perform some single-minded experiments in cyberspace, talk to your partner about it—see what her attitude is.

"If she has no problem with it, then explore away," says Tamosaitis. "But consider that you're taking the first step down a slippery slope. Online affairs are a form of acting out, she believes. "There's always the possibility that what starts out as a virtual relationship could lead to a real face-to-face meeting. And then you're really over the line," she warns.

Ginkgo

 New research suggests that the herbal remedy ginkgo might be just the ticket for fixing erectile dysfunction. Already considered a conventional drug in Europe for circulation problems, ginkgo's been proven to improve circulation. When circulation problems are impairing your manly pipes—say, years of poor eating habits have clogged your arteries, including the ones in your penis—there are some indications that ginkgo might come to the rescue.

In one study, 240 milligrams of ginkgo biloba extract (GBE) were given to 50 impotent men for nine months. Some of the men also received shots of papaverine, a conventional erection-boosting drug commonly prescribed for impotence. After the study, researchers found that the ginkgo men and the ginkgo men who got the papaverine, too, all saw significant improvements in their erections. A previous study had similar results: About 30 of 60 men who had not responded to papaverine therapy regained potency after taking 60 milligrams of GBE daily for six months.

GBE is sold in health food stores, typically in 60-milligram dosages. But it won't pay to run off and treat yourself with any expectation of results without first consulting a doctor. If your flaccid fellow is down because of, say, psychological or neurological problems, all the ginkgo in the world wouldn't do you a lick of good.

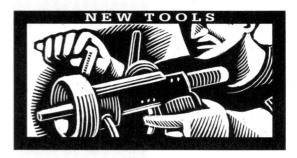

Lasting Longer

Numbing Creams

There are numbing creams on the market to dull the sensations of sex in order to delay premature ejaculation. While we're strongly in favor of building control naturally, keep on the lookout for lidocaine-prilocaine cream in the future if you have problems with premature ejaculation.

Lidocaine and prilocaine are two common topical anesthetics that doctors use for local anesthesia, and they are available by prescription only.

In a small pilot study on 11 men, researchers from Wellesley Hospital and the University of Toronto instructed men to rub 2½ grams of lidocaine-prilocaine on their penises. They then covered the cream with a condom and waited 30 minutes.

After 30 minutes, the men could remove the condom and the cream if they wished. Of the 11 men in the study, 9 of them reported improvement in staying power, with 5 of them ranking it as "excellent."

One man lasted 20 minutes before climaxing, though he complained that his penis was numb and suggested that the researchers reduce the amount of numbing agent a bit.

If these findings are confirmed by larger studies, this could be a breakthrough treatment for premature ejaculation.

Spicier Meals

Cooking in the Nude:
Quickies Cookbook

Looking for something to add some zest to your sex life? Why not heat things up with a new cookbook—and we don't mean Betty Crocker. Try *Cooking in the Nude: Quickies* by Debbie and Stephen Cornwell. They also wrote *Cooking in the Nude: Red Hot Lovers.* Here's a sampling of what's on the menu from the *Quickies* book: Caesar and Please Her; Fondue Me, Please!; Fetish-ini; Tempting Tender Loins; Veal You or Von't You? They can be found in bookstores, gift and gourmet shops. $9.95.

Better Artificial Insemination

In Vitro Fertilization

Low sperm counts account for roughly 20 percent of all fertility problems among couples trying to start a family. But now, experts have devised a type of in vitro fertilization to improve the odds. Instead of subjecting the woman's egg to a blast of sperm, doctors harvest a single whip-tailed warrior from the man's semen and inject it directly into the egg using a microscopic needle. The egg is then transplanted into the woman's uterus. The entire process, very much akin to the sharpshooting of a high-powered rifle as opposed to the scattershot of a shotgun, is called intracytoplasmic sperm injection, and it's being performed at the Robert Wood Johnson Medical School in New Brunswick, New Jersey, where officials report a success rate of 43 percent—one of the highest in the country.

Cozier Cuddling

Polyester Long Johns

Let's say that you and yours want to cuddle on a cold winter's night, but it's too cold to go *au naturel*. High-tech undies beat the pants off the old cotton jobbers. Polyester long johns are high-performance pajamas that wick water away from your skin and push it through the material into the air. These futuristic space suits look cool, keep you warm and keep you high and dry, not wet with sweat.

MontBell's new DriOn, for example, is made of a special polyester yarn that pulls moisture away from your skin and kills odor-causing bacteria. To order, call 1-800-683-2002. Cost for a top and a bottom: $36 each plus shipping. Or try the Full Moon Suit from Not Just Johns. It's a one-piece made of Milliken and Company's Wicked Wick polyester fabric, complete with a four-button backdoor for midnight trips to the latrine. They come in several colors. To order, call 1-800-642-6525. Starting at $56 plus shipping.

A Happier Mate

Sensor Products' HIS 'n' HER Motion-
Activated Night-Light

Okay, this isn't exactly a "new tool" for your sex life, but you can bet your bottom that you might get more if you're looking out for *her* bottom. The Sensor Products company produces a motion-activated night-light that automatically senses your presence in the bathroom and makes the throne glow green when the seat's down and red when it's not. That way, she won't take an unexpected midnight dip that leaves you all washed up the next morning when you try to wake her with soft kisses. The unit also projects a bull's-eye pattern onto the water to help you aim at night. Scorecard not included. Call 1-800-447-6437. $29.95 plus shipping.

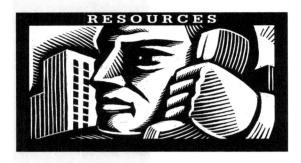

Sex Toys

Good Vibrations Catalog
938 Howard Street, Suite 101
San Francisco, CA 94103
1-800-289-8423

This San Francisco–based outfit calls itself a "clean, well-lighted place" to shop for sex toys, books and videos. The catalog contains a varied selection of lubricants, "safer-sex supplies" and a few things you probably didn't know existed. The catalog arrives in plain packaging with "Open Enterprises" as the return address, and the company pledges not to rent your name to anybody else.

Sexual Health

Yahoo! Sexuality Guide
http://www.yahoo.com/society_and_
culture/sexuality/

The aficionados at Yahoo!, a search engine for the World Wide Web, have collected and linked many of the sexuality Web sites in one convenient place. Dive in here, and all fetishes, interests, questions and ideas will be explored.

Health Advice

Go Ask Alice Service
http://www.columbia.edu/cu/
healthwise/alice.html

Go Ask Alice is an all-purpose health-advice service, but since it was created for Columbia University students, it's not surprising that the Sexual Health and Relationships forum is the most lively part. Alice fields questions on topics such as "flirting," "dating first cousin," "tired of his foreskin" and "cleaning cat-o'-nine-tails." Her thoughtful responses (which are actually suggestions from health experts) and uniformly mild and nonjudgmental language make this a resource worth checking out.

Seduction

The Love and Romance Home Page
http://home.navisoft.com/
loveandromance/index.htm

At a loss for words to tell your loved one how special she is? Then use someone else's. This site has fill-in-the-blank letters, poems and art to "assist you in expressing your love in a special and unforgettable way." The author of these sentiments is said to be a "modern-day Cyrano." Other services provided include a book gallery, personal ads, a travel page and a personal search service. The site is run by the Electric Press, a small publishing company that publishes books on "romantic communication." Its goal is to help you find the love of your life and keep the fires of love burning.

Condoms

Condom Country
http://www.condom.com

If you're looking to expand your repertoire of condoms, this site's for you. Brought to you by the retailer Condom Country, you can "browse" through an extensive catalog, complete with photos, or search the index for your favorite brand. There's even advice on use and safety. The catalog includes such items as male and female condoms, sexual aids, T-shirts, books, boxer shorts and "fun stuff."

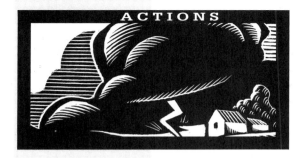

It may be the world's oldest pastime, but we're still coming up with new information about sex. Here are several suggestions for safer, better sex, based on recent research or writings.

1. **Increase sense-a-tivity.** Sex therapists say that "sensate-focus" exercises are an excellent way to relax and build intimacy. They ground you in the present moment so that you and your partner can appreciate touching and feeling at its most exquisite. To do sensate-focus exercises, try this, suggests Cathy Winks, co-owner of Good Vibrations, a retail and mail-order adult bookstore in San Francisco, and co-author of *The Good Vibrations Guide to Sex.*

a. Ask your partner to lie down and relax.

b. Now, ever so slowly, begin to caress her body. Not her genitals. Her body.

c. After 15 minutes of exploring every part of her body but her privates, move on to those pleasures.

d. Remember, you're not fondling her or trying to arouse her. You're *caressing* her. Your goal is to explore her as if it's for the first time. Enjoy the touching itself—don't worry about orgasm, intercourse or anything else. Very simply touch for the sake of touching.

e. Explore her genitals for another 15 minutes. By then she'll either be very aroused or relaxed. If she's relaxed, enjoy the emotional bond by cuddling and relaxing in each other's intimacy. If she's aroused, we trust that you'll know what to do next.

2. **Slow it down.** Although it's still taboo to some people, most sex therapists say that masturbation is an excellent way to relax, relieve sexual tension, explore and refine your own sexual response, improve your staying power and build intimacy with your partner (when, of course, you're masturbating together). The key to good masturbation, however, is to break lifelong habits of rushing through masturbation and feeling guilty about it.

Of course, if you have reservations because of social, religious or other reasons, that's understandable. But if you're willing to take your sexuality in your own hands, here's some advice from Betty Dodson, Ph.D., a New York City sex educator and author of *Sex for One: The Joy of Self-loving.*

• Consider treating yourself to a long leisurely session of masturbation instead of always going for a quickie.

• Make your self-loving sessions as intense and lingering as partnered sex.

• Make a date with yourself. Rent a sexy movie. Play some music. Light some candles.

• Before moving directly to your penis, caress your entire body gently and slowly. Find and concentrate on your erogenous areas, like the nipples. (Did you know that up to 60 percent of men get nipple erections when aroused?) Other hot spots are the chest, thighs, buttocks, back of legs and waist.

• When you get down to pleasure, keep the rhythm slow and sensual. Vary the pacing and remember that your most sensitive spot is your frenulum, that V-shaped piece of skin on the underside of your penis, where the glans meets the shaft. Knowing this can help you speed up or slow down climax, depending on what you had in mind.

3. **Protect your love glove.** If your lubricant's got oil in it, you're in for "condom erosion." According to Stephanie Sanders, Ph.D., associate director of the Kinsey Institute for Research in Sex, Gender and Reproduction at Indiana University in Bloomington, research has shown that within 60 seconds a condom exposed to an oil-based lubricant can develop holes large enough for the AIDS virus and other sexually transmitted disease organisms to pass through. Soon after, the holes are large enough for sperm to penetrate. Which means that you have reason to be afraid of disease or unexpected pregnancy.

A lot of guys make this mistake, says Dr. Sanders, and most times unwittingly, because many people think that if a lubricant washes off easily, it doesn't have oil in it. That's not always the case.

Bad (condom-eating) lubricants include petroleum jelly, Vaseline Intensive Care lotion, baby oil and Nivea. Good lubricants are water-based—no oil allowed. Two examples are K-Y jelly and Lubrin inserts. Want to make sure? Read the ingredients or ask your pharmacist, suggests Dr. Sanders.

4. **Be a handy man.** To be more than just a mediocre masseur, remember that dry, smooth skin can be caressed without painful friction or snagged hair. But serious touching, particularly invigorating and arousing massage, requires lubrication. Use a commercial massage oil, available at health food stores, or make your own, suggests Winks. Just use pure oils, like almond or peanut oil. To increase the ambience, add a few drops of concentrated peppermint or strawberry essence for a delicious lingering aroma. Other scents that work well include lavender, mandarin and Roman chamomile, which some experts claim calm the body.

To use the oil, put a quarter-size dab of it in the palm of your hand, then rub your hands together so that it warms up. Don't use oil on clothing or near the eyes, ears or nose. As for strokes, the most common is *effleurage* (ef-FLER-ahj), which uses the fingers and flat of the hand in long, gliding strokes that go toward the heart. Brisk, assertive strokes are better for invigorating; deep, slow strokes for relaxing; and gentle, nearly imperceptible strokes for sexual stimulation.

5. **Get adventurous.** One of the most important organs you can bring to the bedroom is the one between your ears, not your legs. The more open-minded you are about sex play, the broader your range of pleasure and enjoyment will be, experts say. Once you open your mind to new adventures of the carnal kind, you might actually enjoy them. To do that, realize that, as Arlene Goldman, Ph.D., coordinator for the Jefferson Sexual Function Center in Philadelphia, can tell you, sometimes experiments end in disappointment—but that doesn't mean that you should abandon your research altogether.

Let your creativity shine through but maintain a sense of humor when you're playing around with sexual experiments, she suggests. If you decide to try a new position that's so unworkable you throw your back out, go ahead and laugh about it—after the pain's gone. Keeping such a lighthearted outlook is a tough task for most of us to master, because we get so caught up in the need to make every sexual experience the best one possible. Let the games begin.

6. **Practice your stripping.** As part of one of the largest, most rigorously controlled sex surveys of all time, researchers asked women to name their favorite turn-ons. A whopping 81 percent said that watching their partner undress was somewhat to very appealing. It even beat out receiving oral sex.

Disrobing with pizzazz isn't something that comes naturally to most of us. After all, we're more likely to be the ones doing the looking. But if you want to treat your partner to her own private striptease, here are some moves to keep in mind, gleaned from *The Intimate Touch: A Guide to More Active Lovemaking for You and Your Partner* by Dr. Glenn Wilson, one of Britain's best-known psychologists, and *Sex Secrets* by Brian Chichester, Kenton Robinson and the editors of *Men's Health* Books.

   a. Undo your tie slowly and deliberately. While maintaining eye contact, drape it around her neck and pull her close for a passionate kiss.

   b. Unbutton your shirt lingeringly, revealing half your chest at a time. Turn your back, slip your shirt half off and show her your shoulders. Then turn around, slip your shirt off and let it drop to the floor. (If it's a pullover, practice taking it off smoothly in one move by crossing your hands and grabbing the left side of the shirt near your waist with your right hand and the right side with your left hand. Then pull up in one smooth move.)

   c. Never, ever fold clothes as you undress. This isn't the time to keep your wardrobe neat.

   d. Kick off your shoes with flair, but watch windows and mirrors. And don't forget to remove your socks before jumping into the sack. A naked man wearing socks looks silly, not sexy.

   e. Let her unzip your zipper—but don't let her touch anywhere else. At this point, the pot should be simmering, not boiling over.

   f. Pull your pants down one leg at a time. Or let them fall naturally by thrusting and gyrating.

   g. Consider doing all the above to music. Or keep it quiet and sultry. G-strings for you and $50 in singles for her are optional.

7. **Be a dream lover.** Find out what your lover wants most by asking her what she dreams about, suggests Gayle Delaney, Ph.D., author of *Sexual Dreams: Why We Have Them, What They Are*. Next time you both have a chance to talk privately without interruptions, ask your partner to describe her most sensual, arousing dream experiences. Ask simple questions to encourage her to provide detailed feedback, but don't impose your own interpretations on her responses. Then ask her questions that would connect your own sex life with her dream sex life. Dr. Delaney found that most women dream of a lover who takes his time, enjoys foreplay and expresses his emotions during sex. Finding out what your lover's dreaming of might be the best way of making both your dreams come true.

8. **Keep your semen clean.** Here's something you don't hear too much about: The odor of sperm can be offensive to your partner, depending on what you've eaten recently. Normally, semen is described as having a musky odor, says Mark Sigman, M.D., assistant professor of urology at Brown University School of Medicine in Providence, Rhode Island. But if you've eaten beets, asparagus or brussels sprouts—all of which can give urine a characteristic smell—you could be tainting the bouquet of your ejaculation. That's because ejaculatory fluids could be coming in contact with the odor as they pass through your penis. Here's another cause for foul-smelling ejaculation: not ejaculating frequently, which can allow bacteria to build up.

4

WEIGHT LOSS

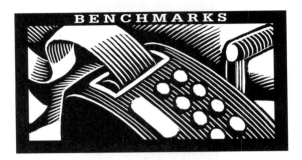

AVERAGES

■ Percentage of people who said that they would rather be rich than thin: 82

■ Amount of fat consumed by an American adult each week, expressed in sticks of butter: 6

■ Pounds of fat that cosmetic surgeons remove from Americans annually: 200,000

■ Year in which, at the current rate of increase, all Americans will be overweight: 2059

■ Percentage of American adults who are obese: 25

■ Estimated amount spent annually on weight-reduction products: $33 billion

■ Approximate percentage of American adults who go on a diet each year: 44

■ Change, since 1986, in the number of Americans who say that they are on a diet: 17 million fewer people

■ Most important reason for losing weight, according to one poll: 67 percent said better health, 21 percent said looking better, 6 percent said having a better love life and 3 percent said getting a better job

■ Caloric adjustments needed to lose one pound per week:
decrease food intake by 250 calories a day and increase exercise to burn 350 more calories a day

■ Percentage of total daily calories most people eat in the evening: 48

■ Number of times an American opens the refrigerator each day: 22

■ Amount of additional time that a man spends eating per week compared to a woman: 30 minutes

EXTREMES

■ Heaviest person: six-foot-one former taxi driver who weighed more than 1,400 pounds at his heaviest

■ Greatest dieting weight loss: loss of 920 pounds in 16 months, bringing the dieter down to 476 pounds

■ Greatest sweating weight loss: 21½ pounds of 239 pounds within a 24-hour period

■ Largest recorded waist: 119 inches

■ Smallest waist for someone of normal stature: 13 inches

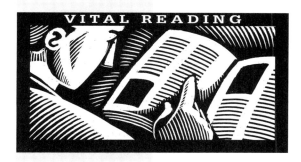

A New Angle on Weight Loss

A recent diet promises to help you shed pounds, feel more alert, and stave off heart disease and diabetes. Learn how to reap the most benefits with the least effort.

In a diet world dominated by low-fat chocolate shakes and no-cal sodas, we're always on the lookout for a manly approach to weight loss. So when *The Zone*, a diet book with an emphasis on eating lots of protein, hit the shelves, we were excited. Author Barry Sears, Ph.D., promises that tightly restricting the ratio of fat to carbohydrate to protein can slim you down, add years to your life and even help you think more clearly.

But there's a hitch. To reap all these benefits, you have to spend an enormous amount of time and energy (at least up front) calculating, weighing and apportioning everything you put into your mouth. A sampling from Zone dieters on the Internet confirmed our suspicion. The majority of people posting remarks reported having given up in frustration.

How could a diet be that daunting? Dr. Sears characterizes his philosophy thus: "You're treating food as if it were a prescription drug, delivering a controlled amount of protein and carbohydrate at every meal." When he says controlled, he means it. *The Zone*'s cardinal rule is that you must maintain a 0.75 ratio of protein to carbohydrate. In other words, for every four grams of carbohydrate, you must eat three grams of protein at the same time.

To hold to this ratio, you must break down everything you eat into specific blocks. You always eat a protein block (say, a piece of turkey breast) with a carbohydrate block (maybe a cup of broccoli). Compared to current Food and Drug Administration recommendations, you'd be eating twice the protein and half the carbohydrates with his diet.

While we like the promised benefits, we couldn't see ourselves spending time "blocking." So we took Dr. Sears's diet to the experts in the field and asked them to sift the solid claims from the bunk and recommend the simplest way to lose weight and prevent heart disease. Here's what they told us.

Claim: It takes fat to burn fat. Insulin interferes with fat-burning. Since dietary fat slows the body's production of insulin, fat consumption actually encourages the burning of fat stores (such as those love handles you'd like to lose).

Consensus: Our experts agreed, with a few reservations. To understand Dr. Sears's system, you must first have a handle on something called insulin resistance. As we age and/or gain weight, the insulin in our bodies begins to work less efficiently. It takes more insulin to process sugar normally. More insulin in the bloodstream sets off a heart-threatening cascade of events: decreased HDL (high-density lipoprotein, or "good") cholesterol, increased triglycerides and higher blood pressure—all of which can lead to clogged arteries.

With insulin resistance in mind, the recent advice to adopt high-carbohydrate diets takes on a different cast. Although reducing saturated fat (the kind in whole milk and fatty meat) has been shown to reduce LDL (low-density lipoprotein, or "bad") cholesterol, the carbohydrates that take its place may trigger an unhealthy insulin response. "A diet rich in monounsaturated fat solves both problems: It neither elevates LDL cholesterol nor triggers an insulin response," says Gerald Reaven, M.D., a researcher at Stanford University. And monounsaturated fat, the kind predominant in olive oil, avocados and nuts, additionally has been shown to elevate HDL cholesterol.

Action to take: If you're overweight or over age 50, you're probably somewhat insulin-resistant. It makes sense to eat a balanced diet, with 30 to 40 percent of your daily calories largely from monounsaturated fat. Replace butter with olive oil, fatty meat with nuts, and sour-cream dips with guacamole.

Claim: Carbohydrate is a drug, and when eaten in abundance, it can be toxic.

Consensus: If you're insulin-resistant, eating lots of carbohydrates that enter the bloodstream quickly can overtax your pancreas (the organ that produces insulin). Researchers aren't sure if this might lead to diabetes, but it's possible, says Paul Lachance, Ph.D., chairman of the food science department at Rutgers University in New Brunswick, New Jersey.

How do you know what kind of carbohydrate to be wary of? Researchers have devised a way to categorize the speed at which sugar from various foods enters the bloodstream. Foods with a high glycemic index (G.I.) are thought to produce a larger insulin response than those with a low G.I. A simple rule is that any food containing refined sugar or syrup (most cookies, breads and crackers, for example) is likely to have a high G.I.

Action to take: Favor low–G.I. foods, such as beans, peas, lentils, skim milk, yogurt, apples, cantaloupe, grapefruit, cherries and peaches. Not only will they keep your insulin swings in check because they contain lots of fiber, but also they'll make you feel more satisfied or full. And look past the "no-fat" labels to the calorie listing. If you're an average-size man trying to lose weight, you'll want to ingest less than 2,500 calories a day. Save high–G.I. foods for postexercise snacking (they refuel the muscles if eaten within two hours of your workout). Good postworkout snacks include bananas, raisins, bagels and cereal.

The Glycemic Index of Selected Foods

The following chart lists the glycemic index (G.I.) of some common foods. High–G.I. foods enter the bloodstream and elevate insulin faster and more abruptly than lower–G.I. foods, thus setting off a series of heart-threatening events.

Low G.I.	Medium G.I.	High G.I.
apple juice	All-Bran	bagels
apples	cereal	baked
black beans	bananas	potatoes
butter beans	bran muffin	breads
cherries	chocolate	carrots
chick-peas	grapes	cola
dried	green peas	corn chips
apricots	ice cream	corn flakes
grapefruit	kiwifruit	doughnuts
kidney beans	mangoes	hard candy
lentils	new potatoes	honey
lima beans	oatmeal	jelly beans
peaches	orange	pineapple
peanuts	orange juice	raisins
pears	pasta	rice cakes
plums	pizza	taco shells
skim milk	popcorn	waffles
split peas	rye bread	watermelon
yogurt	sweet corn	white rice

SOURCE: *American Journal of Clinical Nutrition,* **Vol. 62, 1995: pp. 871S–890S.**

Claim: Protein triggers the hormonal system to produce chemicals that keep insulin levels under control.

Consensus: It's this cornerstone of the Zone diet that makes many experts we spoke with uncomfortable. "I don't know of any studies that support the claim that protein triggers less insulin production than carbohydrate," says Thomas M. S. Wolever, M.D., Ph.D., associate professor of nutritional sciences at the University of Toronto.

In fact, the amount of protein that an active man would have to eat on the Zone diet is far higher than any recommendations we've seen in other dietary plans and may significantly tax the kidneys. And unless you're willing to use a lot of protein powder or eat only a few low-fat, high-protein foods (such as egg whites), it'll be tough to get the recommended protein without taking in too much saturated fat.

Action to take: Eat a reasonable amount of protein; if you're not very active, 56 grams a day should be plenty. Add an extra daily serving or two (10 to 30 extra grams) if you're exercising hard.

Claim: Regular exercise will help keep insulin resistance in check.

Consensus: While Dr. Sears seems to prioritize his diet over exercise, most experts feel that working out is still the critical factor in warding off insulin resistance. "Exercising will substantially reduce insulin resistance in everybody all of the time," says Dr. Reaven. "Weight loss and activity levels are much more powerful in improving insulin sensitivity and thereby lowering insulin levels than changes in diet."

Action to take: Every little increase in activity helps. If you're not up to running, walk. If you don't want to lift weights, clean your garage or work in the garden. Anything active is good for insulin control.

Claim: Eating a bedtime snack that meets the Zone criteria may prompt the release of a vital stay-young hormone.

Consensus: Nobody knows. High levels of insulin do block the release of human growth hormone, an important substance that helps your body burn fat and consolidate muscle.

Action to take: Eating a Zone-favorable snack before bed appealed to us as an option. You just need a little protein (a dollop of cottage cheese, tuna salad or sliced turkey) and a little carbohydrate (half an apple or a few chunks of melon). Dr. Sears says that after eating such a snack, you'll be rewarded with an especially deep sleep and a high level of alertness upon awakening. Although the scientific jury is still out, this one can't hurt to try.

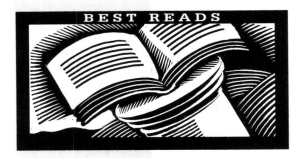

Our Obsession with Fat

It's a foible of life that the innocent often get blamed for things that they didn't cause. In this excerpt from the book Smart Exercise *(Houghton Mifflin, 1994), author Covert Bailey comes to the defense of fat, explaining why it is so essential to life.*

Americans are so obsessed with their desire to get rid of body fat that they blame the fat itself. "Fat is terrible!" they say. "I hate fat! Why do I have all this fat?" The truth is that fat is the most efficient gas tank ever designed.

We can make fat out of almost anything we eat. All the carbohydrate in bread, pasta and potatoes, if it's in excess of what the body needs, can be turned into fat. If we eat more protein than we need, the liver converts it into fat. And we all know that eating too much fat just makes us fatter.

The liver can convert bread, carrots, avocados, potatoes—you name it—into fat. It's actually miraculous. Let's invent a car engine that can turn everything we put into the gas tank to gasoline. Put in avocados, and the engine simply converts the avocados into gas. Put in hamburger, and our beautiful car converts it into gasoline. Wouldn't that be fabulous? People would respect such a wonderful invention.

"Why Did God Make Us Have Fat?"

The human machine is just as wonderful. It can convert almost anything you put in your mouth into fat. If your gas tanks are bulging, don't blame the gas tank and don't fault the fabulous fuel-making system. Instead, ask, "Why did God make us this way?" It's as if God said, "Today I am going to design an upright running machine. I've designed foxes, coyotes, deer and antelope, all of which run fantastically well. But now I want to design a creature that can run on two feet so that the other two feet can be used to hold things. I need to design a special fuel system for this creature, since it's only going to have two legs to run on. Its fuel tank must be so perfectly distributed over its body that it won't tip over frontward or backward. I'm going to design this creature so that anything it eats can be converted into its primary fuel."

By now you should be saying, "Holy smokes! I didn't realize that fat is our primary fuel." I want you to stop blaming your fat. That's where most of the energy comes from when you run, play tennis or dance. Show some respect for your unbelievably efficient primary-fuel-producing, -storing and -burning machine. Instead of going on bizarre diets whose entire intent is to pervert the system God gave you, learn how to use this fuel.

Fat: The Primary Fuel

I have a friend who likes to barbecue on his back deck. He puts charcoal in the grill, squirts some lighter fluid on the charcoal and throws a match on it. The lighter fluid goes "BOOM," but somehow his charcoal never starts burning. So he squirts more lighter fluid, lights another match and watches it blow up again while his wife and I make fun of him. He makes frequent trips to the store for more lighter fluid. One day his wife commented, "Charlie's charcoal grill runs on lighter fluid."

In a way, muscle is like that grill. Muscle burns both fat and sugar: The sugar burns instantly like lighter fluid, yielding only a small amount of energy, but the fat continues to burn for a long time, like charcoal once it gets started. You get lots more calories, or energy, from a fat molecule than you do from a sugar molecule. When you're playing active sports you may run out of sugar; you never run out of fat.

We now know that even people who are starving never, never, never use up all of their body fat. This may surprise you, since starving or anorexic people look so emaciated, but there is fat even on the bodies of people who weigh only 75 pounds. They look like skeletons when they die because they lose so much muscle, but autopsies show that they still have 10 to 15 pounds of fat hidden inside. These people do not, in fact, starve to death.

Nobody in the history of the Earth has ever actually starved to death. At some point during starvation, as the body runs out of glucose it starts using protein for fuel. In the process of burning protein, it taps the immune system antibodies, which are proteins. Starving people become highly susceptible to bacteria and viruses; they die of infectious diseases precipitated by lack of protein in their bodies.

People Worry Too Much about Vitamins, Proteins and Carbohydrates— It's FAT That Runs the Body

Like starving people, those who are very fit occasionally have lighter-fluid problems. During long, rigorous sports events, their muscles run out of sugar. When that happens, their energy drops abruptly because the burning of fat, triggered by sugar's spark, has ceased. Athletes think they run out of energy because their sugar has run out; in reality, they have plenty of "fat energy" left but no way to draw from it. They constantly look for ways to store more sugar in their muscles, mistakenly thinking that sugar is their primary fuel. But it is only the starter fluid; fat is the primary fuel.

The Failure of the Low-Fat, High-Carbohydrate Diet

In February 1995 the New York Times *ran a front-page article that caused huge ripples in the health community. The article discussed the research of a few doctors who believe that our current thinking about nutrition was all wrong: that we need much less carbohydrate and far more protein in our diets than the "establishment" was advocating. Several books have emerged on the subject, and the debate rages on. In the following excerpt from* Protein Power *(Bantam, 1996), Michael R. Eades, M.D., and Mary Dan Eades, M.D., lay out the arguments against the federal Food and Drug Administration's current eating guidelines.*

Yes, doctors today are aware that diet plays a significant role in the development and progression of the major diseases afflicting modern man—heart disease, diabetes, obesity, high blood pressure and many kinds of cancers. As a consequence, dietitians, nutritionists and physicians constantly exhort us to eat properly to avoid these disorders. By their definition, eating properly means rooting out fat from our diets and replacing it with complex carbohydrate.

Ever since the surgeon general recommended in 1988 that Americans severely reduce their consumption of fat, especially saturated fat, the race to zero-fat products has been on. Eggs, red meat and other superior protein sources have been virtually drummed out of the American kitchen. Reduce fat intake to almost nothing, we are told by battalions of nutritional experts, and good-bye obesity, heart disease, diabetes and all the rest. Sounds great in theory, but—and here's why physicians a hundred years from now will be shaking their heads—it doesn't work.

The low-fat, high-complex-carbohydrate

approach has proven a failure. It doesn't reduce cholesterol levels to any great degree unless followed to an almost ridiculous extreme, in which case it can actually cause other equally sinister problems. It gives diabetes sufferers endless grief in trying to regulate their blood sugar levels. It doesn't reduce high blood pressure unless it brings about significant weight loss. Its success rate for weight loss is almost nonexistent. (You may be surprised to learn that we've treated many people who have gained weight on the low-fat diet.) The result of the current no-fat mania has been a fatter and less healthy America, thanks in part to the zeal of food manufacturers who have given us an endless variety of fat-free high-carbohydrate junk to replace the fat-filled junk we were eating before.

In the face of this dismal record, what do we as medical professionals do? Do we write off the low-fat diet as something that sounded good on paper but didn't work in practice, abandon it and begin searching for something better, as we would a new drug that had failed? No. Instead we say, "Bring on more of the same. Let's try harder, let's try longer, let's be more diligent." We tell our patients that it must be their fault if their condition doesn't improve on a low-fat diet; they must not be following it correctly. But such thinking flies in the face of metabolic reality because dietary fat alone is not the problem. The problem lies in the biochemical structure of the low-fat diet and the mixed signals it gives to the body's essential metabolic processes. Ironically, not only does the low-fat diet fail to solve the health problems it addresses, it actually makes them even worse.

The human body is a remarkably resilient, reactive, regenerative piece of biochemical machinery. Like any piece of complex equipment, it functions best when treated properly. The proponents of low-fat dieting believe that the best way to treat the body is by restricting the amount of fat, particularly saturated fat, that the body takes in and replacing it with complex carbohydrate. Their flawed thinking goes like this: Too much fat accumulation in the arteries causes heart disease and other problems, too much fat accumulation in the fat cells causes obesity and too much fat intake exacerbates diabetes, so if we reduce fat intake, we'll solve all these problems. Although it seems logical, it doesn't work because it doesn't take into account the body's biochemistry and the ways our metabolic hormones cause us to store fat. When we understand and control these potent body chemicals, we can achieve our health goals by controlling fat from within rather than trying to eliminate it from without. To begin to understand how this works, let's first examine food from a biochemical perspective.

What Is This Thing Called Food?

All food, from pancakes to sushi, is composed of macronutrients, micronutrients and water. Aside from water, which makes up the lion's share of everything, food is made primarily of the macronutrients protein, fat and carbohydrate. These three macronutrients are the only food components that provide energy—measured as calories—to maintain life. The micronutrients—vitamins, minerals and trace elements—provide no caloric energy but are nevertheless essential for life. They perform a multitude of cellular functions, many of which involve the efficient use and disposal of the macronutrients. Without macronutrients we would suffer malnutrition, starvation and death; without the micronutrients we would suffer deficiency diseases, a precipitous health decline and death. The nutrients from both groups are necessary for life.

Balancing the Big Three

Since the entire caloric content of food comes from the three macronutrients, it is obvious that decreasing any one macronutrient—fat, for instance—requires increasing another (carbohydrate or protein or both) to maintain any given caloric level. If your metabolic needs for a day require 2,000 calories and, in accordance with the recommendations of the nutritional establishment, you reduce your fat intake, what happens? You increase your intake of carbohydrate and protein to make up for the calories lost by removing the fat, right? Actually, it's a little more complicated than that. You don't go to the grocery store and buy three scoops of protein, five scoops of carbohydrate and two scoops of fat; you buy meat, eggs, vegetables, fruits, dairy products. Some foods—meat and eggs, for instance—contain only protein and fat, while others such as apples and grapes are practically all carbohydrate with only a trace of protein. You can trim the visible fat from cuts of meat to reduce fat content, but otherwise it's difficult to extract just one macronutrient from a particular food item. So the only way to change the ratios of fat, protein and carbohydrate is to change the types of foods eaten. If you want to decrease your fat intake, you simply eat less meat, eggs and dairy products and replace them with fruits and vegetables. Sounds reasonable, but is it?

Not really, and here's why. Humans don't require equal amounts of the three macronutrients for optimal health. The average person requires at least 70 to 100 grams of protein per day, or about 300 calories' worth, and 6 to 10 grams of linoleic acid (a type of fat that is essential to health), about 75 calories' worth. What about carbohydrate? The actual amount of carbohydrate required by humans for health is *zero*. We haven't made these figures up; they represent the consensus of scientific wisdom today. Now, this doesn't mean that as long as you get 75 grams of protein and 6 grams of fat, you'll do fine. You need more calories to provide energy for your bodily functions. It does mean that if you got

enough energy from either protein or fat and maintained your minimum intake of each, you would do fine. Eskimos eat very little carbohydrate, in fact no carbohydrate during the winter, and survive nicely to a ripe old age. Although their traditional diet is composed of a large quantity of protein and an enormous amount of fat, Eskimos suffer very little heart disease, diabetes, obesity (despite the cartoons), high blood pressure and all the other diseases we associate with a more civilized lifestyle. Furthermore, Eskimos don't have metabolic systems from an alien planet; they have the exact same biochemistry and physiology that we do. Yes, you could eat the same diet and tolerate it nicely.

Bearing in mind that protein and fat are essential to health and carbohydrate isn't, what happens when we cut back our fat as the nutritional establishment recommends? Since we can't for the most part remove the fat from the food, we end up replacing foods that contain fat with those that don't. Since most sources of good-quality protein—meat, eggs and dairy products—contain a fair amount of fat, to cut back on fat we end up cutting back on protein as well and replacing them both with carbohydrate. Most vegetable sources of protein—beans and grains—are incomplete unless combined carefully and contain far more carbohydrate than protein. In the end if we strictly follow the low-fat prescription, we can end up deficient in protein (it's difficult to be deficient in fat because the only essential fat is linoleic acid, which is found in vegetable oils).

But possibly the worst news of all is that eating more carbohydrates stimulates your body's fat storage. In attempting to reduce fat intake, you wind up actually getting fatter, because some macronutrients stimulate profound metabolic hormonal changes. Surprisingly, fat doesn't do much. If you were to swill down a dish of lard while hooked up to a laboratory device to measure the levels of your metabolic hormones—chiefly insulin and glucagon—you wouldn't see much activity, because fat is essentially metabolically inert. Carbohydrate, however, would set off a Mad Hatter's tea party of metabolic activity. Eating a handful of grapes while hooked to the same device would initiate a wild swinging of gauge needles indicating a rapid increase in insulin and a decrease in its opposing hormone glucagon, all perfectly normal metabolic responses kindled by the consumption of carbohydrate. It follows logically that the constant consumption of large quantities of carbohydrate would then produce large quantities of insulin, which indeed it does.

Even complex carbohydrates stimulate the response because all carbohydrates are basically sugar. Various sugar molecules—primarily glucose—hooked together chemically compose the entire family of carbohydrates. Your body has digestive enzymes that break these chemical bonds and release the sugar molecules into the blood, where they stimulate insulin and the other metabolic hormones. This means that if you follow a 2,200-calorie diet that is 60 percent carbohydrate—the very one most nutritionists recommend—your body will end up having to contend metabolically with almost two cups of pure sugar per day.

What's Insulin Got to Do with It?

So, what does insulin have to do with anything other than diabetes? And if you don't have diabetes, why should you care about insulin at all? Because it's important to your health.

Insulin, a hormone produced and released into the blood by the pancreas, affects virtually every cell in the body. Insulin occupies a chapter or two in every medical biochemistry and physiology textbook, entire sections in endocrinology texts and even two pages of tiny print in our 15-year-old *Encyclopaedia Britannica*. Whole textbooks are devoted to its myriad activities. Insulin regulates blood sugar, yes, but it does much more. It controls the storage of fat; it directs the flow of amino acids, fatty acids and carbohydrate to the tissues; it regulates the liver's synthesis of cholesterol; it functions as a growth hormone; it is involved in appetite control; it drives the kidneys to retain fluid; and much, much more. This master hormone of metabolism is a substance absolutely essential to life; without it, you would perish—quickly.

But insulin is also a monster hormone. It has a dark side. In the proper amount it is life-sustaining. Too much of it causes enormous health problems. Reams of scientific studies, with more added to the stack daily, implicate excess insulin as a primary cause of or significant risk factor for high blood pressure, heart disease, obesity, elevated cholesterol and other blood fats, and diabetes (yes, insulin itself can cause diabetes).

How do you go about controlling insulin? With a carbohydrate-restricted, moderate-fat, adequate-protein diet that modulates the body's metabolic hormones, including insulin. Diet is what makes insulin levels go haywire in the first place, so it stands to reason that dietary changes should be able to reverse the problem. Diet is, in fact, the only way to solve this problem.

The foods we eat exert a profound influence on what happens within our bodies hormonally—both for good and for bad. By eating the correct balance of foods we can almost medicinally alter what goes on inside us in a healthful way. By eating the wrong foods we can precipitate health disasters. We can more easily dig our graves with a fork and spoon than with a shovel.

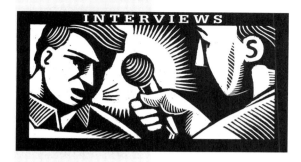

Kelly Brownell on
The Sociology of Weight Loss

Though your weight is ultimately your own responsibility, others have a lot to do with how—or whether—you'll get in shape. That's why when Kelly Brownell, Ph.D., put together his LEARN weight-control program, he included relationship tips with his advice for nutrition, exercise and motivation. (For more information on the LEARN program, call 1-800-736-7323.) In this interview, the Yale University psychology professor explains how the people around you affect your habits and how you can take control.

Should you listen to what other people have to say about your physical condition?

If people tell you that you look good, then you probably do. You should accept that and not drive yourself crazy dieting. Very often, the way people look doesn't match up with the way they think they look. There are far too many people dieting when they don't need to. People enter into a conflict with their own bodies. Instead of being friends with their bodies and seeing them as allies, they become enemies with their bodies.

If you can't trust your own judgment but you don't trust anyone else's, how will you ever know if you need to lose weight?

The knee-jerk response is to look at height-weight tables to see if there's a health reason to lose weight. But there's controversy about just how much above the norms you have to be before you have increased health risk. Generally, though, if people are 20 percent or more above their ideal weights, it would be healthier to lose.

Being overweight is not a dichotomous variable. It's not that you're either overweight and have massive health risk or you're perfect weight and have none. Risk increases in a pretty linear fashion with weight: If you're a little bit overweight, you have a little bit of risk; if you're a lot overweight, you have a lot of risk. People at weights closer to normal have to make a decision whether it's worth the effort and restriction to lose weight.

What if you want to lose weight, but feel like you're surrounded by people who can eat anything and never have to exercise?

It's like any other area of life: You have to take your lumps. You might be envious of people who are taller or smarter or have more money than you, but that's the hand of cards you're dealt. You have to learn to make the best of it.

It's easier said than done, because our society places so much emphasis on the way you look, so people who don't match up to the ideal can feel like they're failures. It's horribly unfair. What we need to do is accept differences in body shape and size like we accept differences in eye color and hair color.

Is it a bad sign if you decide to lose weight but are uncomfortable talking about it? If nobody's in on your plans, are you more likely to fail?

We classify people as either solo or social dieters. One style is not better than another—what's important is that a person approach it in a way consistent with his own needs. There are some people who really like to do this privately: They don't like other people knowing that they're in a program or that they're attempting to lose weight. They don't want people to notice or get too involved.

A solo dieter would make a mistake by joining a weight-loss group. There's no rule that people have to know what you're doing. But if you're going to lose a fair amount of weight, people are going to notice. You'd better prepare yourself to deal with that sooner or later.

What about the social changers?

They respond much more positively to social support. They can get it from friends, family, co-workers or other people in a program. We consider support from others to be a latent resource—it's like mining for gold. It's there, but you have to go get it.

There's a series of steps and procedures that you should follow to elicit support: First, ask for it, rather than just expect it to happen. Be specific in your request so that others know *how* they can help. Instead of saying, "Please help me in my program," say, "Can we take a walk together every night after dinner?" or "Can you try to eat your ice cream when I'm not around?"

The final big step is to reinforce the supporter, to encourage their behavior so that they know they've helped.

Going on a weight-loss program sometimes adds a lot of tension to the atmosphere at home. Is there anything you can do to prepare your family for the transition?

There's no substitute for talking to people. Alert them to the fact that your eating will change, that there are specific things they can do that will be helpful and that you're going to be spending more time exercising.

These things can disrupt the routine of the family. Sometimes people are envious when you're making a positive change in your life. Sometimes the spouse is jealous because she needs to do the same thing but isn't. Some

spouses are threatened when their partner is about to become more attractive. Sometimes you just have a destructive relationship, and this becomes part of the negative interaction.

So how do you handle it?

One way is to have an honest talk, where you discuss your feelings and describe helpful ways of being supportive. Another is to be assertive: Don't yield to the pressure that others put on you. The final option is to ignore it. Just put up with it and do the best you can in the face of it. Of course, the best thing is if you can talk openly with your partner, but sometimes that's not possible.

A lot of men have the opposite problem: Their families pester them about diet and exercise so much that they end up resisting the changes.

That happens a lot. Family members do it in a well-meaning way, but it comes across as nagging. The response—especially for men—is that you either ignore it and deny it or you get angry and pick fights about it.

The best thing to do is to be straightforward and candid with people and tell them how it affects you. Give them ideas of how they can be more helpful. Instead of saying, "You're a jerk for saying this to me," you can say, "It would help me a lot more if you said. . . ."

What if your wife does most of the cooking, and her specialties are high-fat and high-calorie foods?

There are so many prepackaged prepared foods available now that are low in fat and low in calories that if your wife wants to make traditional meals, it's easy to go the store and buy some alternative so that you can eat alongside her.

There may be cases where the wife feels threatened by her husband losing weight and has a subconscious need to subvert his efforts. That may be the real issue, but it gets fought out over food. Be assertive. A really good way to bring people around is to ask for their help. You have to decide how strongly you should push it.

What do you do when you visit your mother and she's baked a triple-layer, double-fudge cake just for you? How can you say no?

You don't have to say no. Eat a little bit. Unless you're visiting your mother three times a day, what difference does it make? In the big scheme of things, it makes no difference at all.

Is your advice the same for Thanksgiving dinner or a big Super Bowl party?

Go ahead and do what you would've done otherwise. Eat the food and write it off as an unusual day. Nobody's perfect. These are special days, so why not eat and have fun?

You're reaction is much more important than the event itself. Let's say that you really pig out—how much are you going to gain? One pound? So what? Just make sure that you don't react to it in a really negative way and let down afterward.

What can you tell yourself when it's over so that you won't starting thinking that *every* day is a special occasion?

"I deserve to have a treat once in a while. This is not a sign that I'm falling apart. I've been doing wonderfully on my program. I know from the past that I can bounce back."

Is it natural to distance yourself from friends and family while you're losing weight?

It depends on how important eating and weight were to your social group. If you were connected to people because of eating, and your eating changes, then it might be natural to move to a new group. But there's no reason why friends shouldn't be friends and relationships shouldn't remain intact.

Daniel Kosich on
Weight Management

Don't expect any easy answers regarding weight loss from fitness consultant Daniel Kosich, Ph.D. Unlike many diet gurus, he's up-front about the physical and emotional work of weight loss—and prepares us to deal with it. Here, Dr. Kosich—who authored the book Get Real: A Personal Guide to Real-Life Weight Management—*tells us how to appreciate ourselves, whatever our size, and accept weight management as a part of our everyday lives.*

You say that people have to like themselves the way they are now if they're going to successfully lose weight and keep it off. How are we supposed to be happy with beer bellies and double chins?

It's a difficult concept. The "if-then" mentality is a big part of the challenge. Often people think, "If I can get to a certain weight on the scale, then I'll feel good about myself," or "If I can fit into a certain piece of clothing, then I'll feel good about myself." If you're in that kind of paradigm, the probability of success or of feeling good if you get there is minimal.

Instead, build a perspective that "I like myself so much right now that I'm going to do what I need to do to get to a healthy weight. I really like who I am, and I want to take good care of myself."

That makes sense, but still, most of us would rather eat bean curd than analyze our feelings. Is there any way to make this mental switch without five years of therapy?

It's individual. When you look in the mirror, if the image projected is a negative one, that's a strong signal that you're on the wrong track. Practice looking in the mirror and saying: "I feel good about who I am. I'm a good person. People like me not because of what I look like; they like me because of who I am."

The root of it is to look at weight management as a part of overall health care—the same way we look at brushing our teeth. It isn't necessarily fun, but we do it to be healthy.

Being overweight is unhealthy. It sets the stage for any number of problems that I'm sure you're well aware of. When people realize that losing weight is an issue of caring for themselves, they're more likely to be motivated to change. It really comes down to being able to say, "I'm the one who's responsible for my own health."

That might work for a while, but once the fat's gone, there's a tendency to revert to old habits. Do you have a technique for helping us make a long-term commitment?

I call it acting as if. Today, I do things I need to do as if I were already at a healthy weight. You see, my body weight ten years from now is not going to be a product of what I do for six weeks or six months—or even six years. It's going to be a product of what I do for the next ten years. Do what you're supposed to do 80 percent of the time; the other 20 percent of the time, realize that you're not perfect.

Does this mean that we're going to be counting calories forever?

I used to give people charts and scales and have them weigh things and draw out seven-day menu plans. And I don't do that anymore. It just doesn't work. People can't live with that kind of rigid structure for very long.

But, like any behavioral change, losing weight involves certain lifestyle issues that some people have a very difficult time modifying. The key to getting to a healthy weight and staying at a healthy weight is getting active.

Even better. We're going to be chained to our treadmills for life?

Look, you don't have to like exercise. People say, "If you do it for three months, you're really going to love running or cycling." I don't agree with that. There are a lot of days I don't want to go on a bike ride; I'd much rather sleep in. But I do it, because I know that if I do it, I'll feel better physically—it's energizing. And I'll feel better mentally, because I've kept a commitment to myself.

Getting more active as a part of lifestyle—not just exercise—is really the key. Walk to the store; don't get in your car. Do more with your kids. These are simple activities of daily living that add a few extra calories of expenditure every day.

Shift from looking at diet as the number one priority and get your body moving. Once that happens, it seems to open the door. Often, active people eat better.

I can see how this would affect someone who's obese, but can such subtle changes really help the average guy who just wants to lose 15 pounds in time for his high school reunion?

Focusing on the scale is a real detriment. It creates the impression that weight loss is the number one goal. In my opinion, the goal is health. If you adopt a healthy lifestyle, your body weight will change incrementally, as an adjunct.

The accumulation of body fat has happened over a number of years. Getting to a healthy body weight is not going to be a short process. It is going to be a slow, accumulating process that comes from adopting healthy living habits most of the time. It's not a question of living by a rigid system that no healthy person would adhere to.

I just saw a newspaper ad that said I can lose 49 pounds in 29 days. The reality is that 1 pound, maybe 1½ pounds, a week is a realistic expectation. So, you're looking at 4 pounds a month.

Obviously, people are going to say, "Shoot, I want the 49 pounds in 29 days!" But the people who do that are not going to be successful in the long run. Yes, they might buy this product and lose their 49 pounds, but a year or two down the road, they're going to have it all back again.

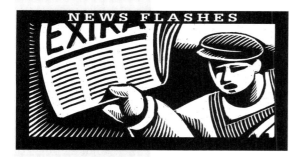

Study Disproves Eat-Late, Gain-Weight Theory

NEW YORK—Consuming a majority of your daily calories during the evening hours does not make you more susceptible to gaining weight, according to a new study based on data from the U.S. Department of Agriculture. The conclusion challenges a widely held nutritional truism.

In recent years, nutritionists have consistently recommended that people meet their daily energy and nutrient needs by consuming three or more meals distributed throughout the day. In particular, they have urged Americans to avoid eating the bulk of their daily calories at the end of the day. The thinking was that calories consumed later in the day would be more readily converted to fat while the body sleeps at night.

However, after analyzing data from more than 1,800 subjects, researchers were unable to find any association between the body weight of the participants and the percentage of calories each consumed after 5:00 P.M.

The researchers calculated that most of the subjects consumed about 46 percent of their total calories in the evening with no effect on their body weight. The findings did, however, indicate that evening eating was associated with some relatively small differences in the quality of nutrient intake. Late eaters, for example, might have trouble getting the recommended servings of fruit and vegetables into their diets.

Repeated Dieting Bad for Mental Health

HOUSTON—"Yo-yo" dieting, in which a person goes through a constantly repeating cycle of gaining and losing weight, has already been associated with a whole list of physical side effects. New research indicates that yo-yo dieting also can be hazardous to your mental health.

In the first study of its kind, psychologists at the DeBakey Heart Center in Houston monitored nearly 500 men and women to document their weight—pounds lost, maintained or gained—throughout one year. The participants also filled out questionnaires that monitored their stress levels, abnormal eating behaviors and weight perceptions.

The results indicate that yo-yo dieting is linked to poor self-esteem and depression. The researchers noted that the subjects who regained weight tended to feel bad about themselves, which then made their self-esteem suffer and their depression worsen. In contrast, the study showed that the people who maintained their weight possessed a much more positive sense of well-being and believed that they had less stress in their lives. Overall, the weight maintainers had better control of their eating habits and were generally more healthy than their yo-yo dieting counterparts.

Free Food, Money Fail to Induce Weight Loss

MINNEAPOLIS—Neither monetary incentives nor providing dieters with weekly food provisions proved to be effective tools for successful long-term weight loss, according to a recent study.

In an effort to identify the best ways to enhance weight-loss maintenance, researchers examined whether providing food and money incentives could add to the long-term effectiveness of standard treatments. The study involved

101 men and 101 women who were provided with one of four treatments for an 18-month period: (1) a standard behavioral treatment, (2) the standard treatment plus weekly food provisions, (3) the standard treatment along with money incentives for achieving weight loss that could total up to $25 per week for each participant or (4) the standard treatment plus the food provisions and the money incentives.

Initially, all four approaches resulted in weight loss, with most participants tending to lose weight during the first 6 months of the program. Those who received the food provisions but not the money lost the greatest amount of weight during the initial 18 months. During the 12 months that followed the end of the program, however, all the groups, regardless of the treatment approach, regained weight. The researchers concluded that four factors—exercising, eating less fat, having better nutritional knowledge and perceiving fewer barriers to adherence—were ultimately the best predictors of successful long-term weight loss.

"Ideal" Weights May Not Be Ideal

NEW YORK—Standard weight tables that are used to recommend "ideal" ranges for individuals may be suggesting weights that are actually as much as 15 pounds too low for most men, say researchers at Cornell University in Ithaca, New York. After analyzing the results of 19 studies that examined mortality and weight, and which involved more than 357,000 men and almost 250,000 women, the researchers concluded that the health risks associated with being moderately underweight are comparable to the health risks of being considerably overweight.

The researchers' findings also led them to believe that the standard weight tables, which imply that any weight higher than the one speci-

fied will result in a shorter life span, may be incorrect. It was discovered, for instance, that White men who were moderately underweight at 50 were more likely to die within the next 30 years than were their counterparts who were moderately overweight.

The researchers are not sure why lower weight is associated with higher mortality. They do, however, believe that their findings suggest that for people who are just moderately overweight, losing weight may not be the answer to increased longevity.

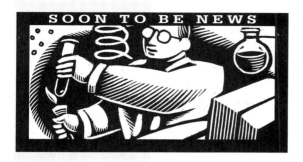

SOON TO BE NEWS

A Safe Diet Pill?

Because of the steady rise in the number of obese people in the United States, drug companies are trying harder than ever to produce a substance that can safely and effectively assist in the process of weight loss.

There are numerous new diet pills currently working their way to market through the Food and Drug Administration's (FDA) approval process. Most of these pills fall under a few broad categories of chemical compounds. One of the categories focuses on suppressing the body's appetite system. Another group aims at increasing the body's fat-burning rate. A third category attempts to replicate the activity of leptin, a protein that is believed to be involved in setting weight levels.

One moral dilemma: If these drugs prove effective but also cause side effects, how should doctors determine who warrants treatment? *As these new diet pills move closer to receiving FDA approval, the medical community continues to debate their pros and cons.*

Shrink Your Belly with Wine?

Researchers at the University of North Carolina speculate that there may be a chemical in wine that keeps wine drinkers' bellies smaller than their beer buddies' bellies.

The scientists measured the circumference of the bellies of over 12,000 men and women. There were several groups represented within the study's population, including beer, wine and hard liquor drinkers at three levels of consumption and a group of nondrinkers.

After reviewing all the abdominal measurements, the researchers found that the wine drinkers had the smallest guts and the beer drinkers had the largest. Lifestyle factors may play a role in these differences. After all, beer and pizza parties can be more damaging to the waistline than wine tastings. The researchers believe, however, that there may be a belly-busting chemical contained in wine. *The hope is that future studies will allow researchers to identify this chemical.*

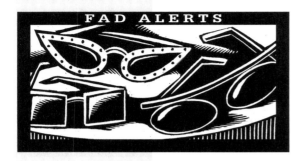

High-Protein, Low-Carbohydrate Diets

 The Zone. Dr. Atkins. Healthy for Life. You've probably met someone at the gym who's on one of those high-protein, low-carbohydrate diets. You hear all the movie stars are doing it. But before you give up your bran muffins for all the steaks and butter you can eat, you might want to examine these new weight-loss plans a little more closely.

While most of the country is busy counting fat grams, proponents of these diets are focused instead on insulin levels, as Michael R. Eades, M.D., co-author with Mary Dan Eades, M.D., of *Protein Power*, explains. Insulin is the hormone that, among other things, promotes the storage of energy in fat cells. It's produced in response to excess glucose in the bloodstream—an excess that occurs when more carbohydrates are consumed than are needed for immediate body functioning.

So, the theory goes, consistently eating too many carbohydrates can eventually lead to chronically elevated insulin levels, which, in turn, cause weight gain, high blood pressure and other health problems.

"The key is not so much protein as it is the metabolic changes brought about by restricting carbohydrates," Dr. Eades says. "We don't advocate eating excessive amounts of protein. We put people at a minimum and tell them that they can have more if they want, because people tend not to binge on protein."

What isn't clear, though, is whether the weight lost using such a system is a product of lower insulin levels, as Dr. Eades theorizes, or simply lower total calorie intake.

"A person eating a high-protein, high-fat meal could eat less food and fewer calories because high-fat food fills one up faster than if he were having a balanced meal," says Michele Trankina, Ph.D., a nutritional physiologist and consultant at St. Mary's University of San Antonio in Texas. "But my question is, over time, if they're eating so much animal-based food, what is all the saturated fat and cholesterol doing to their arteries?"

Another concern is loss of the numerous vitamins and minerals that carbohydrates supply. In their strictest form, these diets can reduce carbohydrate intake to as little as 200 calories a day, the minimum amount for maintaining brain function.

Dr. Eades himself warns that anyone on a serious low-carbohydrate diet needs to take a potassium supplement in an amount that is usually available only in prescription tablets. He also says that implementing his plan can initially cause headaches, feelings of windedness and loss of endurance. After the first few days, these symptoms rapidly go away, and many studies show an increase in endurance after this plan is adopted.

One thing experts on both sides of the debate agree on is that more clinical studies need to be done. In the meantime, Dr. Eades suggests that men with only a few pounds to lose make subtle changes, cutting back a bit on wheat and potato products, for example.

Dr. Trankina offers an alternative method for keeping insulin levels lower: "To avoid storage of excess energy, eat smaller portions more frequently instead of having giant meals a few times a day."

Fat-Simulating Products

 Remember the uproar over olestra? Procter and Gamble spent decades developing the substance with the texture and consistency of fat but no calories, before it was approved for use in snack foods early in 1996. It's made up of fatty acids bound to sucrose molecules, and is not digestible—it simply passes through the body intact.

Some doctors and health organizations objected to olestra, because it has a tendency to absorb fat-soluble vitamins and carotenoids and flush them out of the body along with it. The first olestra-containing chips were fortified with some fat-soluble vitamins, but that didn't solve another problem: In cities where the products were initially test-marketed, some consumers reported stomach cramps and diarrhea.

It remains to be seen whether olestra will be omnipresent or outlawed, but meanwhile, there are other controversial products making use of some of the same theories. And because these food additives—which are designed to prevent real fat from being digested—are not made from synthetic compounds, they do not need government approval.

"The vitamin supplement companies, which are not regulated, are promoting products that are supposed to bind fat in the intestine and carry it out of the body unabsorbed," Dr. Trankina says. "But guess what else they bind? Fat-soluble vitamins A, E, D and K. A person can develop deficiencies in a big hurry."

Cabbage Soup Diet

 Some fad diets never die. Just when you think they've passed on to the realm of amusing folklore, someone brings them back to life—and in the process convinces plenty of people to forgo the benefits of sound nutrition. Which is why it's really not so funny that the cabbage soup diet is making another comeback.

The latest version started making the rounds after a tabloid reported that celebrities were losing more than 15 pounds a week on the diet. The soup recipe calls for cabbage, celery, green beans, green onions, green peppers and tomatoes to be combined with onion soup mix and V-8 juice. In addition, dieters are allowed to eat specific prescribed foods each day—for instance, once a week, they have bananas and milk with their cabbage soup.

People who follow the directions do drop weight, so what's the problem? Bloating, flatulence and diarrhea, for starters, according to Dr. Trankina. And the high sodium content in the soup mix and canned juice can lead to fluid or mineral imbalance, which would threaten the life of anyone on diuretics for a heart or kidney condition.

"It violates the rules of basic nutrition," says Dr. Trankina. "The nutrients aren't there in sufficient quantities. I don't see much potassium or much vitamin A or beta-carotene—unless you add carrots to it. It's even a little too low in fat."

The bottom line is that there's nothing magical about cabbage soup. The reason that pounds fly off with this diet is that you probably consume fewer than 1,000 calories a day. If you want to eat low-cal, there are far more appetizing ways to do it.

"Obviously, you can't live on this stuff forever," Dr. Trankina says. "After a while, the last thing on earth you'll want to see is cabbage soup. It doesn't take a scientist to understand that. Eventually, when you start eating the way you did before, you gain all the weight back."

In-Line Skating

 It first caught on as a fad for fun. But lately, in-line skating has been touted as a great way to get fitter. It turns out that the two are not mutually exclusive. If you're struggling to lose a few pounds and not enjoying your exercise, skating might be an activity to try. It's a lot more exciting than walking, and it's easier on your body than running, says Wayne Westcott, Ph.D., strength consultant to the YMCA of the USA—assuming that you don't crash into an oak tree.

Serious in-liners get a more-than-adequate aerobic workout, according to a University of Wisconsin study. At high speeds, they can burn 19 calories a minute, roughly the same number as someone running a six-minute mile. But moving at a more normal pace, you may not feel like you're working hard enough. That's because you're spending more time gliding than you are stroking, says Joel Rappelfeld, in-line skating instructor and author of *The Complete Blader*. He suggests bending over farther—like a speed skater—to create resistance and use additional leg muscles.

In-line skating really starts to get interesting when combined with team sport. Obviously, it's done wonders for the popularity of hockey, but the latest craze is in-line basketball. There's even a National In-Line Basketball League that organizes play in several cities in the United States and Canada.

Taking your skating to the courts has a few other added advantages: There aren't going to be any cars or sewer grates to trip you up.

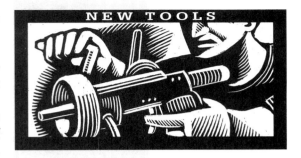

NEW TOOLS

More Efficient Workouts

Precor M9.45 Treadmill

If you're never quite sure whether you're working out hard enough to burn fat, the Precor M9.45 treadmill might help. Its software can calculate your proper target heart rate, based on your age. Then when you put a monitor band around your chest and start your walk or run, the treadmill will automatically adjust its speed and incline to keep your heart pumping at just the right speed. An extra $99 gets you hand weights that serve as remote controls. These weights let you change the speed or incline without breaking stride. $4,000.

Better Weight Management

Anti-Diet Kit

Being overweight is a common problem, but when it comes to shaping up, it's still pretty much every man for himself. An expert may give you the answers today, but will you know how to use them yourself tomorrow?

One tool that will help is the Anti-Diet Kit, from Jack Groppel, Ph.D., a licensed nutritionist and sports scientist with LGE Sport Science, a company that specializes in corporate fitness seminars, personal training and fitness and sports psychology, in Orlando, Florida. Dr. Groppel advocates spreading several small, low-fat meals throughout the day and making use of both aerobic workouts and strength training. Instead of losing pounds, his plan focuses on reducing body fat, not lean muscle mass, and makes use of flexible personal menus and tips for monitoring your progress.

The kit, which comes with a coupon for a $50 nutritional analysis, contains Dr. Groppel's book, *The Anti-Diet Book*, skin-fold calipers by Accu-Measure for determining your body fat percentage, instructional audiotapes, a daily log book and more. Call 1-800-543-7764 to order. $129 plus $5.50 shipping and handling.

Leaner Breakfasts

SnackWell's Toaster Pastries

There are no perfect substitutes for a cream-filled, glazed doughnut with chocolate on top. But if you think that you can't live without your early-morning sugar rush, at least you now have some lower-fat alternatives. Nabisco's SnackWell line has introduced toaster pastries that have one gram of fat per 1.75-ounce serving. They come in four flavors: blueberry, strawberry, apple cinnamon and fudge. The pastries, which have no saturated fat or cholesterol and no more than 170 calories each, are individually wrapped and sold in boxes of six. $1.99.

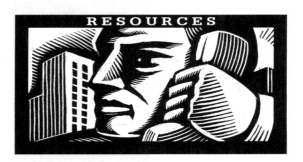

Healthy Eating on the Road

Heart Smart Restaurants International
6617 North Scottsdale Road
Scottsdale, AZ 85250
1-800-762-7819

Someday they'll invent the refrigerated briefcase. Until then, when on the road, getting healthy vittles will always be a challenge. But here's a break: Travelers can receive a free listing of restaurants throughout the country that serve low-fat and low-salt dishes. For more information, call the number above or send a stamped (55 cents), self-addressed, legal-size envelope to the above address for your free copy. Heart Smart Restaurants is a company that does menu analyses for restaurants and will give them their stamp of approval if restaurants agree to do certain healthy things, such as serve margarine rather than butter and skim milk instead of whole milk.

Functional Foods

University of Illinois Functional Foods
for Health
http://www.ag.uiuc.edu/~food-lab/nat/

Getting the biggest nutritional bang for your food buck is important when dieting. To view the latest scientific information on functional food topics (those that deal with food products that have disease-preventive and health-promoting benefits), check out the Web site sponsored by the University of Illinois's Functional Foods for Health program. Here you can find out all about the health effects of foods and food components.

Eating Disorders

National Association of Anorexia

Nervosa and Associated Disorders

Box 7

Highland Park, IL 60035

(847) 831-3438

Although people tend to associate eating disorders with women, these illnesses also affect men, either as the victims or as family members or friends of the victims. For those who need assistance, the National Association of Anorexia Nervosa and Associated Disorders offers free programs to help both victims and families. The information they provide includes listings of support groups and counselors in your area, information packets and some counseling services.

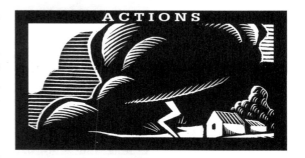

ACTIONS

We've been over the basics a billion times: Lower your fat intake, eat your vegetables and get regular exercise, and you'll lose weight. It *sounds* simple enough. So why are all those extra pounds still hanging around? Maybe you need a few more tips to make your weight-loss program work. Here are some ideas.

1. **Shrink your stomach.** If trying to lose weight always leaves you ravenous, it could be because your days—or years—of overeating have expanded your stomach capacity, meaning that it now takes a lot more food to make you feel full. The process can be reversed—as long as you give up bingeing. Doctors at the Obesity Research Center in New York City put several overweight subjects on a low-calorie diet and found that their stomachs shrunk to a normal size within a month. Lead researcher Allan Geliebter, Ph.D., suggests trading in your huge dinner for several small meals eaten throughout the day. That way, your stomach can adjust without your having to go hungry.

2. **Eat filling foods.** The idea is to maximize fullness and minimize calories. Australian researchers at the University of Sydney fed students 240-calorie portions of specific foods, including potatoes, oranges, white bread, whole-wheat pasta and croissants, then asked them to describe how hungry they felt. They named potatoes the most hunger-satisfying food, at more than three times the satisfaction level of white bread, which, in turn, was twice as satisfying as the worst food, croissant. Some other good choices to satisfy your hunger without too many calories include fish, oranges and whole-wheat pasta.

3. **Be picky about exercise machines.** Many workout tools rely on your body weight to provide resistance. This means that as you lose pounds, the exercise becomes less effective—unless you substantially increase your speed. "Unless your machine has some way of adding weights or resistance to compensate for the weight you've lost, you're kidding yourself," says Charles Kuntzleman, Ed.D., director of the BlueCross Blue-Shield of Michigan Fitness for Youth Program.

4. **Eat breakfast.** You already know that breakfast is the most important meal of the day. But now researchers say that it can keep your weight down, too. In a Spanish study comparing the eating habits of obese people with those of normal weight, researchers found that eating a big breakfast may keep you from becoming fat. In the study, the obese people ate smaller breakfasts with minimal nutritional value, then followed with larger portions of heavier foods later in the day, causing the weight gain. People who ate a large quantity of several different breakfast foods—a variety of breads, fruits and juices—ate less later in the day and maintained more normal weights.

5. **Crack yourself up.** Laughing 100 times burns roughly the same number of calories as spending ten minutes on a rowing machine, says William Fry, M.D., a psychiatrist and associate clinical professor emeritus at Stanford University School of Medicine. Okay, so comedic flair and svelteness don't necessarily go hand in hand—as one look at Oliver Hardy or Roseanne would prove. But at minimum, keeping a sense of humor will certainly help you adjust to your new diet and fitness regime.

6. **Be on guard at work.** Your job has a lot to do with the way you eat, so you had better make sure that your weight-loss strategy can coincide with your career. Fran Grabowski, R.D., co-author of *Low-Fat Living for Real People*, has seen it all: a policeman who had to spend most of his night alone in a patrol car with frequent stops at the only open restaurant, the doughnut shop; a judge who could get called into court—and away from food—for 12 hours at a time; a school bus driver who snacked constantly between his morning and afternoon shifts. The real issue in these cases is not fat grams or fiber, she says. "It's access to food.

"Identify ways to improve your access to healthy food. Often it's hard to find healthy alternatives at night. Brown-bag it or ask a favorite waitress to have some fruit and bagels available. If you don't expect to have time to eat, plan ahead so that you can go for a quick 'real' meal before or after work or on a break. And if you find that you're in a situation where there is just too much food available, your challenge is to find something else to do besides eat. Plan to eat like you plan for retirement, consistent small steps in the right direction," says Grabowski.

7. **Carve time deliberately.** So you're going to start exercising. "But you're already living 24 hours a day!" Dr. Kuntzleman says. "Where are you going to get that extra half-hour?" Well, you could hit your snooze button three fewer times every morning. You could give up *Seinfeld* reruns. Or you could use part of your lunch hour. The answers are pretty obvious—if you ask the question. But if you skip the step of deciding which few minutes of stuff you're willing to eliminate from your life, your exercise program will be doomed from the start.

8. **Be a 24-hour-a-day athlete.** If you have it in your head that the only way to get in shape is to run ten miles a day, you're going to end up doing nothing. "Anything you do to be physically active should count as exercise in your mind," says Kelly Brownell, Ph.D., professor of psychology at Yale University. "If you go to the mall and park far away from the door, that counts. If you rake leaves in the yard, that counts. If you use the stairs rather than the escalator, that counts." Even if you never were to manage to move on to more strenuous exercise, all these small bursts of extra activity would do you good.

9. Use the month-per-year formula. "For every year you've been sedentary, it will take one month to rehabilitate yourself," Dr. Kuntzleman says. So, if you've been a couch potato for 12 years, expect to spend a year building the stamina you'll need to get through a tough workout. Not sure how to start? "I'm a big advocate of walking," Dr. Kuntzleman says. "It's low-impact, it's convenient and you don't feel self-conscious."

10. Rethink serving size. "Everything in our society affirms the value of large serving sizes," Grabowski says. It'll only cost you pennies to supersize your combo meal at a burger joint, for instance. Even fat-free foods contain some fat, and you'll get fat if you eat too much. What is the correct serving size? "If you are overweight, your serving size is presently too large. A good serving size is between the size of an airline serving or frozen convenience food and the amount that you are presently eating," Grabowski says.

11. Can the beer. True, there's evidence that drinking beer has some health benefits, but let's face facts—getting rid of your gut isn't one of them. A University of North Carolina study confirms what common sense told us long ago: that beer drinkers tend to carry more pounds around the middle than wine drinkers do. Canadian researchers may have pinpointed part of the reason why: Men generally don't reduce their food intake to compensate for the calories they consume in the form of their favorite brew.

12. Develop your own eating plan. People are different, and so are the ways that they eat. Some count on three square meals a day, while others would rather eat mini-meals throughout the day. You probably have a good idea of what kind of eater you are. Work with yourself. Do not go against your grain and try to eat in a way that seems unnatural. "Consistency is the key," says Grabowski. "Find the eating plan that works best for you and then stick to it."

13. Lighten up your goals. You need to have reasonable goals—for both eating and exercise. Don't starve yourself on 900 calories a day when you could eat twice that and lose weight comfortably, Grabowski says.

"A lot of people say, 'I'm going to exercise every single day and never take a day off,'" Dr. Kuntzleman adds. "Then as soon as they do miss a day, they say, 'Well, I blew that. I quit altogether.'"

You might not even need to lose as much weight as you think you do. According to researchers at Cornell University in Ithaca, New York, the national weight guidelines for some men appear to be too low, depending on height and build.

14. Get intense. Adding a short blast of hard exercise to an otherwise moderate routine—adding a bit of running to your nightly walk, for example—has big benefits. First, you'll burn more calories and build more muscle. Second, the extra effort will keep your metabolic rate up longer after the exercise is finished. The more intensity you can add to your exercise, the better. "If you're trying to optimize the time invested, you're going to need a serious training regimen somewhere along the way," Dr. Kuntzleman says. "If you're obese, you need to go slow; but if you're lean and want to stay that way, do high-intensity exercise."

5

DISEASE-PROOF

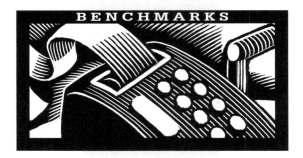

AVERAGES

■ Ratio of Americans who die from smoking-related illnesses each year to those who die as a result of illegal-drug use: 21 to 1

■ Number of Americans who smoke: 49 million

■ Life span of the American male: 72.8 years

■ Percentage of skin cancers that appear on the face, head and neck: 80

■ Number of Americans who die from pneumonia each year: 40,000

■ Number of men who die each year from high blood pressure–related illnesses: 14,000

■ Percentage of American men over the age of 20 who have high blood pressure: 25

■ Number of men who die of heart attacks each year: 250,000

■ Number of men who develop prostate cancer each year: 317,000

■ Percentage of men who know the function of the prostate gland: 42

■ Percentage of American adults who don't drink: 33

■ Number of condoms sold in the United States each year, per adult male: 5

■ Number of cases of food poisoning each year: 80 million

■ Percentage of men who are regular vitamin users: 40

EXTREMES

■ Number of lambs needed to make one lambskin condom: 1

■ Oldest authenticated age: 120 years, 237 days; Shigechiyo Izumi of Tokunoshima, Japan, was born on June 29, 1865, and died of pneumonia on February 21, 1986

■ Fastest speed at which particles expelled by sneezing have been measured: 103.6 miles per hour

■ Highest body temperature: 115.7°F; Willie Jones, 52, was admitted to Grady Memorial Hospital in Atlanta on July 10, 1980, with heatstroke on a day when the temperature reached 90°F with 44 percent humidity

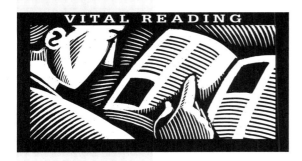

Beneficial Bacteria

Want smoother digestion, a healthier prostate, a stronger heart and greater resistance to disease and cancer? Here's how to restore and keep the good bugs in your body growing strong.

You're born with trillions of beneficial bacteria lining your gut that can feast on carcinogens, sop up dangerous chemicals, manufacture natural antibiotics and help you better absorb vitamins. But as you get older, many of these good bugs can literally fade away, leaving an opening for their disease-causing peers to stake a colonic claim. Courses of antibiotics, bouts of diarrhea, stress and the aging process itself can all tip the bacterial scales out of your favor.

Recent research suggests, however, that you need not sit idly by: Making specific dietary changes can turn back your intestinal clock. "What you choose to eat can make a tremendous difference in whether colonies of beneficial bacteria thrive or perish," says Glenn R. Gibson, Ph.D., head of the microbiology department at the Institute of Food Research in Reading, Great Britain, and co-author of two of the new studies.

To understand the selective feeding strategy, you first have to know who's on your side and what they have to offer. Of the thousands of strains of bacteria, two are standouts: *Bifidobac-*

terium bifidum and *Lactobacillus acidophilus.*

Smoother digestion. When our bodies can't break down a key ingredient in milk, called lactose, bad bacteria break it down into gas and short-chain fatty acids. We burp, we bloat and we pass gas as our bodies try to cope with these acids. But *L. acidophilus* consumes lactose with no unwanted by-products. "No doubt about it, *L. acidophilus* is a definite benefit for those who are lactose-intolerant," says William Sandine, Ph.D., professor of microbiology at Oregon State University in Corvallis. Both *B. bifidum* and *L. acidophilus* have also been shown to alter the transit time of fecal matter so that it doesn't travel too slowly (constipation) or too quickly (diarrhea). It's also thought that the good bacteria consume some chemicals that can cause both gas and bad breath.

Increased natural immunity. In the dog-eat-dog world of your colon, both *L. acidophilus* and *B. bifidum* have had to develop some pretty tough defenses against their competitors to survive. And, since their enemies are *your* enemies, researchers have dubbed the weapons produced for this chemical warfare "natural antibiotics." *L. acidophilus* can make four—acidolin, acidophillin, lactobacillin and lactocidin—all of which have been shown to take down bacteria that will hurt you, while leaving other, beneficial bacteria intact.

The result of this antibiotic action is a heightened immunity. One Italian study has found that older people who downed *L. acidophilus* and *B. bifidum* capsules four times a day experienced a boost in immunity as evidenced by more immune "fighter" cells and less intestinal inflammation.

Food-poisoning protection. Ever wonder why some come down with food poisoning after eating food contaminated with *Escherichia coli* and salmonella and some don't? One factor may be the presence of actively beneficial bacteria.

L. acidophilus has been shown to usher both *E. coli* and salmonella harmlessly out of the body. "They work by so tightly colonizing the intestinal wall that these poisonous bacteria can't settle in and are swept out with the fecal matter," explains Natasha Trenev, co-author of *Probiotics*.

Improved sexual health. One creature that you, your penis and your prostate can definitely get too much of is *Candida albicans*. When this yeast becomes overgrown, it can convert into a form that can, in turn, penetrate your gut and seep into your blood. Once free in your bloodstream (a condition called candidiasis), *C. albicans* can travel to your skin and nails, leaving you more vulnerable to penile yeast infections, rectal itch, jock itch and prostatitis.

In one study, researchers speculate that men may have contracted prostatitis from sexual contact with women who had a *C. albicans*–caused vaginal infection. Another suggests that *C. albicans* alone can create serious prostate infections.

How does *C. albicans* take over? Although a high-sugar diet and regular use of lubricants that contain the spermicide nonoxynol-9 are thought to create conditions conducive to yeast proliferation, a significant factor is likely a lack of beneficial bacteria.

Japanese researchers have shown that, in people receiving drug therapy for leukemia, treatment with *B. bifidum* reduced candida counts from 100,000,000 per gram to 10,000 per gram. *L. acidophilus* has been shown to stop *C. albicans*'s growth in a test tube, and oral administration has been used successfully to halt candidiasis. Researchers speculate that by maintaining healthy levels of beneficial bacteria in the first place, a man may ward off the whole spectrum of yeast-related sexual infections.

Ulcer healing. Two strains of bifidobacteria can help prevent ulcers from forming and repair damage if they do, according to a recent study out of Japan. "The evidence is mounting: Some strains of *L. acidophilus* and *B. bifidum* will inhibit *Helicobacter pylori*, the bacterium shown to cause ulcers," says Trenev.

Cancer prevention. Luckily for us, some beneficial bacteria have a good appetite for carcinogens. When colon cancer patients were fed *L. acidophilus*–fermented milk, levels of two possible cancer risk makers were dramatically decreased. The results were compelling enough to cause the Swedish researchers to speculate that "certain strains of lactobacilli might lower colon cancer risk."

Increased levels of heart-helping vitamins. Low levels of vitamin B_6 may be as significant a risk factor for heart disease as smoking or high cholesterol, according to a recent study. Other studies have shown that 80 percent of men are deficient in another proven B-vitamin heart-helper, folic acid. Some researchers have wondered why men who consume the same B vitamins absorb different amounts. The presence of beneficial bacteria in the gut may be the answer: Not only do they increase absorption of the entire B-vitamin family, they actually produce their own folic acid and vitamin B_6 as a by-product. Lucky us.

Toxin flushing. By chomping down the by-products of man's metabolism, beneficial bacteria lighten the load on the filtration organs, possibly preventing kidney and liver disease. Ongoing research with kidney dialysis patients has shown that *L. acidophilus* can inhibit undesirable bacteria that dialysis may often encourage. Research on men with liver disease has shown that *B. bifidum* is good at sopping up unwanted by-products, making less work for the liver and allowing the organ to heal itself.

Attracting the Good Guys

How do you tip the balance toward the good guys and away from the bad? Diet, diet and diet. Here are two strategies.

Choose bacteria-laden food. Any food that's fermented, by definition, contains bacteria or yeast as an agent. Some fermented foods, like yogurt, pack in lots of beneficial bacteria, while other foods, such as beer, bread and some cheese, boast a fair amount of yeast. To favor beneficial bacteria, opt for foods that contain their kin.

Yogurt. The king of bacterially fermented food, yogurt is a great source of two transient bacteria, *Lactobacillus bulgaricus* and *Streptococcus thermophilus*. These guys are just passing through—they stake no colon-tissue claim—but the by-products of their interaction with milk can feed *L. acidophilus* and *B. bifidum* and ease digestion.

For best results, stick with yogurt that advertises "live cultures" on the label. The claim isn't a guarantee—the cultures can always die before you get around to eating the yogurt (even if that's before the sell-by date)—but it's some measure of assurance, especially if you eat it right after you buy it.

If you're curious whether the cultures have survived from the time of manufacture to the time you eat them in your favorite yogurt, try this simple test: Heat some regular milk (don't boil) and add a couple of teaspoons of your yogurt. Leave overnight (or 12 hours) in a warm-water bath. If the milk curdles, you have a live one.

Kefir. This slightly alcoholic (3 percent) milk is a legendary health tonic from Russia. Containing a blend of three transient beneficial bacteria, kefir offers a substantial amount of the B vitamins as well as special stomach soothers. Look for varieties that include torula on their ingredients list. (*Note:* This kefir is illegal in some states.)

Feed the little buggers. To encourage stability in the *L. acidophilus* and *B. bifidum* colonies, opt for foods high in fiber and low in sugar and fat. High sugar consumption favors *C. albicans*

and other pesky yeasts, while high fat can overwhelm the good guys.

There are also a few super pro-beneficial-bacteria foods.

Heated milk. Warm whole or 2% low-fat milk before bed may do more than just help you sleep. On heating for 20 minutes (without boiling), two sugars present in milk form a chemical called lactulose, which has been shown to dramatically increase levels of bifidobacteria in the stools of babies. So powerful is lactulose that doctors prescribe supplements for people with liver disease.

Special sugars. The key to effectively feeding beneficial bacteria is transporting the food past the stomach—and the stomach acid. In other words, you're looking for stuff that you can't digest. Some of the best bacteria foods are those that contain chemicals called fructooligosaccharides (FOS).

Foods high in FOS include bananas, garlic, onions, artichokes, chicory and asparagus. If you're eating six to seven servings of fruits and/or vegetables a day, you should be taking in at least two grams of naturally occurring FOS, a level shown to improve the growth of *B. bifidum*.

The Heart-Helping Big Four

These critical minerals will go a long way toward keeping your heart healthy. Here's what you need—and what you don't.

There are countless numbers of articles, press releases and broadcasts every month on how women need calcium for strong bones. But what you don't hear enough about is how critical a healthy daily dose of calcium is for a man's heart health. "We are seeing a continued deterioration in the adequacy of the male diet in this country in terms of mineral intake," says David A. McCarron, M.D., professor and head of the Division of Nephrology, Hypertension and Clinical Pharmacology at the Oregon Health Sciences University in Portland. "In fact, half of all American men are not getting enough calcium necessary for basic heart health." Calcium, though, is only one of the big-four heart minerals that men may be coming up short on.

Minerals are profoundly interdependent. Working alone, they're ineffective, but working together, they're regular health powerhouses. Nowhere is that more true than in the interaction of the critical heart minerals: calcium, magnesium, potassium and sodium. The key here is balance.

Calcium. So critical is this nutrient for providing maximum blood flow to the heart, by facilitating the ability of blood vessels to relax, that there's a petition before the Food and Drug Administration to approve new labels on foods rich in calcium. Such labels would say essentially what many scientists have concluded: Adequate calcium intake equals lower blood pressure. Not to mention its bone-strengthening power.

Optimal intake: 1,000 milligrams per day (1,500 milligrams if you're over 65).

How to get it: Drink or eat three servings of something like milk, yogurt or a leafy green vegetable daily.

Supplement alternatives: If you're lactose-intolerant or just don't like milk, you can replace one or two of your food servings with a supplement pill. Choose one that lists calcium carbonate as its key ingredient (such as Tums or Os-Cal), and take 500 milligrams spaced throughout the day for maximum absorption.

Magnesium. You might think of calcium and magnesium as the two arms in a wrist-wrestling match. As long as the two are balancing each other, the knot of fists is in the air—your heart is receiving maximum benefit. Too much calcium, and your heart could spasm. Too much magnesium, and your heart has trouble mending.

Optimal intake: 350 milligrams per day.

How to get it: Replace any white bread with wheat bread and white rice with brown rice. More than 80 percent of a grain's magnesium is lost in the milling process. Top magnesium suppliers include all produce, nuts, beans, unmilled grains, tofu, halibut, wheat germ and soybeans.

Supplement alternatives: If you're eating six servings of fruits and vegetables a day and opt for unmilled grains, you're probably getting all the magnesium you need. If not, you're probably falling about 100 milligrams short of the optimal 350. Consider adding a 200-milligram supplement. If you're also taking calcium carbonate, you may want to pair it with magnesium oxide or magnesium hydroxide. If you're taking magnesium alone, opt for magnesium gluconate to avoid possible diarrhea.

Potassium. By helping the transmission of nerve impulses throughout the body, potassium plays a key role in maintaining a regular heart rhythm. High intakes of this versatile mineral have also been shown to reduce the risk of stroke.

Optimal intake: 4,000 milligrams per day.

How to get it: Fresh fruits and vegetables and fish lead the potassium pack. One baked potato (with skin) provides almost 1,000 milligrams. A cup of orange juice, a tomato, half an avocado and a salmon steak all ring in at about 500 milligrams. If you're eating about six servings of fruits and vegetables each day and favor fish and whole grains, you're hitting the optimum level.

Supplement alternatives: Americans average 2,000 milligrams of potassium a day. If you find yourself eating on the run or taking a potassium-depleting diuretic or have a family history of stroke, you may want to add one 99-milligram supplement (any more supplemental potassium than that and you may run the risk of dangerous side effects).

Sodium. Just as magnesium balances calcium, so sodium balances potassium. The correlation is so strong, in fact, that increasing your intake of potassium can lower blood pressure just as much as taking lots of extra sodium can raise it.

Recent research indicates that very low sodium diets can actually increase your risk of having a heart attack as much as fivefold. And low-salt diets are of proven benefit in reducing blood pressure only in the 5 to 10 percent of the population that is "salt-sensitive."

So if you have no kidney problems, are not currently suffering from high blood pressure and haven't been diagnosed as salt-sensitive, you may be better off just following your instincts when it comes to how much sodium to eat, making sure that you keep up a healthy intake of potassium.

Optimal intake: Nobody knows; most doctors definitely recommend taking less than 12 grams per day.

How to get it: Just add salt when you get the urge.

Unheralded Minerals

Although you won't find these nutrients listed on many labels, a daily dose could add years to your life—and life to your years.

There's something deceptive about food labels. Sure, they're helpful when you're watching fat or calories, but when it comes to nutrients, they can deceive you. Judging from the labels, a handful of peanuts or a spoonful of wheat germ doesn't offer much more of a nutritional advantage than, say, a Twinkie. And processed cereals appear to be the king of healthful foods. What's missing? Trace minerals. These are the chemicals that our bodies need in such small amounts that the government doesn't even bother to track them. But, believe us, your body keeps score.

"Trace minerals contribute to everything from keeping your blood pressure in check to boosting your immune system to strengthening your erections," says James Balch, M.D., a urologist in Greenfield, Indiana, and the author of *Prescription for Nutritional Healing.* Here's a list of these top-scoring minor-league minerals and some tips on how to make sure that they go to bat for you.

Chromium. You may have heard this mineral touted as a muscle-building miracle worker. While it's unlikely that daily doses of chromium will turn you into Mr. Olympia, this trace mineral can dramatically improve the way your body processes sugary foods and may help ward off adult-onset diabetes, according to Richard A. Anderson, Ph.D., a scientist with the U.S. Department of Agriculture's Human Nutrition Research Center in Beltsville, Maryland.

How to get it: Dr. Anderson says that the average man should try to get between 50 and 200 micrograms of chromium daily, which is tough to do from diet alone, since it's present in small amounts in oysters, wheat germ, broccoli and bran.

One solution: brewer's yeast. Taking 2½ tablespoons of this a day will provide about 50 micrograms of a form of chromium that is especially easy for the body to absorb. An added bonus is that you'll get a myriad of other nutrients, including calcium, potassium, magnesium, zinc, manganese and selenium.

When to supplement: If you suffer from unpleasant blood-sugar swings, you may want to consider supplementing—just don't take more than 200 micrograms daily. A controversial new study suggests that taking high doses of chromium picolinate (a common supplemental form of chromium) could damage the genetic information in hamster cells, possibly indicating an increase in the risk of cancer for humans.

Copper. This heart superhero helps regulate blood pressure, balance cholesterol levels and keep blood cells healthy and the heart beating steadily. "Because copper is good for the blood and heart, it's also good for keeping erections strong," says Dr. Balch.

Copper has also been shown to boost immunity, so much so that one study suggests that an adequate daily intake could help to protect against HIV and its progression to AIDS.

How to get it: Good food sources include nuts, cherries, shellfish, lobster, crabs, mushrooms, whole-grain cereals and gelatin.

When to supplement: Two things can block copper absorption: (1) taking more than 50 milligrams of supplemental zinc daily and (2) consuming many foods and/or drinks containing high-fructose corn syrup. If you take zinc for a prostate problem or drink lots of soda and/or eat processed foods, you may want to take a copper supplement of 1.5 to 3 milligrams. Just be sure that you take it several hours apart from any supplemental zinc or natural prostate remedies containing zinc.

Molybdenum. Although a man needs only a trace amount of this mineral (as little as 75 micrograms a day), a deficiency can lead to weakened erections, according to Dr. Balch.

How to get it: Beans, peanuts, whole grains, peas and dark green leafy vegetables all provide molybdenum.

When to supplement: Don't. Excess amounts can hinder the absorption of other key minerals. Just be sure to eat a wide variety of unprocessed, whole foods.

Sulfur. "The most overlooked beneficial mineral is sulfur," says Dr. Balch. "Adequate amounts stabilize blood pressure, de-sludge blood and enhance the immune system."

Sulfur also aids in the synthesis of collagen, a key component in keeping skin moist and wrinkle-free.

How to get it: Flavor your food. Garlic, chives, leeks and onions all have significant amounts of sulfur. Additional sources include Brussels sprouts, cabbage, eggs, kale, turnips and wheat germ.

When to supplement: Don't bother with sulfur supplements per se. If you hate onions and garlic, opt for a garlic supplement to get your sulfur. Studies have shown that other chemicals found in garlic help sulfur do its healthful work.

Silicon. Natural levels of this key "vanity" mineral, which is responsible for healthy-looking hair, skin and nails, decrease with age.

How to get it: Beets, bell peppers, soy foods, brown rice and whole grains all offer silicon naturally.

When to supplement: If your diet is lacking in silicon-rich food, you may want to try a silicon supplement, often marketed as a "hair and skin formula." Just be sure you take in less than 100 milligrams per day.

Nipping Melanoma in the Bud

A simple self-exam twice a year could save your life.

New figures show that the incidence of the malignant form of skin cancer, melanoma, is increasing faster than that of any other kind of cancer. According to a survey by the American Academy of Dermatologists, there are 80,000 Americans diagnosed with melanoma, twice the previous government estimates, making it the fifth most common cancer.

And while both men and women develop melanoma in equal numbers, men account for almost 70 percent of the deaths from the disease. "As a rule, men have tended to ignore their precancerous lesions for longer periods of time," explains Rex Amonette, M.D., president of the American Academy of Dermatologists. But it doesn't have to be that way. Here's your complete guide to stopping skin cancer in its tracks.

Take a look at yourself. Since the cells that form melanoma are the same cells in moles, it's critical to take stock of all the moles on your body twice a year. Make a point to set aside 20 minutes twice a year, preferably with your spouse, to examine each mole.

Count 'em up. First, count the number of moles on your body. Use a hand mirror in conjunction with a full-length mirror to see the ones on your back. If you count more than 20, be aware that your risk of developing melanoma is increased.

Use the ABCD rule. To tell whether a mole may be turning cancerous, apply the following criteria.

- Asymmetry. Look for any differences between one side and another. Is one edge ragged? Healthy moles are usually perfectly round.
- Border. Examine the edges of the mole closely. Melanomas may have one border area that looks different from the others.
- Color. Normal moles often range in color from light to medium brown; melanomas are often closer to black.
- Diameter. A mole larger than six millimeters across, roughly the size of a pencil eraser, is more likely to be cancerous.

If any of your moles exhibit any of the ABCD symptoms, schedule an appointment with your dermatologist. If he thinks it's at all suspect, he can remove the entire lesion—and maybe stop a case of melanoma before it starts.

The Magic of Garlic

Boosting your heart's health and warding off prostate cancer are just two of the many health benefits garlic can bring— you just have to put up with the smell.

For years researchers have believed that garlic contains one or two healthy compounds, but new research reveals that that number may actually run in the hundreds.

Nature designed the garlic clove as a healthy time bomb: When sitting on a grocery-store shelf, garlic is odorless, its chemicals held in different components of the clove. But as soon as garlic is crushed, bruised or chopped, these chemicals powerfully combine to form a substance called allicin, which gives garlic its characteristic scent. Allicin, in turn, quickly breaks down to a whole host of separate compounds that have been linked to everything from preventing blood clots to lowering cholesterol to slowing down prostate cancer growth. The trouble is that these reactive-sulfur compounds, exactly what make garlic so good for us, are also responsible for the notorious odor.

That's bad news for the garlic supplements, recently touted as an odor-free alternative, that have been cropping up on the shelves of supermarkets throughout the country. Although sales have recently topped $10 million a year, garlic supplements can't match the whole clove when it comes to these newly discovered health benefits, according to Eric Block, Ph.D., professor of chemistry at the State University of New York at Albany. "The principal health contributors to garlic are components of sulfur and, to a lesser extent, selenium—both of which smell pretty bad."

And the more compounds scientists uncover, the more health benefits are being laid at garlic's door, with reduction of high cholesterol levels being the most clearly proven. Not only does garlic cause excretion of dietary cholesterol, but it also may actually shut off the production of LDL (low-density lipoprotein, or "bad") cholesterol in the liver, according to Stephen Warshafsky, M.D., assistant professor of medicine at New York Medical College in Valhalla. In a roundup of the best garlic studies to date, Dr. Warshafsky and his colleagues concluded that eating one clove of garlic a day for several months can lower total cholesterol an estimated 23 milligrams per deciliter (a significant 9 percent).

Another heart-healthy side effect of garlic munching is the kind of blood thinning that can ward off such serious conditions as hardening of the arteries, heart disease and stroke. The allicin in garlic can transform itself into a compound that actually prevents the platelets in the blood from clumping. Called ajoene (named after the Spanish word for garlic, *ajo*), this compound may be as potent as aspirin in preventing the formation of blood clots—and a lot more palatable. Once again, the components at work contain sulfur, which is what's mainly responsible for the odor of garlic, says Dr. Block.

What's more, certain chemicals in garlic can actually slow the growth of prostate cancer cells—at least in a test tube—according to promising new findings. Garlic's cancer-inhibiting effects are currently being tried in mice that are genetically adapted to accept human prostate cancer cells.

"Even though we are only in the early observational stages of the study, the mice that were given garlic show less deterioration and more activity. They seem to eat better, too," says John Thomas Pinto, Ph.D., associate professor of biochemistry in medicine at Cornell University Medical College and director of the Nutritional Research Laboratory at Memorial Sloan-Kettering Cancer Center in New York City. "This is very encouraging."

Not only do chemicals in garlic promise to slow the growth of existing prostate cancer; they also may prevent the cancer from beginning, or "initiating," in the first place. Like beta-carotene and vitamins C and E, garlic compounds have recently been identified as antioxidants, scavengers of unstable molecules, called free radicals, that can oxidize cells and damage your body, much as rust ruins metal. Garlic derivatives can help to round up free radicals and carry them out of the body before they can ever start a prostate tumor from forming, says Dr. Pinto.

All of this research points to the wisdom of including garlic as one component of a healthy diet. The scientists we spoke with emphasized that garlic's health benefits can be maintained by eating as little as one clove of garlic a day and cautioned that you can always have too much of a good thing. Excess garlic, either whole or in the form of supplements, can cause heartburn, indigestion and irritation of the entire gastrointestinal tract. Each person has a different tolerance level, so build up your garlic consumption slowly.

And don't even think about taking megadoses of garlic supplements. Excessive amounts of raw garlic can cause damage to antioxidant molecules that occur naturally in our bodies. "There are compounds in raw garlic that are pro-oxidants, too, so you don't want to poison yourself with large amounts of garlic," warns Dr. Pinto. Garlic in large quantities, either raw or in supplement form, may also interfere with the dosage of certain medications, so speak with your pharmacist or physician before downing more than a couple of cloves a day.

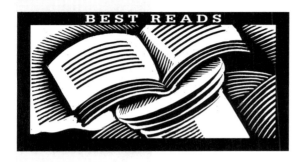

Aging: It's a State of Mind

What are the secrets of long life? Ask Doug Dollemore and Mark Giuliucci and they'll tell you a strong mind. In Age Erasers for Men: Hundreds of Fast and Easy Ways to Beat the Years *(Rodale Press, 1994), they detail the attitudes and approaches that can extend a man's life far beyond his expectations. At the end of this adaptation, there is a quiz to help you get a clearer idea of what your life expectancy is.*

Forget about the birthday candles on your cake or gray hairs on your head. Age isn't a number, say researchers. It's an attitude. Some guys are barely past puberty and already worried about midlife crisis. Other men are pushing 75—and feeling great.

"It's absolutely true that you're as young as you think," says Ben Douglas, Ph.D., professor of anatomy at the University of Mississippi Medical Center in Jackson and author of *AgeLess: Living Younger Longer.* "By having the right attitude, not only will you live longer, but you'll remain younger longer."

He ought to know. Part of his job is to research why some old people remain young in heart, mind and body despite reaching ages usually achieved only by tortoises. And after studying scores of centenarians—including one man who was still enjoying a vibrant and disease-free life at age 110—he concludes that there's no reason why we all can't live through that triple fig-

ure . . . as long as the healthiest part of you is between your ears.

"Regardless of race, religion, socioeconomic background, even their diet, in my research the people who age the best all seem to share similar characteristics," says Dr. Douglas. "They all have a good sense of humor; they don't take life too seriously. They tend to be active, having worked hard every day of their lives. And they also tend to be forward-looking people. Rather than looking back at what they've done or didn't do, they focus on what's ahead, whether it's the election or a baseball game or seeing their grandchildren."

Those findings seem to go along with what other scientists have been saying: How you think about aging may be the most crucial point in how you age.

Improving with Age

That's not to say that you can smoke like a chimney, drink like a fish, eat like a pig and just psych your sofa-slugging self into being the George Burns of your block. You have to practice a healthy lifestyle to avoid most of the conditions that cause us to look and feel old. But even so, why is it that some guys follow the rules and still get old while others age slower than Dick Clark?

It may be a matter of self-perception. "People who live long and healthy lives have a purpose in life; they have a reason to get out of bed each morning," says Walter Bortz, M.D., clinical associate professor of medicine at Stanford University and author of *We Live Too Short and Die Too Long.* "My friend George Sheehan (the late *Runner's World* columnist), used to say, 'Make yourself indispensable.' My granddad used to say, 'Make yourself necessary.' People who live long and productive lives don't feel old because they make themselves necessary."

And so should you.

A good first step is to realize that getting older, while having its drawbacks, also has certain advantages—beyond looking "distinguished" as you gray. So before checking out the sticker prices of red convertibles, keep a few things in mind about middle age and beyond.

Emotionally, you're at your most stable—or you should be. Maybe you can't bench-press as much as some pimply faced teen at the gym, but does your wife or sweetheart care? Maybe your hair is thinning or you need bifocals, but will your kids love you any less because of it? With all due respect to your fraternity brothers, your current support group is probably more loving and understanding than what you got in those bulla-bulla days, and hey, at least you don't have to arm-wrestle for the last beer. Plus, with each passing year comes the added maturity to see things more rationally and with the experience lacking in someone 10 or 20 years younger.

Financially, you're at the prime of your career and earning potential. No longer green and still not ready to be sent to greener pastures, your worth on the job skyrockets and promotions come more readily than they did a decade ago. After all, you're taken more seriously now. And as a result, you're able to buy those finer things in life: a nice car, a nice house or apartment, even bookshelves that don't involve concrete blocks.

And intellectually, you've never been more capable. In fact, practical problem-solving ability peaks during your forties, according to research at the University of Wisconsin. (Yes, it's even greater than in your teens, twenties or thirties.) So even though brain cells are dying, experience and practical common sense—the stuff that only comes with age—more than make up the difference. This seems to hold true well past the middle years.

Case in point: Researchers at the University of Southern California and the University of Missouri timed a group of typists ranging from college age to well into their sixties. They expect-

ed a blowout by the younger folks, since their fingers are more nimble and their reaction times are faster. But everyone typed an average of 60 words per minute. The older typists, it seemed, achieved their speed with cunning: They read ahead in the text and typed smarter, saving a millisecond here and a nanosecond there.

See the Glass Half-Full

There are other studies, all of which prove the same point. Maybe you've lost something in certain aspects, but you've gained so much more in others. And once you realize this and can see your future through optimistic eyes, you'll minimize your chances of feeling old. Not only will optimism help you be a little happier with the inevitable, it may also actually help you live longer.

Another case in point: According to a study at Brown University in Providence, Rhode Island, blaming your aches and pains on age itself, rather than on the actual cause—like playing basketball for too long or the fact that you caught a virus—may make you die sooner. Researchers surveyed nearly 1,400 people over age 70 who were experiencing health problems. Those who blamed their ailing health on "old age" had a 78 percent greater risk of dying in the near future than those who cited a specific, non-aging reason. "Once you say a problem is due to old age . . . you've given up, in a way," explains William Rakowski, Ph.D., assistant professor of medical science at the Center for Gerontology and Health Care Research at Brown University.

Of course, optimists are made, not born. "The right attitude needs to be cultivated," says Dr. Douglas. "It's done so in realizing that the world doesn't come to an end if your team doesn't win the pennant or if the Republicans or Democrats don't get into the White House. It's going out and running the best race you can run."

And that's something to keep in mind as you

are about to run the most challenging laps of your life.

"There are obvious things you can do to look and feel younger and live longer: Don't smoke. Exercise regularly. Eat a good diet and use alcohol in moderation. But most people know about that," adds Huber Warner, Ph.D., deputy associate director of the Biology of Aging Program at the National Institute on Aging in Bethesda, Maryland. "To me, one secret to aging well is the ability to come to grips with a decline in physical function that is real but still being able to use what you have to maintain function as well as possible. Maybe you'll never be a champion pole vaulter, but realize that even though you may be older, you can still do a lot of things—and still do them well."

How Many More Years Do You Have?

The long and the short of longevity is this: You're born with a genetic wiring diagram imprinted on your cells, and that affects your life span. But beyond that, it's really up to you. To get a clearer idea of what your life expectancy may be, try the following quiz. It's based on the work of experts on aging, primarily Robert F. Allen, Ph.D., author of *Lifegain*. Keep a running tally of your score as you answer the following questions.

1. Did your grandparents live to be at least 80? (+1 for each instance) _____
2. Did your mother or father live that long? (+3 for each) _____
3. Did your mother or father die of a heart attack or stroke before age 50? (−4 for each) _____
4. Do any immediate family members (parent, sibling, grandparent) have now or did have cancer, a heart condition or diabetes since childhood? (−3 for each) _____

5. Did any die of the above problems before age 60? (−2 for each) _____
6. Did any immediate family member die of prostate cancer, colon cancer or any other natural cause before age 60? (−1 for each) _____
7. Do you exercise aerobically for at least 30 minutes three or more times a week? (+2) _____
8. Do you play sports or do light physical activities like yard work once or twice a week? (+1) _____
9. Do you almost never exercise? (−2) _____
10. Do you get five or more helpings of fruits and vegetables daily? (+5) _____
11. Do you eat a lot of high-fat foods but rarely, if ever, eat fruits and vegetables? (−4) _____
12. Do you eat a lot of high-fat foods but try to balance these with plenty of fruits and vegetables? (+1) _____
13. Has your total cholesterol always been 200 or less? (+4) _____
14. Is your total cholesterol now 200 or less but once was between 240 and 299? (+3) _____
15. Is your total cholesterol now 200 or less but once was 300 or more? (+2) _____
16. Is your total cholesterol now between 240 and 299? (−1) _____
17. Is your total cholesterol now above 300? (−2) _____

Questions 18 to 22 all pertain to your diastolic blood pressure (the 80 in a reading of 120/80), considered the more important number.

18. Has your diastolic pressure always been 88 or lower? (+3) _____
19. Is it 88 or lower but once was 90 or higher? (+2) _____

20. Is it 88 or lower but once was 105 or higher? (+1) _____
21. Is it 90 to 104? (−1) _____
22. Is it above 104? (−2) _____
23. Did you ever smoke? (If no, +2) _____
24. Did you quit five or more years ago? (+1) _____
25. Do you smoke less than a pack a day? (−1) _____
26. Do you smoke one-half to one pack a day? (−2) _____
27. Do you smoke one to two packs a day? (−6) _____
28. Do you smoke more than two packs a day? (−10) _____
29. Do you smoke marijuana once a week or more? (−1) _____
30. Is the best description of you easy-going and relaxed? (+3) _____
31. Is the best description of you aggressive or easily angered? (−3) _____
32. Do you have a demanding job with little say over how things get done? (−2) _____
33. Do you have four or more years of college? (+3) _____
34. Do you have one to three years of college? (+2) _____
35. Do you have a high school education only? (+1) _____
36. Have you always been within 5 percent of your ideal weight? (+2) _____
37. Are you currently within 5 percent of your ideal weight, but were once more than 30 percent over? (+1) _____
38. Have you always been from 5 to 30 percent overweight? (−1) _____
39. Has your weight fluctuated by more than ten pounds several times since high school? (−2) _____
40. Have you always been more than 30 percent overweight? (−4) _____

41. Do you drink moderately (no more than two beers, two glasses of wine or two shots of whiskey a day on average), but not to the point of drunkenness? (+2) _____
42. Do you abstain totally from alcohol? (+1) _____
43. Do you regularly drink until intoxicated? (−6) _____
44. Do you have an annual physical exam? (+1) _____
45. Do you have a proctological exam every other year after age 40? (+2) _____

How to Score

Begin with 72 (the average life expectancy for men). Adjust for your current age (add one point if you've passed the age of 30; two if you've passed 40 and so forth). Total your score from the questions above. Then add it all up.

   72 Average life expectancy
+ ___ Age adjustment
+ ___ Score from questions above
= ___ Total (estimated life expectancy)

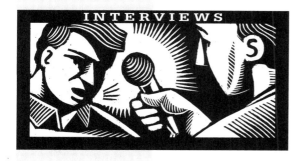

Robert Carney on
The Mind-Disease Connection

You know the mantra: Cut your risk of disease by eating healthy foods, throwing out the cigarettes, getting exercise. But current research suggests that saying good-bye to stress and depression can also play a big role in disease-proofing your body. These mental states increase your risk of heart disease, heart attack and stroke.

To find out how your state of mind can affect your body's well-being, we talked with Robert Carney, Ph.D., professor of medical psychology at Washington University in St. Louis.

Does depression put you at risk for disease?

Yes. It's a significant risk factor for mortality and complications in cardiac patients. That's very well documented. We know that people who've recently had a heart attack and become depressed are about four times more likely to die than people who aren't depressed, regardless of other risk factors such as diabetes or high blood pressure. Actually, depression may be a bigger risk factor for these people than smoking.

But we're also finding some evidence that depression may place you at risk for heart disease in the first place. Depression predates heart disease in many patients.

Of course, it's possible that what we're seeing is how depression affects other areas of a person's lifestyle. If you're depressed, you're more likely to smoke, you may not do what your doctor tells you, you may not eat the right foods and you may not exercise. All these behaviors add to your risk.

But we think that other factors are at work. There's an association between depression and increased autonomic nervous system activity. The autonomic nervous system controls the rate of heartbeat and heart rhythm. We know from studies that people who are depressed have higher levels of sympathetic activity. Their hearts tend to beat faster. If they have heart disease, they're more prone to arrhythmias and complications. We think that's the most important reason for the higher mortality in heart patients who are depressed. And increased sympathetic activity even could have a negative effect on the heart of someone who seems healthy. It could contribute to higher blood pressure and other problems that increase the risk of heart disease, heart attack and stroke.

What about stress?

It's not as significant a factor as depression, but it may contribute to increased cholesterol and hypertension. Plus, a lot of people under stress eat more, don't exercise and eat what they're not supposed to. So you get even more risk of high blood pressure and other cardiovascular problems.

You're more likely to see blood pressure and cholesterol rise due to stress if you're what we call a hot reactor.

This type of person reacts strongly to stress. Researchers use a variety of tests to determine a person's cardiovascular response to stress. Complicated math tests often produce an increase in blood pressure. Having a person role-play an uncomfortable experience can also increase blood pressure.

The rise in blood pressure that these types of stress tests produce is transitory, but we've found that people who react strongly to stress when they're young are more likely to develop hypertension when they approach middle age. So it looks like what starts out as a transitory response to stress becomes the normal condition.

We also suspect—although we need to do more work on this—that cholesterol and triglyceride levels also go up when you're stressed. It's possible that, like high blood pressure, this momentary rise becomes your normal condition as you get older. So, taken together, if you're a "hot reactor" and react physically to stress, you end up with a higher risk of having high blood pressure and high cholesterol, major risk factors for heart disease, heart attack and stroke.

We used to think that type A personalities were the most vulnerable to heart-health problems. Current research doesn't really support the type A theory. Depression is certainly a much more important factor.

So what can you do about depression and stress?

Early identification of depression is key. A lot of the time, this risk factor isn't identified. Symptoms that really indicate depression are often attributed to an illness or go unnoticed. For instance, if you have a chronic illness, everyone seems to think that depression is normal, but that's not the case. In reality, only 20 to 25 percent of people become depressed over chronic illness, so depression clearly isn't a "normal" reaction.

As for practical things you can do: Well, we know that people who exercise and adhere to a healthy diet are less likely to be depressed. So if you can get back on track with the rest of your life, your depression may also be reduced. But that's easier said than done.

It helps many people, especially those who've had an illness or injury, to remember that depression isn't a permanent state. The depression is often tied to that one event. It can go away. It's also important to know that it can happen to anyone—people may be fine for weeks, months or even years. Then, perhaps during a stressful time, they have a depressive episode. You don't have to live out the rest of your life in a depressed state.

How can you spot depression?

Depressed mood, loss of interest in things that normally you find interesting, problems concentrating, sleeping problems, loss of appetite. You may feel less hungry and lose five pounds or more. You may feel hopeless, helpless, cry for reasons you can't explain. It tends to last for a period of time, usually two weeks or more. That may be clinical depression, as opposed to feeling low, which may last for a couple of days and usually has fewer symptoms.

What can you do about it?

Often depression, especially if it's in response to a medical problem or something specific in your life, doesn't require extensive intervention. Unfortunately, we really don't understand the process involved in depression. Many people get over depression on their own. But we do know that emotional support speeds recovery. Sometimes just knowing that you're depressed and getting emotional support from friends and family can be enough to help you recover. But you need to talk with your doctor. We find that there are times when short-term intervention is required. In that case, you may need psychotherapy and/or antidepressants. It'll be faster and easier to treat depression if you get help early. If you get depressed and don't seek treatment for several months, treatment may take longer and may be less successful.

There's a lot you can do to help minimize depression. Work on feeling secure in relationships. People who are isolated are more likely to be depressed and stay depressed longer.

And put the rest of your life in order. If you're depressed, you don't feel very motivated.

Try to focus on simple tasks and goals, since you probably don't feel in control. For example, if you smoke and have tried repeatedly to stop, there's not much point in trying again when you're depressed—you'll be more likely to end up with one more failure to add to your list of things gone wrong. Instead, work toward a more achievable goal. If you smoke 30 cigarettes a day, work on cutting down to 25. That way, you can feel that you're making progress toward your ultimate goal and you're meeting concrete goals along the way.

Make lists of daily tasks so that you can check them off when you're done. (Keep the lists fairly short. If you make a long list and get to only a few of the items on it, this could backfire and make you feel like you haven't accomplished anything.) This also helps if you're depressed because you probably have trouble with memory and concentration.

Make a list of reasons for living. When you're depressed, you may feel that life has no meaning. For instance, an older person recovering from a heart attack may write down things like "I can still enjoy my grandchildren" or "my wife and I play cards." The point is to figure out the things that you enjoy and can do. When you feel really low, pull out your written list and read it. Basically, it contradicts the idea that life is over or meaningless, a feeling common to people with depression.

Bear in mind that you are depressed, you're not coping very well but you can get better. Reminding yourself of this helps you focus on depression as a short-term problem.

Don't be overwhelmed—small steps, small goals are most important in helping you recover.

About stress? A popular technique is to learn how to step back and analyze a situation. Is it worth the stress? For instance, if you're a hot reactor and you get cut off in traffic, ask yourself, "Is it worth getting upset about?" Is it worth letting your blood pressure shoot up? Does it really make any difference? Will the other driver get to his destination any faster than you will?

Pay attention to what really bothers you and what causes stress and try to eliminate those things from your life. Make sure that you have time to relax.

Harinder Garewal on
Understanding Antioxidants

A lot of scientists believe that free radicals are the culprits that help diseases get off the ground. These little molecules generally wouldn't be a problem, except that they're lacking one of their two electrons. Since electrons tend to pair up, the shortage makes them highly unstable. They're always looking for another substance to interact with so that they can get that extra electron. Their search wreaks havoc on the body. Free radicals can help set the stage for heart disease, heart attacks and strokes. They can damage your DNA, making your cells more susceptible to cancer.

The solution? Antioxidants. These molecules provide the missing electron. They stop free radicals in their tracks. Your body makes its own supply, plus you get them in healthy foods or supplements.

To find out how antioxidants can help disease-proof your body, we talked to an expert in the growing field of antioxidant research, Harinder Garewal, M.D., Ph.D., assistant director of cancer prevention and control at the Department of Veterans Affairs Hospital and a cancer specialist at the University of Arizona Cancer Center in Tucson.

How do free radicals do so much damage?

There are a number of possible chemical reactions that can occur. Not all are necessarily harmful, but several probably are. For example, they can oxidize certain fats in the bloodstream, changing their chemical structure. Through a variety of mechanisms, oxidized fats are attracted to your artery walls, where they attach and cause cells to proliferate. (Unoxidized fats are much less of a problem.) This eventually leads to a thickening of the artery walls. You end up with narrowed arteries and an increased risk of heart disease, heart attack and stroke. Other chemical reactions involving free radicals result in DNA damage that can help cancers develop.

What role do antioxidants play?

They are part of the body's defense against free radicals. For example, they interact with the free radicals, so that the fats in the bloodstream are protected from oxidation. Oxidative free-radical damage is very likely involved in many disease processes. The connection between staying healthy and consuming foods rich in certain antioxidants is very strong, although more research needs to be done in identifying precisely what individual agents are more important than others.

One problem is that just about anything that interacts with oxygen or oxidized free radicals can be called an antioxidant. So the term is not very precise. A lot of products that are claimed to be antioxidants are, in the technical sense, but they may have no role in disease prevention. Examples of antioxidants that are probably important and are being studied are vitamin E, vitamin C, selenium and a group of substances called carotenoids, one of which is beta-carotene.

We're also finding that these antioxidants often work together—vitamin C, for instance, is important in helping vitamin E stay effective.

What happens is that when vitamin E interacts with a free radical, it gets oxidized and loses its antioxidant capabilities. If the transformed vitamin E then interacts with vitamin C, vitamin E reverts to its original form. Vitamin C then becomes oxidized, but it's restored by enzymes in the body as well. Therefore, intake of several different antioxidants may be more effective in the prevention of oxidative damage and disease than trying to consume very high doses of a single compound.

Is there any way to avoid taking in free radicals in the first place?

They're produced as part of the body's metabolism. Plus, they're in pollutants, cigarette smoke and all kinds of things you encounter every day. Furthermore, oxygen and oxidation are not all bad. In fact, they are essential for life. It is the damaging oxidative reactions that need to be countered. Thus, one can't avoid free radicals, but the goal would be to neutralize the harmful ones, perhaps by consuming adequate amounts of antioxidants.

How do you know if you're getting enough antioxidants?

That's hard to say. Researchers have been looking at large populations, their diet and their risk of disease. Most such studies have simply looked at the relationship between intake and disease. More recently, we have begun to think in terms of blood and tissue levels of these agents. Researchers are trying to define levels below which there is an increased risk of disease and above which there is no added benefit and perhaps even harm.

In Western populations, some of the most interesting results are with vitamin E and its effects on heart disease. Increasing vitamin E by dietary changes is very difficult because it is present in fatty foods whose intake may be associated with problems of its own. If ongoing trials turn out to be as positive as the study of populations has been, supplemental intake of vitamin E might well be of great benefit.

This is actually a very difficult area for researchers. There's no practical way of doing a perfect trial for disease prevention, especially with readily available, nontoxic agents such as these. In contrast, you can test the effectiveness of antibiotics, for instance, just by administering them to reasonably small numbers of sick people and looking at how they respond to treatment. However, when you're trying to evaluate how disease is prevented, you just have to pick a population, which must be representative of the target population, and wait for the disease to show up. And then try to show that the agent you are testing is associated with a reduction in disease. And often the study that you do has problems resulting from compromises made in its design.

For instance, a study of beta-carotene in Finland showed higher rates of lung cancer among people who took supplements. But the study focused on heavy smokers, the average cigarette use being over 20 cigarettes a day for more than 30 years. Clearly, this is small minority of the general population. Furthermore, the follow-up of almost 5 to 6 years is too short. Remember that the positive population studies are based on decades of dietary and intake habits.

As you can see, the data we have on antioxidants are not perfect. This is because perfect studies are practically impossible to complete successfully. It is easy to say that "randomized, blinded, placebo-controlled trials in the right population"—that is, perfectly designed trials—are needed. Ideal trials are easily designed on paper, but doing them is a different matter.

In several formal and informal surveys, about 40 to 60 percent of physicians, including cardiologists, either take antioxidants like vitamin E or recommend them to patients and relatives at risk for heart disease.

How can an individual tell if he's getting enough antioxidant protection through his diet?

If you eat the recommended five to nine servings of fruits and vegetables per day, you are probably getting enough of the most important antioxidants. However, daily compliance with this regimen has been very poor in our population.

What antioxidant supplements do you recommend for prevention, and in what doses?

Let me back up a bit to emphasize that supplements aren't substitutes for things like smoking cessation, a healthy diet and regular exercise. And it would probably never be a good idea to take massive doses of any supplement. Supplementation must be viewed as an addition to other healthy lifestyle activities.

This field is rapidly evolving. One of the most exciting antioxidants in our population is vitamin E, with its potential for preventing heart disease, among other possible benefits. As mentioned earlier, given its nature and the foods where it is found, increasing vitamin E by dietary changes is very difficult.

As we cut fat from our diets, which is good, we also reduce intake of several sources of vitamin E. Most people's levels aren't so low that we can call them deficient in the classical sense, but if 150 IU or greater is needed daily for disease prevention, they're much too low to receive the benefits of disease prevention. You have to take a supplement to reach such intake levels. Clinical trials using vitamin E generally use 400 to 800 IU per day. From a side effect standpoint, there is really no reason to be concerned with these doses—there are no major side effects, nor problems with significant toxicity.

Because it's fat-soluble, your body stores vitamin E in fatty tissues located all through your body. Once you have taken supplements for a few weeks, if you forget to take it one day, there's no reason to panic—your blood levels will stay high enough for a few days as the vitamin stores in your body provide the needed amount. Similarly, beta-carotene also stays in body stores.

As there is unlikely to be a single, perfectly designed trial to prove conclusively whether vitamin E or the other antioxidants prevent disease, for reasons I discussed earlier, the decision to use one or more of these must be made by balancing all the evidence for or against a benefit versus the risk of side effects or other harm. Clearly, research needs to continue, and I strongly urge people to participate in studies if they can. However, in the absence of that option, I would personally recommend vitamin E, particularly if there is a history of increased risk of heart disease. I would also urge discussing this with your physician to be absolutely sure that there are no problems to be expected with its use.

What about the other antioxidants, particularly water-soluble ones?

The situation is different for water-soluble vitamins, like vitamin C. These are promptly excreted in the urine, thereby requiring frequent intake to maintain blood levels. Thus, dosing three or four times a day has been suggested.

How much should you take?

The most convincing studies for disease prevention looked at proper dietary intake with five or more servings of fruits and vegetables daily. This would be my first recommendation. Beyond this, and especially if doing this regularly is a problem, one can consider supplementation. A well-balanced multivitamin is not unreasonable, but avoid unnecessary extra iron intake.

If you wish to take antioxidant supplements, then reasonable doses for beta-carotene are about 10 to 15 milligrams per day; for vitamin C, 250 milligrams three or four times daily; and vitamin E, 200 to 400 IU per day. A little selenium, especially if you live in areas where selenium is low in the soil, is also reasonable. Once again, I want to emphasize that this is not an alternative to other health-promoting behavior such as exercising and smoking cessation.

How do you pick a quality product?

Among scientists, there is some argument about whether it's better to use the so-called natural or synthetic versions of some antioxidants. A lot of the studies involving beta-carotene, for instance, use pure trans-beta-carotene, which is never found in natural foods as the sole carotene. There are more than 300 types of carotenoids in nature. Beta-carotene or carotenes extracted from a natural source will have these other carotenoids. The debate right now is whether these other carotenoids are just carrier molecules or whether they have additional roles. The rationale for the natural products is that it is the form they have in fruits and vegetables that confers protection. Nevertheless, convincing proof that this is indeed important is lacking.

Synthetic vitamin E (alpha-tocopherol) has been used in many trials that suggest possible beneficial activities. However, some data suggest a role for gamma-tocopherol and other related compounds, which exist in nature and in the natural extract products. In general, the natural extracts are a bit more expensive than the synthetic compounds. If you don't mind the cost, there is probably nothing to lose by using the natural extracts, as they generally contain enough of the synthetic compound. But conclusive proof of benefit of one form over the other does not as yet exist.

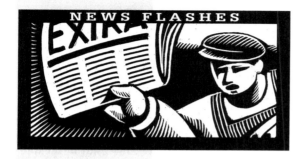

Folic Acid Effective against Heart Disease

DALLAS—Heart disease patients with high levels of a chemical linked to heart disease respond best to an increased intake of folate, a vitamin that is folic acid's natural form found in food. Folate can be found in many fresh vegetables and fruits.

Folic acid has been most widely touted in recent years for its critical role in preventing birth defects when taken by pregnant women. Folate is found in green, leafy vegetables—such as spinach, asparagus, beans and peas—and in many fruits, including apples and oranges. Folic acid is also available in most multivitamin supplements.

Researchers at the University of Utah in Salt Lake City found that in heart disease patients, a low folic acid level goes hand in hand with a high level of homocysteine in the blood. Homocysteine is a chemical that narrows vital arteries that carry blood within the heart and to the brain. Researchers found that men with the highest homocysteine levels were 14 times more likely to have coronary artery disease than those with low to average levels.

Other studies have pointed out how excess homocysteine worsens artery disease: Large amounts appear to be toxic to cells that line the interior of blood vessels and to increase the stickiness of platelets and other clotting factors.

Researchers conclude that raising folic acid levels high enough can reduce homocysteine levels in the blood. Ongoing research focuses on determining optimal folic acid levels. Megadoses probably won't be needed, researchers say. Just adding a reasonable amount of folic acid to your diet can have a positive health impact.

Researchers Find Genetic Cause for Infertility

CAMBRIDGE, Mass.—New research into male genetics suggests that the ability to create healthy sperm is at least partly linked to genes passed on by fathers.

Scientists at the Whitehead Institute for Biomedical Research in Cambridge, Massachusetts, have been exploring the Y chromosome—the piece of DNA that determines what sex a newly fertilized egg will become. Previously, scientists thought this chromosome was mostly devoid of genes. However, the researchers have discovered that this masculine chromosome contains at least a few dozen genes, in addition to the one that enables a developing embryo to become male.

In particular, the researchers have presented evidence that some cases of male infertility result from specific regions being "deleted" within the Y chromosome. This finding suggests that the deleted area contains a gene or genes crucial to the production of healthy sperm, they say.

The new studies add another explanation, besides those of chemical exposure and infections, for why an estimated 3 to 4 percent of men generate no sperm or so few that they are infertile. Just how often a low sperm count can be attributed to deleted areas of the Y chromosome is still unclear, but researchers report that infertility problems, in some cases, can be passed from father to son.

Tomatoes Topple Prostate Cancer Risk

BOSTON—A study of 47,849 men over five years found that those who ate the most cooked tomato products were the ones with the lowest risk of prostate cancer.

Men who had 10 servings a week had a third of the risk that men getting 1½ servings a week had. While more was better in this study conducted at Harvard Medical School, even 4 servings per week was associated with a 22 percent reduction in risk of prostate cancer, researchers said.

Tomatoes are high in lycopene, a chemical found extensively in red and orange vegetables such as carrots and sweet potatoes. Researchers think that lycopene may help prevent cancer by mopping up free radicals, highly reactive molecules in your body that can cause cell damage. The study suggests that lycopene may be twice as potent at ridding the body of free radicals as beta-carotene, one of the most commonly touted free-radical destroyers.

Although eating tomatoes right off the vine is a good way to get lycopene, cooking the tomatoes in a little oil actually increases the lycopene count. During the cooking process, tomato cell walls break down with the heat, and the lycopene gets absorbed into the cooking oil. For protection from prostate cancer, researchers conclude that tomato sauce should be in your diet.

Artificial Flavorings Good for the Heart

HYATTSVILLE, Md.—A new study from the National Center for Health Statistics in Hyattsville, Maryland, suggests that natural-food enthusiasts may be missing something. Artificial flavorings in everything from barbecue potato chips to toothpaste may be good for your health.

Many artificial flavors contain salicylates, chemical cousins of aspirin. Aspirin, of course, is known to reduce heart attack risk by preventing blood clots. Researchers from the National Center for Health Statistics found that many Americans consume the equivalent of one baby aspirin a day from the artificial flavorings put in processed foods. That's about 80 milligrams, the amount of aspirin often recommended as a daily dose to ward off heart attacks.

Americans' growing taste for artificial flavorings may be one reason why fewer people are dying from heart attacks, the researchers noted.

Skin Cancer Protection

HOUSTON—Eating a diet high in fat may promote the development of basal cell and squamous cell carcinomas—the two most common forms of skin cancer in the United States.

In a two-year trial conducted by researchers at the Baylor College of Medicine in Houston, 101 people who had basal cell or squamous cell carcinoma were assigned either to a control group, in which they ate an average of 38 percent of calories from fat, or to a group in which they kept fat intake to 20 percent of calories. Numbers of new skin cancers were assessed at eight-month intervals during the two-year study. During the last eight months, 1 out of 51 people in the low-fat group had a new skin cancer, compared to 8 who developed lesions during the first eight months of the study. Researchers at Baylor also found that people who ate more fat were nearly five times as likely to have one or more premalignant lesions as those on the special diet.

Baylor researchers point out that avoiding sun exposure is still the best way to prevent skin cancer. But it now appears that eating a low-fat diet may be the second line of defense.

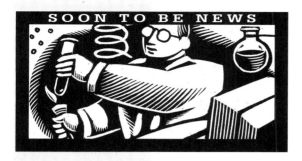

A Drug to Stop Aging?

Scientists have identified a hormone that appears to play some role in the aging process. Studies are beginning to suggest that taking supplements of the chemical—called dehydroepiandrosterone, or DHEA for short—might stall age-related breakdowns of the body.

From youth through early adulthood, the adrenal gland secretes DHEA in steadily rising quantities. But production tapers off as we age. By age 80, people have between 80 and 90 percent less DHEA in their blood than they had at the age of 25.

A team of scientists from the University of California, San Diego, treated 16 people (ages 50 to 65) for six months with either the hormone DHEA or a placebo. The 8 study participants receiving DHEA had a 75 percent increase in their overall well-being, compared to the other volunteers. Although the study was small, team leader Samuel S. C. Yen, M.D., reported that volunteers showed improved ability to cope with stress, greater mobility, improved sleep and less joint pain. Men, in particular, reported increased muscle strength and decreased body-fat mass. Better yet, the doctors didn't see any adverse effects.

The Food and Drug Administration (FDA) has classified DHEA as a dietary supplement and not a drug, so it is available through mail order or over the counter. *Some doctors, though, think that the FDA will look into regulating DHEA if they feel there is potential for abuse.*

A Better Test to Detect the Spread of Prostate Cancer?

A procedure being tested by Cytogen, a Princeton, New Jersey, company, is up to six times more accurate than older tests in detecting cancer cells that have spread from the prostate. By the time prostate cancer is detected, there's a 30 percent chance that tumor cells have traveled to another part of the body. Conventional tests often miss these wandering cells, leaving doctors in the dark about the best treatment course.

The test, called ProstaScint, involves injecting patients with a radioactive particle that seeks out and binds to a molecule found mainly on prostate tumor cells. A gamma camera then scans the torso for the now-radioactive cancer cells.

Although the FDA has yet to approve ProstaScint, it usually follows advisory board recommendations. *Expect the test to be available this year.*

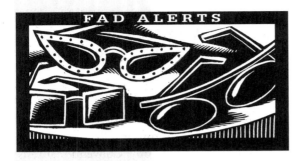

Melatonin

 Melatonin is a chemical that regulates your body's timekeeping. It helps your brain establish the rhythms that keep you up during the day and put you to sleep at night. It also helps keep your body from going off kilter when the days shorten during the winter months, says Ronald R. Watson, Ph.D., professor of research at the Arizona Prevention Center, University of Arizona in Tucson.

People have been taking melatonin supplements for years to fight jet lag and cure occasional insomnia. But these days, it's getting credit for doing a lot more than keeping your body on schedule. People say that it may slow down the aging process. Or work as an antioxidant to protect cells from damage by free radicals, unstable molecules of oxygen that wreak havoc in your system and can help get cancer and heart disease off the ground.

In animal studies, melatonin has helped to control cholesterol and improve the function of the immune system in elderly mice. In the lab, it has protected rats from carcinogens.

But opponents point out that the amount of the hormone that the brain produces to put you to sleep at night is 0.3 milligram. The typical supplement sold in health food stores contains ten times that amount (or more). And no one really knows how high levels of melatonin affect the body.

Few scientific studies have been done on how these high levels of melatonin affect humans, but two completed studies show that it can impair mental functioning and cause headaches.

Plus, melatonin's disease-fighting capabilities just haven't been borne out in human studies. "Melatonin works well as an antioxidant in the test tube, but we still do not know whether it is effective as an antioxidant in the body," says Lawrence J. Machlin, Ph.D., president of Nutritional Research and Information in Livingston, New Jersey.

Also, melatonin is not a regulated drug, so there is no assured quality control in its manufacture and distribution, says Michael D. Myers, M.D., a family physician and obesity specialist in Los Alamitos, California, who frequently treats patients with sleep disorders.

"What are you buying? Are you buying something from a cow's pineal gland? From a pig's brain? Something manufactured synthetically? You really don't know what you're getting. You don't know where it comes from," Dr. Myers notes.

Beta-Carotene

 Beta-carotene's disease-preventing properties have been called into question. Once heralded as the miracle antioxidant, able to protect against all kinds of ailments, beta-carotene recently fell from grace. In a recent major study, researchers from the National Cancer Institute followed 29,133 Finnish men ages 50 to 69 who were long-term smokers. Many also drank more than their fair share. The men who took a high-dose beta-carotene supplement showed an 18 percent increase in lung cancer risk. Overall death rates went up by 8 percent.

Despite the fact that sales have plummeted and a lot of guys have thrown their bottles of beta-carotene out the window, most researchers still believe that lower-dose beta-carotene protects. They point out that, even in that study, the men with the highest blood levels of beta-carotene had lower risks of both cancer and heart disease.

"They did find more lung cancers in smokers. That was actually a big surprise," says Robert Russell, M.D., director of human studies for the U.S. Department of Agriculture in Boston. "We don't know if, in very high amounts, beta-carotene is broken down into products that promote tumors or if beta-carotene at high doses may have interfered with absorption of other beneficial substances in the diet. The people in the study got 30 milligrams of beta-carotene a day, way over the amount that I recommend, which is 5 to 8 milligrams. The high dose made sense at the time because we've seen a relationship between diets and blood levels high in beta-carotene and protection against cancer. It seemed safe, and we thought that if we used more, we might see results faster."

Dr. Russell notes that the next step for researchers is to "take a step backward, take a look at what happened in the Finnish study and try to find out why beta-carotene had a detrimental effect, but only in smokers. We can carry out experiments in cell cultures to examine the interaction between substances in smoke and beta-carotene. We need to know what went on so that the next time a fashionable molecule comes around, we don't jump on the bandwagon. In any case, I suspect that, in the future, the emphasis in research will be much more on diets rather than single nutrients and supplements."

Coenzyme Q$_{10}$

 "Coenzyme Q$_{10}$ is the biggest medical discovery of the twentieth century, bigger than the Salk polio vaccine," says Stephen T. Sinatra, M.D., director of medical education and former chief of cardiology at Manchester Memorial Hospital in Manchester, Connecticut. As an antioxidant, it keeps fats from oxidizing into free radicals that would congregate in the walls of your blood vessels. Some studies suggest that coenzyme Q$_{10}$ may be involved in the first line of defense against oxidation, because it's the first antioxidant to bite the dust in laboratory scrimmages against free radicals. Coenzyme Q$_{10}$ works hand in hand with another antioxidant, vitamin E. It has been shown that coenzyme Q$_{10}$ will help regenerate oxidized vitamin E and keep it active longer.

Coenzyme Q$_{10}$ is present in just about all cells. When the body's healthy, it produces coenzyme Q$_{10}$ from food sources. But when you get older, or if you're sick, your body doesn't make enough. Major deficiencies over time could lead to heart disease, says Dr. Sinatra.

Researchers at the University of Texas Medical Branch in Galveston added coenzyme Q$_{10}$ to the treatment of 424 patients with various kinds of heart disease. They found that 87 percent had an improvement in their heart function. In addition, 43 percent of the patients were able to reduce their other medication. According to Dr. Sinatra, cardiologists who use coenzyme Q$_{10}$ on a regular basis in their practices find that they can reduce their patients' other medications usually up to 50 percent of the time.

Coenzyme Q$_{10}$ is also one of those nutrients that doesn't like to work alone. In addition to reactivating vitamin E, it seems to help power up selenium, a mineral long linked with heart health. In one study by researchers at the Klinikum Sudstadt in Rostock, Germany, of the patients who took a combined supplement of selenium and coenzyme Q$_{10}$ for a year after a heart attack, only one died—but not from a cardiac problem. The control group, on the other hand, had six cardiac deaths in the same time period.

As if that weren't enough, coenzyme Q$_{10}$

may help speed up your metabolism and help you lose weight. Some studies also suggest that coenzyme Q_{10} may fight periodontal disease and combat allergies and asthma.

According to Dr. Sinatra, almost anyone except young children and pregnant or lactating women can take low doses of coenzyme Q_{10}—30 to 90 milligrams—to prevent disease. But if you have serious disease, such as heart disease or cancer, and you are under your doctor's supervision, you might consider a larger, therapeutic dose of 180 to 360 milligrams.

You'll need to work with your doctor to determine the dose that's right for you, says Dr. Sinatra. He adds that "a lot of doctors aren't familiar with coenzyme Q_{10}."

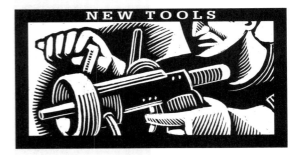

NEW TOOLS

More Convenient Testing

Cholesterol Home Test Kits

As with your blood pressure, a good-quality cholesterol reading is composed of two numbers. LDL (low-density lipoprotein) cholesterol is the stuff that gunks up your arteries, and HDL (high-density lipoprotein) is the good, or "helpful," stuff that keeps the LDL in check. Sure, knowing your total cholesterol count is useful, but increasingly, it's the two separate numbers that doctors are interested in. The problem is that to get a two-number cholesterol count requires a few drops of blood and a laboratory analysis.

A home test kit can now give you the total count (LDL plus HDL) but not the individual levels of HDL or LDL cholesterol. It provides an overall assessment of your cholesterol picture—important because cholesterol levels fluctuate in response to stress, illness and other factors.

The scientists who developed the tests caution that these products are intended for people who are on cholesterol-reducing drugs or who already know that they should watch their fat intake. However, according to Robert DiBianco, M.D., director of cardiology research at Washington Adventist Hospital and associate clinical professor of medicine at Georgetown University School of Medicine, both in Washington, D.C., "these are very good screening tests. Everyone should know their cholesterol level and have at least a screening test done for total cholesterol. It is as important as knowing your blood pressure. Maybe even more so." In general, he notes, anyone with a screening test of over 200 should get a complete analysis that shows HDL, LDL and triglyceride levels. This test is run on blood drawn after fasting and is analyzed in a regular lab. Unless you have hemophilia or take anticoagulants, the tests are safe.

The test, called CholesTrak, like those your doctor gives, requires just a couple of drops of blood, pricked from your finger. You place the blood on a pad in a plastic device. The blood filters through the pad to a series of chemically treated strips of paper that analyze the cholesterol content. After about 15 minutes, you can read your cholesterol level. Available at grocery stores and drugstores, between $10 and $13.

Earlier Detection

Colon Cancer Home Screening Kits

Colon cancer is the third leading cause of cancer death in the United States for men, even though this cancer often starts out as a benign polyp. That's why screening is so important.

Once available only from a doctor's office, a fecal occult blood test can now be found at the corner drug store. Unlike the older tests where you wiped a stool sample on pieces of special paper that was then analyzed by a laboratory, these new home test kits avoid the need to handle the stool, and the results are immediately obvious. You just take a specially treated pad and put it in the toilet after you have had a bowel movement. If a blue-green cross appears, the test is positive for the presence of blood.

Some fecal occult blood tests are affected by certain foods, but according to the manufacturers, the EZ-Detect test is not, so there is no need for dietary restriction. For two days before and during the test, you should avoid medications that contain aspirin, anti-inflammatory medica-

tions and rectal ointments. If you are taking medications, including prescribed iron, check with your doctor. Also, if your hemorrhoids are flaring up or you are constipated, wait until you feel better before doing the test.

A positive test does not mean that the blood in the feces is caused by cancerous lesions. It could also be the result of hemorrhoids, diverticulosis or a host of other conditions. No fecal occult blood test picks up nonbleeding cancerous lesions. If the test is positive, consult your physician for follow-up tests. Even if the test is negative, the manufacturers of the EZ-Detect suggest that you see your physician if you have any symptoms that concern you, such as diarrhea or constipation lasting longer than two weeks or an unexplained weight loss. Available in drugstores, $6.

Private Screening

Confide HIV Testing Service

One of the biggest worries with HIV testing has always been the fear of medical records getting into the wrong hands. The new HIV home test, Confide, allows you to get tested without anyone ever knowing anything at all about you. For starters, the test can be ordered by telephone or purchased over the counter at drugstores, clinics and college health centers.

You test yourself, taking a small blood sample from a finger, placing a few drops on a test card and using a prepaid protective mailer to ship it to the medical laboratory.

Each kit is identified by its own 14-digit number. That's the code you give when you call a toll-free number for test results. All positive results are conveyed over the phone by trained counselors. They also provide referrals, information and general support. If the test results are negative, a recording or counselor will give you information about HIV protection.

For more information, call Confide at 1-800-THE-TEST. $40 retail price, $50 if ordered by phone.

Better Skin Protection

IvyBlock

Soon you may be able to spread a lotion called IvyBlock on your skin and frolic naked in a patch of poison ivy or poison oak, if you're so inclined. The main ingredient in IvyBlock is a cosmetic and paint-thickening agent that forms a barrier against urushiol, the rash-triggering chemical found in the leaves of these poisonous plants. "It's worth an ocean of calamine lotion," says the poetic James G. Marks, Jr., M.D., professor of dermatology at the Milton S. Hershey Medical Center in Hershey, Pennsylvania. In an experiment he conducted, the lotion prevented reactions in 98 of 144 people who were sensitive to urushiol. The others had only mild rashes. An application to market IvyBlock is before the Food and Drug Administration.

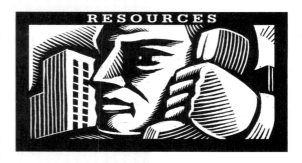

General Health

Good Health Web Site
http://www.social.com/health/index.html

If you want to find an extensive combination of health products, news groups, organizations and libraries, the Good Health site is for you. This Web site provides information on over 1,000 health organizations in the United States, the "Let's Talk Health" discussion page and links to health sites around the world. The most valuable resource here may be the Good Health Library. Readers can find articles on nutrition, cholesterol, mental health, food allergies, prescription drugs and more.

Cancer Awareness

The Cancer Information Service (CIS)
1-800-4-CANCER

A program of the National Cancer Institute, this is a nationwide service for cancer patients and their families, the public and health care professionals. CIS information specialists have extensive training in providing up-to-date information about cancer and cancer research. They answer questions in English and in Spanish and can send printed material. CIS offices also serve geographic areas and have information about cancer-related services and resources in their region.

Heart Health

American Heart Association

http://www.amhrt.org

1-800-AHA-USA1

The American Heart Association has an amazingly comprehensive Web site, offering a mini-encyclopedia on all heart topics. You can also find information about support groups, free brochures and the latest news in the areas of coronary disease and stroke.

Alternative Medicine

University of Pittsburgh

Falk Library of the Health Sciences

http://www.pitt.edu/~cbw/altm.html

Looking for information on alternatives to conventional medicine? Then this is the site for you. This information-packed site sponsored by the National Institutes of Health in Bethesda, Maryland, can link you to research on everything from acupuncture to vegetarian cooking.

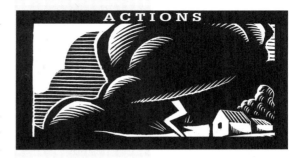

Much of medical research is focused on better ways to cure or fix the human body. But there's a lot of study going into how to prevent health troubles altogether. Much of it is confirming what we always knew—a good diet and plenty of exercise makes you more disease-resilient. But science is uncovering some surprises, too. Here are several things that you can do to keep healthy, based on recent research and writings.

1. Get frequent blood pressure readings. Heart attacks and strokes don't come out of the blue. A lot of the trouble that leads to these killers starts in the arteries. When you have high blood pressure, the blood circulates too vigorously under too much force. The pressure tears up the artery walls, which allows the harmful LDL (low-density lipoprotein) cholesterol to attach and form plaque. "High blood pressure wouldn't be such a serious problem if it didn't do so much damage to artery walls," says Bryant Stamford, Ph.D., director of the Health Promotion and Wellness Center at Kentucky's University of Louisville.

Blood pressure goes up and down over the course of the day, so the random reading your doctor took at your last office visit might not have given you the true picture. Here's how to get the best reading, says Lawrence LaPalio, M.D., medical director of geriatrics at Columbia La-Grange Memorial Hospital in LaGrange, Illinois. Steer clear of stimulants, such as coffee or alcohol. Some prescription medication also gets in the way. For some people, just being in the doctor's office causes nerves to surge and blood pressure to rise. Sit quietly in your doctor's office with your arm resting at heart level for five minutes. Ask the doctor to take several readings.

For moderately high blood pressure, take readings over several weeks to a month. For very high blood pressure, take several readings at the same time and average them. Get one just before you head for home—you may be more relaxed then. If you have mild to moderately elevated blood pressure, you can also get a more accurate picture of your blood pressure by monitoring your own for a month or so.

2. **Have one glass of wine a day.** Part of the reason for the French paradox—the fact that rich French cuisine accompanies an unexpectedly low risk of heart disease—may lie in the vine, researchers believe. Or, more precisely, in the ethanol, the main ingredient in alcoholic beverages that can make you light-headed. Scientists also have found that some of the plant chemicals in wine provide protection from disease. While you're getting happy and relaxed, they go to work blocking the formation of harmful oxidized LDL cholesterol and warding off cancers.

"Light drinking may lower your risk of dying," says Michael Gaziano, M.D., director of cardiovascular epidemiology at Brigham and Women's Hospital in Boston. "People who drink light to moderate amounts of alcohol (a drink or two a day) have the lowest mortality—even lower than nondrinkers. But more than two drinks a day may make your blood pressure go up," says Dr. Gaziano. Heavy drinkers—people who put away three or more drinks a day—increase their risk of a variety of problems, including heart disease, stroke, breast cancer, esophageal cancer and liver disease.

3. **Screen your skin.** Minute changes in the moles and freckles that dot your body's surface can signal the onset of malignant melanoma, a skin cancer that can be cured easily in its early stages, but that quickly spreads.

Examine your skin decorations—from the top of your scalp to the bottom of your feet—twice a year. Look for the ABCs—and Ds—of skin cancer detection as outlined in "The ABCDs of Moles and Melanomas," a brochure from the Skin Cancer Foundation of New York, in New York City.

- A is for asymmetry. An irregular shape is a sign of trouble.
- B is for border. Beware of irregular, scalloped or notched borders.
- C is for color. Different shades of brown or black signal a problem.
- D is for diameter. Anything larger than a pencil eraser may indicate a melanoma.

4. **Muscle up for immunity.** Even if you haven't exercised for years, don't be put off: "As soon as you start to exercise, your risk of cardiovascular problems drops by 25 percent," says Gerald Fletcher, professor of medicine at the Mayo Clinic in Jacksonville, Florida.

"We think exercise lowers blood pressure because it opens up the small vessels and capillaries and helps blood flow into the working muscles that need the extra nourishment," says Dr. Stamford. An added benefit for the muscles is that they become better able to absorb oxygen and glucose.

Moderate amounts of exercise may boost your immune system, some researchers believe. A stronger immune system makes life more pleasant on a day-to-day level. "We notice fewer colds and coughs and less bronchitis in people who exercise," says Dr. Fletcher.

5. **Take a brisk walk to the store.** Or mow the lawn, play tennis or paint the house. These everyday exercises can be an important part of the 30 or more minutes that the Centers for Disease Control and Prevention and the American

College of Sports Medicine suggest you get on most, if not all, days of the week. You don't need a structured, rigorous exercise program. Even small changes in your activity level can help reduce your risk of chronic disease.

6. **Fight disease with fresh fruits, vegetables, grains and seeds.** When you get right down to it, the best recipe for disease-proofing your body is right in your own kitchen—in foods you can buy cheaply and prepare easily. Why? Fresh fruits, vegetables, grains and seeds are high in phytochemicals, natural substances that fight disease. Strive for variety in fresh foods. You'll get a wide assortment of protective substances from a diversified diet.

In a study begun in 1973, researchers kept track of 1,883 men ages 35 to 59 who had high cholesterol levels. Over the next 20 years, the men who had the highest levels of carotenoids—one of the phytochemicals—in their blood had 60 percent fewer heart attacks and deaths.

If you eat a lot of plant foods, you have a lower risk for cancers that attack the lungs, bladder, cervix, mouth, larynx, throat, esophagus, stomach, pancreas, colon and rectum. Scientists also believe that plant foods may help protect you from prostate cancer. In fact, according to the National Cancer Institute, up to 33 percent of potential cancers may be prevented by eating a diet rich in fruits and vegetables.

7. **Stomach trouble? Think bacteria.** Studies suggest that stomach cancer may be tied to a common bacterium, *Helicobacter pylori.* Antibodies that your body produces to fight the bacterial infection may actually stimulate cancer cells in the stomach.

The bad news is that in a study by researchers at the University of Tennessee and the Baptist-Healthplex Family Practice Center in Memphis, about half of the people with indigestion who did not respond to standard treatment with medications like Pepcid had been infected with *H. pylori.* The good news is that the infection can be treated with antibiotics.

8. **Help your insulin.** Insulin makes it possible for sugar to get into your cells and provide important nourishment. If you are "insulin-resistant," your pancreas has to work overtime to produce extra insulin. In time, your body may not be able to keep up with the extra production, and you'll end up with a shortage of insulin—that's when insulin resistance becomes diabetes. With insulin resistance, the extra insulin in your blood raises levels of triglycerides, fats in the bloodstream that help clog up the works. High triglyceride levels are usually associated with low levels of helpful HDL (high-density lipoprotein) cholesterol, which carries the bad LDL cholesterol out of your system. "Insulin resistance and the abnormalities associated with it accelerate atherosclerosis, which leads to heart disease and stroke," adds Gerald Reaven, M.D., a researcher at Stanford University.

Fight the effects with exercise, weight loss and throwing away cigarettes.

9. **Get enough potassium.** Low potassium intake can increase blood pressure, says Frank Barry, M.D., a physician in Colorado Springs and author of *Make the Change for a Healthy Heart.* This automatically puts you at risk for a wide range of cardiovascular woes. Get it from your diet: fresh fruit and vegetables, particularly potatoes and bananas.

10. **Stop smoking.** How could we not mention it? Quitting is at the top of the list for disease-proofing your body. "Quitting will significantly reduce your risk of stroke, heart disease and cancer regardless of your age and improve the quality of life," says Thomas Brandon, Ph.D., a smoking-cessation expert and associate professor of psychology at the State

University of New York in Binghamton. Look at it this way: Within eight hours of quitting, your pulse rate and blood pressure drop, and oxygen levels in your body rise. Within 24 hours, your risk of heart attack dips.

11. **Spice it up.** You know low-fat is synonymous with better health. But what do you do when the low-fat stuff you cram into your face tastes like cardboard? You're used to the taste and consistency of fat.

Turn low-fat from bland to mouthwatering by spicing things up, suggests Maureen Boccella, R.D., from the outpatient nutrition department at Thomas Jefferson University Hospital in Philadelphia. Put salsa, not sour cream, in your baked potato. Sauté in tomato juice or wine, not oil. Use mustard instead of mayonnaise. Make your spices more potent by lightly toasting them in a no-stick pan before adding them to your food.

6

MENTAL
TOUGHNESS

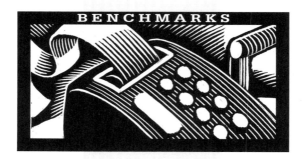

BENCHMARKS

AVERAGES

■ Percentage of men who get their sense of success from how they feel about themselves: 64

■ Percentage of Americans who say that they work 50 or more hours a week: 33

■ Chances that an American "always feels rushed": 1 in 3

■ Percentage of Americans who would rather have more free time even if it means less money: 51

■ Percentage of doctors who say that their patients show increased stress (from their last visit): 42

■ Percentage of Americans who say that "riding in the car" is the biggest waste of time: 28

■ Percentage of Americans who say that they have a good sense of humor: 85

■ Age at which an American develops a phobia: 13½

■ Percentage of Americans who say that they have a "strong belief in a higher power": 74

■ Percentage of Americans who wish they had more time by themselves: 31

EXTREMES

■ Hiroyuki Goto, 21, of Tokyo, recited pi to 42,195 places at the NHK Broadcasting Centre on February 18, 1995.

■ Working on the premise that a joke must have a beginning, a middle and an end, Mike Hessman of Columbus, Ohio, told 12,682 jokes in 24 hours on November 16 and 17, 1992.

■ Longest continuous speech made in the United Nations: 4 hours, 29 minutes, on September 26, 1960, by President Fidel Castro of Cuba

■ Longest working career: Shigechiyo Izumi began work goading draft animals at a sugar mill at Isen, Tokunoshima, Japan, in 1872. He retired as a sugar cane farmer in 1970 at the age of 105 after working for 98 years.

■ Dominic O'Brien memorized and then recalled, on a single sighting, a random sequence of 40 separate decks of cards (2,080 cards in all) that had been shuffled together, with only one mistake, at the British Broadcasting Company studios, Elstree, Great Britain, on November 26, 1993.

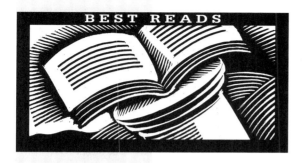

Emotions

Never bought into the "sensitive man" bit? That's because you were following your instincts. In this excerpt from The Male Body: An Owner's Manual: The Ultimate Head-to-Toe Guide to Staying Healthy and Fit for Life *(Rodale Press, 1996), authors K. Winston Caine and Perry Garfinkel provide some other interesting insights into men's emotions, along with some expert advice on how to rein in potentially destructive feelings and bring out beneficial ones.*

Men: cold, calculating, logical, rational, steady, invincible, steely, gritty, oblivious to pain, not swayed by emotion.

Aren't we something?

Truth is, we are expected to exhibit all of the above traits at times. And truth is, none of us is any of these things all of the time. But we are different. Different from women. And that's what makes the male-female dynamic so fascinating and frustrating, says John Gray, Ph.D., author of *Men Are from Mars, Women Are from Venus: A Practical Guide for Improving Communication and Getting What You Want in Your Relationship.*

All of those snips and snails and puppy dogs' tails in male DNA do make us feel and react differently than women. This is why being in touch with our feelings, and understanding how they influence us to act, is so crucial. Our feelings—or lack thereof—govern our relationships, our ability to succeed and navigate the storms of life and our health and overall well-being.

We must express our emotions if we are to maintain health and vigor; we can't bury them. But, notes Dr. Gray, much of the advice that men have been given in the past 20 years about how they need to open up and talk things out is fundamentally wrong. In fact, it's hogwash, he says. The advice is based on studies of what works well for women and ignores the fact that men are different.

Men, Dr. Gray says, instinctively—by nature—tend to express their emotions through actions rather than through words. We need to understand and respect that, he says. Men sometimes need to talk, but only when they're ready. And that's usually after they've mulled over a situation and come to terms with it, he says.

In other words, don't take the "sensitive male" persona that pop culture has promulgated in the past decade too seriously. If you have the typical male genetic coding, you are not going to be kind and gentle and open and sharing—at least not all of the time.

We'll explore specific ways that men can best manage their emotions. But first, let's look at what emotions are and how they affect us.

Understanding Emotions

Emotion, says *Dorland's Illustrated Medical Dictionary*, is "any strong feeling state, such as excitement, distress, happiness, sadness, love, hate, fear or anger."

Emotions are complex. They cause changes in body chemistry. And changes in body chemistry bring on certain emotions. It works both ways, usually without any conscious effort on our part. Often, we can consciously change our emotions by changing our posture, our type and level of activity and our thinking. A physical problem or defect, though, that causes an abundance or a deficiency of certain brain chemicals can create extreme moods that we cannot effectively control consciously, according to Larry J. Feldman, Ph.D., director of the Pain and Stress Rehabilitation Center in Newark, Delaware, and author of *Feeling Good Again: The Most Powerful Medicine Is What You Can Do for Yourself.*

Much mental illness is biological in origin—that is, it's caused by physiological flaws that create chemical imbalances. But much mental illness is simply the result of poor learned responses to life, says Michael J. Norden, M.D., in his book *Beyond Prozac.* Startlingly, Dr. Norden reports, a major study revealed that nearly half of us between the ages of 18 and 54 have met the criteria for psychiatric illness at some point in our lives, and for a third of us, the illness lasted more than a year.

Is there a benchmark for you to measure your emotional health? Science fails us here, if only because emotions are unquantifiable. But Dr. Feldman does offer this simple list of skills that an emotionally healthy man should have.

• He can manage his thinking.
• He is optimistic.
• He can focus on the needs of others.
• He has self-esteem.

Beyond biology, what determines our emotional balance? There are a number of factors, says mind-body medicine pioneer Bernie Siegel, M.D. Chief among them is our basic learned approach to life: our attitude, how we respond to situations. And tied in to that, he says, are our sense of self-worth and our sense of purpose.

Fortunately, says Dr. Siegel, it's never too late to build a better attitude and stronger self-esteem, to find and focus purposefully on a positive mission and to learn better ways to respond to life's stressors.

Develop a Winning Attitude

For a man to feel positive about himself and the world, "he needs to feel he is accomplishing things, doing things, achieving, providing con-

structively," says Dr. Gray. And as we make the transition from youth to maturity, "what we do needs to have a constructive benefit for others."

Do good deeds. We need to engage in activities that help others in order to develop and maintain a balanced, positive outlook, says Dr. Gray. It can be something as simple as chopping wood for somebody, he adds.

Focus on your greater purpose. "We have bodies," says Dr. Siegel, "so we can do things. And we should ask, 'What can I do, more than just earn a living, to contribute love and compassion to the world?' . . . Decide why you're here, what's important to you, what's the point of all of this. And then go and accomplish it."

Quiet the noise. "You are a satellite dish," says Dr. Siegel. "There are many messages coming to you. You have to decide what to focus on. So you pick up the remote and you pick out a channel and manifest it on your screen. Now, the trouble with men, they never focus on one channel. They sit there and fly from one thing to another. They don't focus on 'What has meaning?'"

Pick a positive path. When you are faced with choices, it's important to look deep inside and ask, "What feels right?" says Dr. Siegel. Don't ask, "What will make me the most money? What will most impress the neighbors?" What's important, he says, is "What will truly make me happiest as my way of contributing to life?" This is not selfish.

Cultivate caring. "If you look at men who are depressed—who have no pride, no self-esteem, no motivation—the most important symptom is that they've stopped caring," says Dr. Gray. "Caring is a very delicate feeling for a man to culture. A man must continue finding things that he cares about, that he's interested in, or he loses his energy and becomes depressed."

Try, try again. "The test for being a successful man is, do you care again? Do you try again?" says Dr. Gray.

"Life is a labor pain," says Dr. Siegel. We get rejected, we fail, we feel pain—all on the way to giving birth to great, fulfilling achievements and to ourselves. "It hurts a lot less," he says, "if we decide, 'These are difficulties I choose to confront.' Then we realize that it's not someone else inflicting pain on us but pain we are choosing to go through."

Sweat it out. We can't say it too many times: A program of regular vigorous exercise makes us feel better, helps us think more clearly and causes the brain to release chemicals that make us feel better and make us more resilient. Find an activity you like and do it.

Dealing with Feelings

The war of the sexes: Shakespeare managed to build a five-century-long career out of it. Men and women think, feel, react differently. We know this, and yet at times we still get extraordinarily frustrated and confused by the differences.

This is not a unisex world. It is important for men to deal with their emotions in a manly way and for women to understand what men are doing, says Dr. Gray. And never is this more important than when dealing with anger, he adds.

Men, says Dr. Gray, need to retreat to their caves. To be alone. To be quiet. To reflect. To chop wood, to shoot hoops, to work out aggressive feelings and transform them into positive action. It may take a couple of days, he adds.

Women, says Dr. Gray, need to talk, and through talking, they release their energy.

But if a man who is angry is prodded to talk about it, he may become physically destructive, says Dr. Gray. If he's forced to talk before he's ready, "he will stay angry longer than if he had taken some quiet time to think about what's making him angry," says Dr. Gray. Male anger "wants to be put into action," he explains.

"At those stressful times when there is anger, a man should stop talking, and a woman should stop asking him questions, because asking him questions baits him. It pulls him out. It gets him talking about his feelings, which intensifies his feelings, and he tends to act on those feelings. Men put anger into action much faster. Men have much less impulse control than women.

"That's why 90 percent of the people in jail are men," Dr. Gray says. "It's not because women are somehow nobler; it's just that when women hate somebody, they talk about it. When men hate somebody, they hit that person. They steal from that person. They do something based on those feelings of being mistreated."

What to do about it?

Back off. "A wise man," says Dr. Gray, "is able to take emotional energy and back off and think about what those feelings are and what is the most constructive thing he can do with those feelings."

Get active. When you are emotionally upset, do something constructive. "Take your focus off the thing that is upsetting you and shift your energy somewhere else," Dr. Gray suggests. "It could be just throwing a basketball through a hoop, or watching a football game, or working on a hobby—any activity through which the energy can be transformed and redirected." This is how men think about and figure out what they're feeling, he explains.

Overcome fear. Men tend to turn fear into procrastination, says Dr. Gray. "Engage in a hobby or an activity that you have no fear around, one that generates positive feelings," he suggests. "Then when you're feeling confident, come back to the problem at hand."

Give hurt a break. Feelings of hurt can easily move into feelings of anger and revenge, says Dr. Gray. Treat hurt like anger. Mull it over quietly and work it out with constructive physical activity, he says. If you act out your hurt by hurting others, you will always lose.

Don't wait for "I'm sorry." Men want to be

right about everything. It's prehistoric, says Dr. Gray; it's a survival thing. And it means we're very, very defensive about our emotions when we express them to the person we are upset with. We tend to remain upset until we receive an apology or an assurance that the offending act won't be repeated. This, however, can sabotage our relationships with women. Instead of waiting for a woman to apologize, says Dr. Gray, we need to learn to dissipate the emotional energy through recreational activities and then forgive and forget.

Even though they complain about it, says Dr. Gray, women want us to be right. "Women don't go around looking for guys who are incompetent," he says. What women don't like, he adds, is when we refuse to apologize for our mistakes or when we demand apologies from them.

Express pride. Let others know you admire them. The best way to support a man is to let him know you appreciate something he does or has done. Men, much more than women, need and appreciate recognition of accomplishments.

Keep a log. Jot down things that evoke strong emotions as they happen throughout the day, urges Dr. Siegel. Then, he says, in the evening or before retiring at night, write out some thoughts about the experience. "I call it writing a poem every day," says Dr. Siegel. This is a healthy way for a man to gain greater awareness of his inner feelings, he says.

The Law of Lifetime Growth

In an excerpt from The 22 (Non-Negotiable) Laws of Wellness *(HarperCollins, 1995), author Greg Anderson, founder of the Cancer Conquerors Foundation, writes about aging and the importance of keeping a positive, curious outlook on life.*

The most up-to-date research in gerontology has uncovered a shocking conclusion: As much as 80 percent of what we now call "old age" is not related to biology. Instead, it has its roots in expectations and attitudes. True, the 20 percent that is a product of biology may incapacitate us and even result in our death. But the good news is this: If we concentrate on improving and changing the unnecessary 80 percent, we stand to profit beyond our most optimistic expectations.

The Law of Lifetime Growth is at the heart of this approach.

Everyone—young, old, rich, poor, healthy, diseased—absolutely everyone has the capacity to change, to learn, to evolve and to grow.

Yet we succumb to a set of cultural beliefs that classify and restrict people to roles that create anything but total wellness. It's high time to take seriously the Law of Lifetime Growth.

I was fortunate to be raised in a household that treasured lifetime growth. It was important in our home that we all had an understanding of world news—not just the story, but the history and the people behind the stories. My mother and father made us think. What were the alternatives to a border fight in Pakistan? How could inflation be kept in check? What about civil rights in our own state?

We were encouraged to read, to study, to think for ourselves. In both high school and college I was active in speaking and debate. My parents encouraged me to choose topics that stretched the mind and challenged the thinking and then to reduce those subjects to clearly understandable terms that anyone could grasp. Since the earliest days, I was primed for lifetime growth. Today, I have an insatiable curiosity.

The Law of Lifetime Growth is inextricably intertwined with the idea of vital curiosity. It works for children, young adults, career trackers and seniors. The idea is to constantly explore, to seek, to have an attitude and bearing that says, "I'm interested in finding out what life holds."

Lifetime growth is much more than a classroom issue. Its boundaries spread far beyond academe. Lifetime growth is the cornerstone of successful parenting, of career satisfaction—of fulfillment in all of life.

Nowhere do I need the Law of Lifetime Growth more critically than in my work with senior citizens. In our programs at retirement communities, we view with a critical eye any activities that aim to pacify the residents. Such activities come out of a kind of babysitting model of elder care; they create dependency. I bristled when one social director recently described her intent as "to keep the natives quiet."

Such attitudes stand as cultural roadblocks to lifetime growth. We limit and categorize people based on age and our own beliefs about aging. Our words betray a deep cynicism regarding older people: "Old means no longer productive"; "A senior citizen should just enjoy the golden years"; "He has earned a rest."

No more! The Law of Lifetime Growth must come to the forefront. This law is a far-reaching idea, one that shakes the very foundations of modern society. And it is filled with promise.

Governments and citizens must commit to the concept of lifetime growth. We must recognize that growth is always possible, no matter what our age or ability. Are disabilities limiting? Sometimes. Is growth still possible? Of course. We must redouble our efforts to honor the potential of each life throughout its span.

This law is violated constantly at every level of society. To put an end to this, we must shift the beliefs of massive numbers of people in all cultures. We must strike the category of age off documents except for statistical and record-keeping purposes, in the same manner that the Constitution prohibits us from discriminating on the basis of race or religion. No person should ever again be forced to retire simply because of age.

A commitment to lifetime growth is the key.

Attitude-altering attempts are not the exclusive domain of government. Ultimately, we are each responsible for creating and satisfying our curiosity about life. Our efforts make all the difference! The list of great men and women who have committed themselves to this law is long and inspiring.

Thomas Alva Edison, who attended school for only three months and was deemed mentally slow by his teachers, patented a total of 1,033 inventions! His work spanned a lifetime, with his first patent issued at age 21, his last at age 81. Much of the technology of the twentieth century derives from his achievements, of which the electric light bulb and the generation of electricity are but two.

The lessons: Genius does not depend on advanced degrees or the approval of others; pursue your God-given talents throughout your life. That's the Law of Lifetime Growth.

The comedian George Burns, born on New York's Lower East Side, after the death in 1964 of his beloved wife, Gracie Allen, was expected to retire. Instead, he became even more involved in his work and in life. At the age of 80 he won an Oscar for his role in *The Sunshine Boys*. That's lifetime growth.

The lessons: Overcome loss; rise to new and greater possibilities; never let age be an excuse. That's the Law of Lifetime Growth.

Anna Mary Moses, better known as Grandma Moses, the much-loved painter, farmed until her late seventies. For many of her years she also embroidered, but when she turned 78 her fingers had become too stiff to handle a needle. She began to paint in oils instead. Her pictures of rural America were soon on exhibit internationally. In the hundredth year of her life, she illustrated an edition of *A Visit from St. Nicholas* ("'Twas the night before Christmas . . . "); it was published in 1962, one year after her death.

The lesson: Keep seeking even after defeat. Your greatest work may yet lie ahead. That's the Law of Lifetime Growth.

George Bernard Shaw, the British playwright, remained active and immensely productive until his death at 94. A seminal thinker who sparked thoughtful debate, Shaw wrote about the arts and politics, penning his last play when he was in his late eighties. His work has stood the test of time.

The lessons: Cultivate ideas. Respond to issues that intrigue and motivate. Pursue these interests daily. That's the Law of Lifetime Growth.

The social anthropologist Margaret Mead, at age 72, made a trip to study the Arapesh people of New Guinea. In 1975, a television documentary traced a typical week in her life. She was constantly busy—contributing and exploring. Her week was so packed with work that it exhausted the television crew, most of whom were less than half her age.

The lesson: Find your passion and pursue it. That's the Law of Lifetime Growth.

Benjamin Franklin, writer, scientist, inventor and one of the greatest statesmen of the Revolutionary era, achieved his most notable victories in later life. At 70, he was a member of the committee that drafted the Declaration of Independence, as well as one of its signers. He was 75 when he negotiated the end to the War of Independence. Called the wisest American, Franklin was 81 when he effected the compromise that brought the Constitution of the United States into being.

The lessons: Work, contribute, find a higher cause, give of self and devote your life to the well-being of others. The qualities that drove such activities did not disappear when Franklin died. Perhaps they are out of style. But the great life can be ours by pursuing those ideals. That's the Law of Lifetime Growth.

Edward "Duke" Ellington never retired—although he "retired from booze" when he was in his mid-forties. For nearly 50 years he had a band, always performing, circling the globe. He made his first recording in 1924 and his last in 1974, not many weeks before his death. He left a great legacy—the most distinctive single body of composition in the history of jazz.

The lessons: Never retire—except to put personal excesses to rest. Always aspire—for the greater goal. That's the Law of Lifetime Growth.

The Law of Lifetime Growth demands both a cultural change and a megashift in our own thinking about all that life can be.

This law of wellness represents a great hope for people of all ages, all states of wellness, all cultures.

Grow. Learn. Pursue. Contribute. Enjoy. Make the commitment. You'll know fulfillment as never before. It's the non-negotiable Law of Lifetime Growth.

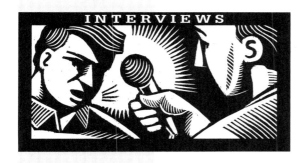

Phil Jackson on
Building Personal and Team Mental Toughness

Phil Jackson is coach of the NBA's Chicago Bulls, one of the winningest basketball teams of the 1990s. To inspire such stars as Michael Jordan, Scottie Pippen and Dennis Rodman to new levels of performance, he has drawn on his years of experience as a player, a coach and a longtime practitioner of Zen meditation. Here he shares some of his tips on building both personal and team mental toughness that have won him coaching kudos—and greater control of his life.

Newsweek magazine lauded you for your "masterful handling of the team's disparate egos and temperaments." What's your management secret?

It starts with trust. Players have to trust that everybody is going to be called on to account for their mistakes. In coaching, there's a rule of thumb. Everybody may not need to hear the fact that they made a mistake but the rest of the team sometimes needs to know that you know that they know they made a mistake. It's my responsibility to call it. After that, it's a juggling act between keeping the guys productive, conforming to the group and making it something more than just making money and being on an ego trip. I remind them that the reward has to be in the group process.

How do you reinforce that group process?

We like to do a variety of things. For example, rather than taking a 180-mile charter flight from Houston to San Antonio, we ride in a bus. This builds a strong group mind-set because it forces the players to at least share the space of a bus together for three hours. I also brought the team to visit my old friend and New York Knicks teammate Bill Bradley (then senator from New Jersey) in Washington, D.C., to show them that the bonds you develop with former teammates, based on some shared key moments, endure.

We know that you've been a meditator for more than 20 years. How does meditation build mental toughness?

Meditation is a discipline first and foremost. It's an awakening process. One reason I enjoy doing it first thing in the morning is that instead of jumping fast forward into life, and getting immediately stressed about the 101 things you have to do in a day, it allows you to sit and let the mind realize who's in control, that thoughts come and go and they're not going to possess us. The other reason is to wake up, to be alert and conscious. I like Zen meditation so much because it's a very wakeful practice. It's about alertness. One of the things that's part of my teaching regime in basketball is that alertness is the key. So meditation keeps my mind aware and alert, conscious of my thoughts but also not holding on to them. And then, again, there's the discipline of doing it every day. And the stillness that it gives you allows you to be peaceful, and *that* allows you to have compassion for others.

More specifically, how do you apply what you learn from the practice of Zen meditation to basketball?

Basketball requires shifting from one objective to another at lightning speed. To excel, you need to act with a clear mind and be totally focused on what everyone on the floor is doing. The secret is not thinking. That doesn't mean being stupid; it means quieting the endless jabbering of thoughts so that your body can do instinctively what it's been trained to do without the mind getting in the way. One of the points of Zen is to perform every activity, from playing basketball to taking out the garbage, with precise attention, moment to moment.

That's fine, but out on the court in the middle of some intense moment—like when Dennis Rodman head-butts a referee, for instance—how do you keep your Zen cool?

One of the things I did early, specifically with Dennis, was just sit out. In other words, I decided that as a coach I was just going to have to be much calmer and not involved in the game to the extent that I was doing confrontational things with the referees or emoting anything that could be taken as a negative from Dennis or anyone. It kept him calmer on the court. He responded in a way that let me know that I was on the right track. As for myself, as soon as I feel tension in my shoulders or neck, that's a signal that I'm holding my breath. I breathe. Breathing is the key, in my estimation. That's one of the things you learn in meditation: to follow your breath. I breathe, then I release it. Then I go on, I keeping going on. I move past that moment, and I'm in the next moment.

In basketball, you're constantly going from one potential crisis to another, literally holding your breath all the time. You have to keep letting go and moving on. Basketball, like golf, is a game in which you can do a tremendous amount of self-abuse over errors and ruin a real nice day and, in the process, probably cause your team to lose. No one plays this or any game perfectly. It's the guy who recovers from his mistakes who wins.

We notice that you protect your back when you walk. Is that still from the double-herniated disk injury you suffered as a player back in 1969?

Yes. I lost a nerve in my leg from that injury, and my leg is atrophied. Ironically, I think the biggest asset to my basketball life was that injury. It's unfortunate the way things happen sometimes, but the injury took me out of the realm of being able to get by on athletic talent. It's hard to come to terms with inadequacy, but I realized postsurgery that I was going to be limited in my athletic abilities and that I was going to have to focus on what I *could* do to compete well. That's probably the thing that not only woke me up but started me a little on this path to coaching. I had to play smarter.

How does the injury affect your ability to stay in shape?

My exercise is limited to walking and meditating, depending on my pain threshold that day. When I'm forced to choose between mind or body, I usually choose mind. Usually, the meditating wins out. Actually, sitting Zen does a lot more for our bodies than we give it credit for. The discipline and regimen of sitting erect for up to an hour has a very positive effect. It calms my digestion and gently tones my muscles. Though I can't do yoga myself—except for a simple sun salutation before I sit—I strongly believe in it as an integral part of exercise.

What's the major stress in a coach's life, and how do you deal with it?

The major stress in a basketball coach's life is getting the best performance, or energy, out of his team. That's achieved through striving for a compatibility and workability within the group and your acceptability as a coach. Beyond that, everything else—losses, wins—can be worked out. That all comes together if the team plays hard and likes to work together.

How about in your personal life? What's the biggest stressor?

The biggest stress has to be balancing between family and work. We play 41 games on the road. That converts to 90 to 100 days, or almost one-third of the year. Even when I'm home, the energy that the job requires puts distance between me and my family. It's not just the obvious stuff. There's the stress of the little things that put a little more pressure on the job: trading deadlines, a few extra hours of work or just working at home watching a game or videotape to get prepared for the next day. All of a sudden, you don't know your kids' teachers, you're unfamiliar with their classes and you realize that you're not participating in their lives.

What's the secret to your strong marriage?

My marriage has prevailed for 20-some years. I think the secret is working at making it work. That's the secret. At one point, we had a situation where we had four kids under the age of five in five years. It was the end of my career, so not only did I have these parenting responsibilities but I also had to deal with the loss of a role or livelihood. That's when I basically got away from basketball for a couple of years and did householding and became immersed in the family aspect. That brought me right back to a base level. It required me to be absolutely aware in every moment. It was very healing for me. Then I gradually got back into basketball and coaching, at first on a part-time basis in the minor leagues. That ran itself into this career.

With such a busy life, how do you find time to meditate?

Well, that's been the hardest thing over the years, to continue to keep the practice of medita-

tion together. I try to sit first thing in the morning. At home, I'm the first person up. I'm the breakfast maker in our house. So sometimes I have to get up at 5:30 or 6:00 in the morning to be able to fit in meditation. On the road, we usually start the day at about 8:30 or 9:00 in the morning, so there's still ample time even if we get in the night before at 2:00 or 3:00 in the morning. The most difficult thing is getting rest and keeping the determination to make sure that you don't let it slide. That's my resolve. I need to know that it's a necessary part of my life.

Finally, we've read that you're a big fan of the Grateful Dead. How do they fit into your philosophy of building team mental toughness?

The Dead are the same thing as a basketball team. Like I tell my guys, they're just "playin' in the band," as Jerry Garcia sang it. Garcia was like Michael Jordan, with the band creating a wonderful thing all around him. They knew each other's licks, and they made beautiful music together. The fact that the group performed together for 30 years—just their longevity, knowing each other that long—knocks me out. For me, the whole Dead thing is a metaphor back to basketball. Basketball is a game, a journey, a dance—not just a fight to the death. It's life just as it is. I emphasize to the players that when they like to work together, good things basically happen for the team.

James Loehr on
Toughening Your
Mental Muscles

James Loehr, Ed.D., is president and chief executive of LGE Sport Science in Orlando, Florida, and author of 11 books, including Toughness Training for Life. *As a motivational sports psychologist, he has trained more than 100 world-class athletes, including tennis star Jim Courier, boxer Ray "Boom-Boom" Mancini, speed skater Dan Jansen and golfer Mark O'Meara. The key to mental toughness, he tells us here, is knowing how to balance increased levels of stress and breaks for recovery.*

What have you found is the best way to motivate people to new levels of mental toughness?

I have found that the ability to get connected emotionally is the single best predictor of what motivates people to become mentally tough. Look at what it takes people to get on an exercise program or lose weight or quit smoking or improve their nutritional habits. Something moved them emotionally in a way that it hadn't happened before. It could be a speaker, an audiotape, a family tragedy, a shaky report, something that moved their spirit in a direction it hasn't been moved before. Motivational speakers, for example, give us a sense of hope and belief. So first, we have to ignite and inspire your emotions.

The next problem is sustaining that initial motivation. All great things happen in a moment of inspiration but follow with progressive achievable steps. That's where you break down your journey into digestible bites of incremental success. Therein lies the key to success: breaking down ultimate goals to successive steps that are attainable right now. That represents the beginning of systematic change, so that what you need and want become one and the same. Then you've gone beyond discipline. It's become part of your life, part of your way of being. Then you experience a great sense of triumph. This has nothing to do with personality styles. Whether you're an introvert or outgoing is irrelevant.

What role does stress play in building mental toughness?

I've spent 22 years trying to understand the impact of stress on performance, health and emotional strength. Stress is a biochemical response that involves energy expenditure. Working with athletes and in the field of sports science, I have witnessed that without stress, the growth process comes to a screeching halt. It's only with exposure to it that life is sustained. In your body, without stress we see an erosion of the muscle's capacity to function, like when your arm is in a cast. The only way to get muscles back—we call it rehabilitation therapy—is to progressively expose it to increased doses of stress. Toughness and rehabilitation are measured in terms of how much the arm can withstand without damage or injury. That understanding of toughening in the physical realm applies to the mental and emotional as well. The strongest people have not been protected from the storms of life but fully immersed in them.

The problem, I've found, is not excessive stress but insufficient healing time, not enough recovery time. Recovery is when growth takes place. Recovery is healing. We've developed a model we call toughness training. It involves periodic exposure to progressively increasing cycles of physical and/or emotional stress alternating with regular periods of recovery.

How about pain threshold? Is there some analogy between physical and emotional pain that can help us understand how to become more mentally tough?

First of all, we've dispensed with the old notion of "no pain, no gain." Toughness is measured not in how much pain you can take but in your speed of recovery. Pain is just a signal that you're getting close to your limit. If you exceed your pain threshold, your body will break down. We've noticed that people usually go through levels in physical training: First you feel good, then winded, then uncomfortable, then pain. Then there's recovery. The pain goes away, your heart returns to a lower rate. You stabilize.

Psychologically, it's the same mechanism. You see, the mind and body are united in every way. Physical and emotional stress share common biochemical and neurochemical foundations, and because of this, physical toughening often leads to automatic increases in emotional toughening.

Low stress, like breaks from physical exercise, is okay for short periods of time. It allows the recovery of energy and affords you some relief. But when low stress becomes chronic, the result is emotional pain in the form of boredom, low motivation, laziness, depression, confusion or apathy. We've put a new spin on the old saying "All work and no play makes Jack a dull boy." We say, "All play and no work makes Jack useless." Avoiding mental effort for long periods will prevent Jack from functioning at his intellectual peak. His emotional toughness is likely to decline as well.

So how much recovery time do you need?

Too much recovery time can be lethal because it's the absence of stress in your life. If you relax too long, you shut down the system of arousal. The signals that you've had too much recovery time are there. You just have to watch for them. But it's a little confusing because the signs of emotional overtraining and undertraining are the same: fatigue, lack of motivation, poor performance, negative thinking, confusion, poor problem solving, absence of passion, depression, low sex drive. They'll tell you that you're undertraining or spending too much recovery time. The exact amount of recovery time needed fluctuates with each person. One thing is true, however, and that is that the fitter you are mentally, physically or emotionally, the faster you recover. Only when stress and recovery are in balance do the mind and body realize that they can safely work harder. When this happens, passion returns to your life.

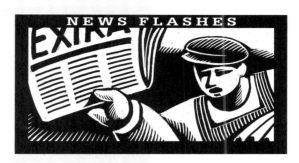

Reaction to Stress Could Predict Heart Trouble

DURHAM, N.C.—The way a person's body responds to mental stress can be a strong predictor of whether that person is vulnerable to heart problems, a study at Duke University Medical Center has revealed.

Wei Jiang, M.D., and colleagues studied 126 outpatients with histories of coronary artery disease who were prone to exercise-induced myocardial ischemia (reduced blood supply to the heart). At the beginning of the study, participants took both mental and exercise stress tests. Researchers followed up with questionnaires and telephone contact after four and ten months, and also at yearly intervals for up to five years.

Patients with mental stress–induced ischemia had higher rates of cardiac occurrences over the follow-up period. They had almost three times the risk of having a cardiac event compared with patients who didn't show any indications of mental stress–induced ischemia, researchers found.

As a direct result of their findings that mental stress–induced ischemia is potentially more dangerous to heart patients than exercise-induced ischemia, Dr. Jiang and his colleagues recommend mental stress testing as a complement to the traditional exercise stress testing for heart patients. Future research in this area will focus on the development of stress-management programs targeted specifically for cardiac patients.

Men Lose Brainpower as They Age

PHILADELPHIA—Men may gain wisdom with age, but they have less brain to store it in, according to University of Pennsylvania researcher and professor of psychology Richard C. Gur.

Men's brains shrink as they age, curbing memory, concentration and abstract reasoning, he concluded after studying the brain functions of 24 women and 37 men over the past ten years. He found the most shrinkage in the frontal lobe of the brain, the area responsible for planning.

Besides measuring brain volume with a magnetic resonance imaging (MRI) machine and looking at metabolism rates in the brain, Gur and his team also conducted a series of tests to see how patients' minds functioned. Patients were told to press a button after they saw a number 7 on a screen followed by the number 9. Over the ten-year period of the study, the men made more mistakes as they aged, he found. Even as early as age 23, men pushed the button when they shouldn't have, or didn't push it when they should have. There wasn't even a hint of a problem in the women, the study showed.

In another test, university researchers read aloud 16 items from a shopping list. Subjects then repeated what they had just heard. Because the men again performed poorly over the ten-year period in comparison to the women, Gur concluded that men lose intelligence as they grow older.

Gur suggests that men may be able to save brain cells by picking hobbies that allow them to rest the gray matter they normally use at work. Lawyers, for example, might avoid chess and crossword puzzles and take up painting or playing a musical instrument in their spare time. Accountants might rest their brains by bird-watching or painting. A bus driver would benefit from gardening.

Marital Spats Weaken Immunity

COLUMBUS, Ohio—Marital spats can be deadly. That's what researchers at Ohio State University found in a study of 31 couples ages 55 to 75.

The study found that abrasive arguments between husbands and wives—married an average of 42 years—caused a weakening of their immune responses and increased levels of stress hormones. This combination can make people more susceptible to illness, such as infectious diseases and, in the worst cases, cancer.

The couples filled out questionnaires that measured their levels of marital satisfaction (only 13 percent rated in the "distress" category). Patients were then hooked up to an intravenous tube that took blood samples at regular intervals. While the couples discussed topics that both agreed caused problems, researchers measured immune function and changes in hormone levels.

The results? The more negative behaviors the couples showed toward each other, the more immune measures were weakened.

B Vitamins Good for the Memory

BOSTON—Mussels, oysters, chicken, asparagus, brussels sprouts, spinach, oranges, bran cereal, whole-wheat bread and rolls.

Read that? Now close your eyes and repeat it. Can't do it? Maybe you can't remember because you haven't had enough of them on your plate.

When researchers in Boston tested the mental abilities of 70 men between the ages of 54 and 81, they found that men with the highest levels of vitamins B_6, B_{12} and folate in their blood did better on certain tests than men who weren't so high in those vitamins.

Men with high levels of B_6 did especially well in the "activity memory" test—a test that measures how well you can remember a sequence of things you did in a day. Men who faltered in B_{12}

had performances slightly below their peers in a test of copying increasingly complex shapes onto a paper.

Researchers have two main theories on how these nutrients are linked to thinking. One is that B vitamins directly help produce neurotransmitters in the brain. Another theory is that lack of these vitamins can actually hurt the brain, causing mini-stroke-like conditions that decrease blood flow and brain function.

Foods high in B vitamins include those mentioned in that first paragraph.

Dogs, Not Spouses, Offer Most Stress Relief

BUFFALO—In times of high stress, your dog—not your spouse—may be your best friend. Even supportive partners can't equal a pet's ability to lower blood pressure and heart rate when you're under performance stress, say researchers at the State University of New York at Buffalo School of Medicine and Biomedical Sciences.

The researchers asked 240 married couples (half of them dog owners) to perform three stressful tasks—mental arithmetic, giving a speech and placing a hand in ice water. Each of the tests was performed under four conditions: alone, with dog or friend, with spouse and dog or friend, and with spouse only.

Results showed that physical stress was highest with just a spouse present and lowest with just a dog. The researchers' reasoning? Dogs aren't in a position to judge or criticize.

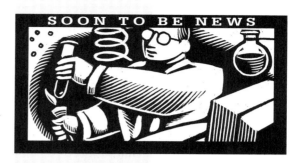

SOON TO BE NEWS

Fruit Fly Yields Clue to Memory?

Researchers have shown that it's possible to improve the long-term memory of fruit flies through genetic manipulation. In a privately funded laboratory on Long Island, New York, Timothy Tully, Ph.D., and his research team are studying the formation of long-term memory, which fades with natural aging and collapses in those suffering from Alzheimer's disease.

Dr. Tully and his colleagues have zeroed in on the role of a gene known as CREB that, in fruit flies, has both an "activator" and a "repressor" protein. Changing levels of these two proteins within nerve cells regulate the conversion of short-term memory into long-term storage, the researchers believe. When levels of CREB repressor cancel out activator, this conversion doesn't occur. If activator levels overpower the repressor, long-term memory is formed.

Tubes of fruit flies are attached to computer-controlled coils and pumps, allowing the researchers to measure the learning capacity of the flies. The batches of flies are given an electric shock in the presence of an odor. Researchers then observe whether they later choose to move into a test tube containing that odor or another. Avoiding the odor associated with shocks is taken as evidence of memory formation. The researchers found that after ten training sessions, the fruit fly has "learned" the lesson and has committed it to long-term memory.

Dr. Tully used biotechnology tools to rig a

CREB repressor so that it could be "turned on" by warming a test tube of flies in a tub of warm water. During electroshock training, the warmed fruit flies failed their long-term memory test—showing that the excess CREB repressor prevents development of long-term memory.

In a second experiment, when the CREB activator was turned on by warming, the flies formed the long-term memory after only one training session, instead of the usual ten.

Dr. Tully predicts the future development of a drug that stimulates CREB activator, thus bolstering formation of long-term memory or a CREB repressor to be administered to trauma victims to prevent formation of disabling traumatic memories.

Does a Full Stomach Improve Memory?

If you can't remember where you left your glasses or keys, an empty head may not be the cause. It could be an empty stomach—one that allows levels of blood sugar to fall too low—a recent study from the University of Virginia in Charlottesville suggests.

After an overnight fast, healthy people 60 to 80 years old drank lemonade sweetened with either sugar or sugar substitute. Those who drank the lemonade with sugar did much better at retelling a short story they read, both a few minutes later and even the next day, after their blood sugar returned to a baseline level.

Psychologist Paul Gold, Ph.D., says that his work indicates that the right level of blood sugar enhances memory storage, especially for older people, whose brains are most affected when levels fall. Too much sugar doesn't work, he says, but further research is needed to see whether eating many small healthy meals or snacks during the day may help—by keeping blood sugar steady.

Research is continuing in this area, and the final payoff may be memory-boosting drugs—for healthy people or even those with Alzheimer's.

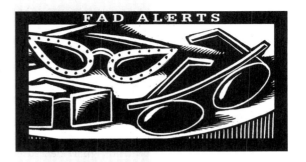

FAD ALERTS

BioDots

 What if you could gauge exactly how stressed out you were at a given moment? And what if, knowing that, you could effectively decrease your stress level by *thinking* your way into a more relaxed state?

That's the concept behind BioDots. Made of liquid crystals that change color in response to changes in your body temperature, these inexpensive adhesive dots, which are a quarter-inch in diameter, stick onto your skin, usually in the soft area between your thumb and first finger.

Sales have increased every year since they first appeared in 1977, according to their manufacturer, Robert Grabhorn, president of BioDot International in Indianapolis. "We've never advertised—just word of mouth," he says. His clients include schools, hospitals, biofeedback centers, stress-management trainers and many other health professionals. They are sold in health food stores and college bookstores, he adds.

"They were considered a gimmick at first," says John Picchiottino, president of Bio-Feedback Systems in Boulder, Colorado, one of the early companies to order the product. "They were called mood dots in those days. Now we sell them all over the country as an aid for people who are phasing out of using temperature biofeedback apparatus."

Here's how they work. One of your body's natural responses to stress—called the fight-or-flight response—may be to divert the flow of blood from your extremities to your heart and torso. Naturally, without blood flow, your hands get cold, turning the dot's color from violet (more relaxed) to blue, turquoise, green, yellow, amber and finally black (more tense). By focusing your attention on your hands, imagining them turning warm, using imagery or just reminding yourself to relax a little, you can lower your stress level. By monitoring the change in the color of the dot as your hands warm, you can measure decreased stress.

"I've been using them with patients for 15 years," says Kirk Peffer, Ph.D., a psychologist at Integrated Health Management in Denver. "Used appropriately, factoring in room temperature and other variables like your own normal circulation, they can be an effective tool in stress management."

Smart Drinks

 The idea of chugging your way to higher intelligence is just too irresistible. But drinker beware: All you gulp may not make you a genius.

Called smart drinks or, more precisely, cognition enhancers, these "cocktails" are offered at trendy spas and health bars. They are made with fruit juices, club soda or water and mixed with herbs and nutrients that, some claim, can improve your memory, concentration, alertness, problem-solving ability, ability to learn and retain information, sexual performance and overall health.

Smart drinks came into vogue in the late 1980s and early 1990s, says John Morgenthaler, co-author (with Ward Dean, M.D.) of *Smart Drugs II*, as a popular phenomenon of the baby-boom generation. "The baby boomers were the drug generation," says Morgenthaler, who claims to have coined the term *smart* in reference to such drinks and other "drugs." "This

wasn't a foreign notion to them. Plus, they were starting to notice that they weren't as quick mentally as they once were. And it also came at the tail end of the government's so-called war on drugs."

Typically, a smart drink will contain such herbs as ginkgo biloba, which is said to help blood flow to the brain and, therefore, aid memory and mental functioning; ginseng, a mild aphrodisiac that herbalists say enhances memory, learning, productivity, physical stamina and immune function; kola nut, a stimulant that some say has more caffeine than coffee; and dandelion, a weed that has anti-inflammatory properties.

Among the vitamins a smart drink may contain are vitamin C; B_6, important for the formation of serotonin, the so-called feel-good brain chemical; and choline, a B vitamin associated with improved memory that increases the brain's ability to produce acetylcholine, which is involved in mental performance.

"You will probably notice a short-term lift from some smart drinks," says Linda Prout, a nutritionist at the Claremont Resort and Spa in Berkeley, California, where smart drinks are served. "The combination of herbs in our drinks definitely packs some punch. But some smart drinks are so diluted or use herbs that require use for about three months before you would notice any difference."

Meanwhile, the Food and Drug Administration (FDA) puts little stock in such claims.

"There is no evidence that such preparations can do anything to increase a person's intelligence and thinking," says Arthur Whitmore, a spokesman for the FDA's Center for Food Safety and Applied Nutrition, the agency's branch that regulates dietary supplements. "Depending on the product, you catch a little buzz and experience a feeling of increased energy that could make you *think* you're thinking smarter. But the agency regards this whole idea as specious. There is no peer-reviewed science to substantiate any of these claims. In fact, we think that it's a marketing ploy and suggest that people are getting ripped off if they have any hopes that such drinks will increase their intelligence quotient."

Bald-Headed Men of America

 The membership requirement is simple: a bald pate. But the honor roll of past or present members is impressive if not downright intimidating: the actors Yul Brynner and Telly Savalas, former Soviet leader Mikhail Gorbachev, former President Dwight D. Eisenhower, basketball legends Michael Jordan and Charles Barkley, rock group REM's Michael Stipe, boxer George Foreman and weatherman Willard Scott.

These are men with attitude, men who stand out in a crowd, men who had better be mentally tough—or else.

"We're not wimps," says John T. Capps III, a printer and founder of Bald-Headed Men of America, based in Morehead City, North Carolina, which has amassed a membership of 20,000 since its founding in 1973. "We're the butts of lots of jokes because we're seen to be at some physical disadvantage, but that experience only makes us tougher.

"Bald is a sense of pride," he adds. "It's a badge of distinction. It takes a type A person to be able to take it and then dish it right back."

The organization's motto is "Bald Is Beautiful." Lately, the number of bald men seems to be growing, as less hair has become more fashionable. Whether by hair loss, male pattern balding, disease or the bold stroke of a shaver, there are more than 30 million men in the United States who are bald or balding, according to the American Hair Loss Council in Chicago.

Now, it seems, it's hip to bare your head.

Shiny scalps are a statement of masculinity, not a reason to feel insecure or vulnerable. The new popularity "had to happen," explains Capp. "Fashions swing from one end to the other. Hair was long back in the 1960s. Now skin is in. Anyway," he adds with a certain balder-than-thou attitude, "everyone will be bald eventually."

So trash the toupee. Never mind the Minoxidil. Blow off the baseball cap. Shave it off. Shave it *all* off. It didn't seem to hurt Michael Jordan's game.

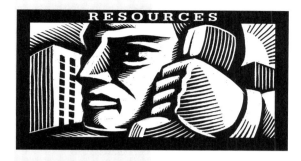

Stress Control

American Psychological Association's
Help Center
http://helping.apa.org

If you're feeling under pressure and need help, the American Psychological Association's Help Center Web site offers easy access to information on coping with workplace stress, family crises and chronic illness. You'll also find tips for handling everyday problems such as a difficult boss or a rebellious child.

Laughter

The HUMOR Project
110 Spring Street
Department MH
Saratoga Springs, NY 12866

Research suggests that the best way to treat stressed-out friends is to make them laugh. But what can you do if you're the one who needs help? One source is the HUMOR Project. It publishes a magazine called *Laughing Matters* that contains suggestions for getting humor into your life. For a free packet of information on the benefits of humor, send a legal-size, self-addressed, stamped ($1.01) envelope to the HUMOR Project.

Massage Therapy

National Certification Board for
Therapeutic Massage and Bodywork
1-800-296-0664

A massage is a healthy way to iron out the wrinkles from a rough day. But don't let just anyone knead your muscles. Find someone recognized by the National Certification Board for Therapeutic Massage and Bodywork, which sets standards for training. Call for a therapist near you.

Sore-Muscle Relief

Chicago Institute of Neurosurgery
and Neuroresearch
1-800-560-2225

Too many hours hunched over a computer can make your neck and back stiff. So call the Chicago Institute of Neurosurgery and Neuroresearch and request a free copy of "Healthy Office Maneuvers," which details ten simple, at-your-desk stretches to loosen you up.

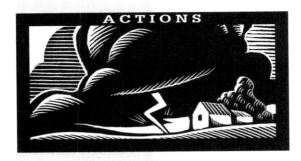

"Mental toughness means everything to a team that would be champion," Greg Gumbel, NBC sports commentator, told TV viewers watching the 1996 NBA Western Conference finals between the Seattle Supersonics and the Utah Jazz. The Supersonics must have been tougher. They won. Staying on top of life's game today requires more than the ability to jump higher, run faster, shoot better, go further. You have to have an agile mind as well as an agile body. Here are tons of tips to improve your mind game.

1. **Dream your way to success.** Nocturnal subconscious fantasies about crossing the finish line may help you win the race—even if you're not a runner. That's the conclusion of Steven Ungerleider, Ph.D., a psychologist at Integrated Research Services in Eugene, Oregon, a member of the U.S. Olympic Committee Sports Psychology Registry and the author of *Mental Training for Peak Performance.* He and colleagues studied the dream patterns of 656 athletes competing in the National Masters Championships. They found that some athletes who dream about sports report personal bests during subsequent competition. "The great news about dreams is that they may lend a helping hand to mental practice and skill development in any sport," Dr. Ungerleider reports in his book. "It seems clear, however, that in some cases, waking performance is directly related to dream performance." The implications for non-athletes trying to win life's race are clear. If you dream it, you can make it so. So dream on.

2. **Master the three Cs to combat stress.** Have you noticed that some people just seem to deal with stress better? Don't you wish you knew their secret? It turns out that researchers have wondered the same thing. To find out, Suzanne Ouellette, Ph.D., professor of psychology at the Graduate School of the City University of New York, studied business executives, lawyers, bus drivers, telephone company employees and others who lead high-stress lives. She found that the healthiest among them all exhibited high levels of three characteristics: control, commitment and challenge. Together these traits are called psychological or stress hardiness. Here's what each means.

Control: This means having a strong belief that you can exert influence on your surroundings, that you can make things happen.

Commitment: This means feeling fully engaged in what you're doing from day to day and giving it your best effort.

Challenge: This means seeing change as a natural part of life that affords at least some chance of further development, seeing new situations more as opportunities and less as threats.

"There are many things a person can do to increase his own levels of stress hardiness," says Jon Kabat-Zinn, Ph.D., director of the Stress Reduction Clinic at the University of Massachusetts Medical Center in Worcester and author of *Wherever You Go, There You Are* and *Full Catastrophe Living.* Among them:

- Come to grips with your own life by being willing to ask yourself hard questions about where your life is going.
- Make a list of specific choices and changes you can make in the three Cs.
- Restructure roles and relationships within your business and social contexts to promote greater control, commitment and challenge among family, friends and people you work with.

3. **Focus on a plan of action.** Rather than being "result-focused, be action-focused," says Shane Murphy, Ph.D., a clinical psychologist in Trumbull, Connecticut, president-elect of the Division of Sport and Exercise Psychology of the American Psychological Association and author of *The Achievement Zone: 8 Skills for Winning All the Time from the Playing Field to the Boardroom.* "The results are outside your control," he says. "You can do all the right preparation, but you still can't predict if you'll win the race or close the deal."

Instead, concentrate on getting the job done in small, doable increments. "Being action-focused tells you what to do to get to where you want to be," says Dr. Murphy. He identifies five steps to get you there.

- Focus on concrete, specific actions.
- Set daily and weekly goals as stepping-stones to your long-term goals.
- Set hard goals rather than easy goals.
- Keep your goals clear and positive.
- Get regular feedback on your progress by keeping a journal or logbook of your progress.

4. **Think creatively.** Use *all* your senses to imagine whatever it is you want to happen, says Dr. Murphy. "Visualization, a popular approach, is limiting," he says. "Using your entire imagination is richer." To get richer quicker, he suggests following these three steps:

- Develop imagination. Practice drawing on all of your senses—sight, hearing, smell, touch and taste—and then actively put yourself in situations that force you to use those senses.
- Imagine how you'll reach your goals. Plan ahead, rehearse the event in your head, devise creative solutions to problems that may obstruct you from reaching your goal.
- Create a successful self-image. "You become the person that you imagine you are," says Dr. Murphy. "If you imagine that you are successful, you'll be successful." In other words, walk the walk and talk the talk.

5. **Build your emotional power muscles.** Too often men respond to emotions by suppressing them, says Dr. Murphy. "We think mental toughness means putting on this invisible armor that will block out all unpleasant emotional encounters. But you cannot completely avoid emotional experiences," he says. The key is learning how to bounce back from emotional setbacks. He suggests this four-step strategy:

- React. If your first reaction to a mistake or an upsetting event is anger, let it out—but in a controlled fashion, says Dr. Murphy.
- Relax. Then calm down quickly. Deep abdominal breathing helps. Various muscle-relaxation exercises also cool you down.
- Reflect. Ask yourself what you've learned from the experience. What was the mistake, and how do you rectify it?
- Renew. Recommit to getting it right. Take the emotional energy and direct it toward constructive results. That way, you can turn a negative emotion into a positive outcome.

6. **Eat breakfast for brainpower.** You can't drive a car from home to work without fuel. You can't think brilliant thoughts at that morning staff meeting without feeding your brain. Fuel up on whole grains and a small amount of protein to charge into the day, suggests Linda Prout, a nutritionist at the Claremont Resort and Spa in Berkeley, California. Avoid high-fat bacon and other meats; digesting all that fat will distract blood from your brain to your stomach—and nobody has gotten a promotion by flaunting his intestinal wisdom.

7. **Get to like lecithin.** This substance helps the body secrete the enzyme choline. The brain turns that enzyme into a neurotransmitter called acetylcholine, which keeps our memory bank accounts full. Lecithin is found in liver, egg yolks and peanuts—all no-no's to people trying to avoid fats. It is also found in soybeans, the stuff of tofu. If that's not your idea of edible food, you can buy lecithin in granulated form and sprinkle it on cereal, suggests Steven Zeisel, M.D., Ph.D., chairman of the nutrition department at the University of North Carolina at Chapel Hill.

8. **Eat boron, think better.** Boron is a micronutrient found in fruits, nuts and vegetables that may help boost brainpower. One study found that people who ate about 3.25 milligrams of it a day scored better on manual dexterity, hand-eye coordination, attention, memory and perception tests than those who didn't. An apple has about 1 milligram of boron, so "these findings would argue that eating more fruits and vegetables might be beneficial," says James G. Penland, Ph.D., the author of the study and a research psychologist at the U.S. Department of Agriculture Human Nutrition Research Center in Grand Forks, North Dakota.

9. **Drink coffee for a quick pick-me-up.** Say what you will about the downside of caffeine, but the chemical *can* be a mind- and mood-booster when taken in moderation, says Judith Wurtman, Ph.D., a nutrition research scientist in the Department of Brain and Cognitive Sciences at Massachusetts Institute of Technology in Cambridge and author of *Managing Your Mind and Mood through Food.* Dr. Wurtman suggests that your body is most sensitive to the slap-in-the-face effect of caffeine when it hasn't had it for a while. That's why that first cup in the morning works so well.

10. **Let music move you to mental heights.** Bring your favorite tapes and compact discs to work when you're on deadline. They may help you get the work done better and faster. Researchers from the State University of New York at Buffalo reported that listening to music while working under stressful conditions may improve concentration and overall performance. In the study, psychologists tested the ability of 50 surgeons to do math calculations with and without musical accompaniment. The doctors were faster and more accurate with the music—and they performed even better when they selected the music themselves. Their pulse rates and blood pressure were also lower. If you don't want to raise your co-workers' pulses, however, be courteous and don't pump up the volume.

11. **Think hard, ward off Alzheimer's.** Mental exercise may be good for your health. That's the conclusion following a Columbia University study in which the mental capacities of 593 volunteers age 60 and over were tested. Researchers found that people who spent their lives in more intellectually demanding occupations had half the risk of developing Alzheimer's disease as those employed in less stimulating positions. One explanation is that an active mind may develop a reserve of brain cells that resists the debilitating disease.

12. **Get brainpower from protein.** A small amount of protein for lunch may help keep mental performance at its peak for the rest of the day, says Elizabeth Somer, R.D., in her book *Food and Mood.* Eating protein prompts the creation of two chemical neurotransmitters in the brain, dopamine and norepinephrine, which keep you more alert. To enhance brainpower, she suggests combining a little protein with a lot of carbohydrates in a light low-fat lunch.

13. **Rediscover your hidden talents.** To unearth your hidden brainpower, return to the past, suggests Thomas Armstrong, Ph.D., author of *7 Kinds of Smart: Identifying and Developing Your Many Intelligences.* "Childhood is the original spawning ground of intelligence," he says. "Visit the place where you grew up or look over old memorabilia from early school days. It'll trigger forgotten memories of the time you won a spelling contest, painted a great picture, got laughs from your friends for hamming it up or spent hours taking stuff apart and putting it back together. All of those are clues about what you find rewarding." Then, he says, build time into your life to cultivate these long-forgotten talents. "Write down five specific things you're going to do in the coming months and years to achieve your goal," he notes. "And then do it. No excuses."

14. **Find focus in rituals.** Take a lesson from world-class athletes who participate in personal little ceremonies before they take the field. Baseball pitcher Dave Stewart fasts on game day. Another pitcher, Bill Swift, listens to Frank Sinatra tapes for 20 minutes in the locker room. Football wide receiver Jerry Rice meticulously chooses exactly the right pair of socks and pants for each game. "Elite athletes use these rituals to become centered so that they can focus on performance," says Bruce Ogilvie, Ph.D., who pioneered the field of sports psychology in the 1960s. "(Athletes) have characteristic ways of getting back into the center of themselves, mainly to eliminate distractions. Home life, issues with the wife or the children, coaching, management—all of these are potential distracters, and it's distraction that causes the slump or inappropriate performance."

15. **Remember to K.I.S.S.** That's Keep It Simple, Stupid. That, in effect, is the advice of Chicago Bulls coach Phil Jackson. A longtime practitioner of Zen meditation, Jackson quotes from Japanese Zen master Suzuki Roshi's book *Zen Mind, Beginner's Mind*: "If your mind is empty, it is always ready for anything; it is open to everything. In the beginner's mind there are many possibilities; in the expert's mind there are few." Keeping a beginner's mind, says Jackson, allows you to be mentally prepared to respond to any situation without preconceived notions.

16. **Meditate on it.** Meditation is one of the oldest disciplines for developing mental toughness known to man. "Meditation is a discipline first and foremost." That comment comes not from some Zen monks in robes sitting crossed-legged in a Himalayan cave. It comes from Coach Jackson of the Bulls. "Meditation allows you to sit and let the mind realize who's in control," he adds. "It gives you a chance to enter the day with peacefulness and also with compassion. It teaches you to wake up, to be conscious and alert."

A large body of research has shown that practicing meditation or any number of other relaxation techniques slows heart rate and calms your whole system, adds Dr. Kabat-Zinn.

17. **Take a breath.** When anger or tension gets the best of you, one of the best techniques is right in front of your nose. Literally. It's your breath. And, again, it's Coach Jackson who best describes how he utilizes it in practical terms. "In tense moments, when anger or frustration comes up, I usually feel tension in my shoulders and neck," says Jackson. "That's a signal that I'm holding my breath. The key for me in getting through those situations without blowing my top is breathing. I take a deep breath, let it go and keeping going on. That's one of the things you teach yourself through meditation—watching your breath."

18. **Take B to beat depression.** A healthy intake of the B complex vitamins is important for anyone who wants to keep depression at bay, recommends Harold Bloomfield, M.D., a psychiatrist in Del Mar, California, and co-author of *How to Heal Depression*. He suggests the following daily supplement program.

- 100 micrograms of folic acid
- 10 milligrams of riboflavin
- 10 milligrams of thiamin
- 10 milligrams of vitamin B_6

7

CURES

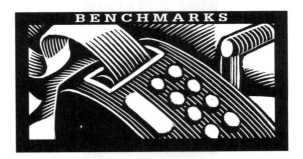

AVERAGES

■ Percentage of Americans who will undergo invasive surgery this year: 12.5

■ Most popular plastic surgery among men: rhinoplasty, or nose reshaping

■ Number of aspirin tablets Americans consume in a year: 80 billion

■ Number of Americans who say that they have quit smoking: 40 million

■ Percentage decrease, since 1970, in the death rate from strokes: 40

■ Percentage decrease, since 1970, in the death rate from heart disease: 14

■ Percentage of men losing their hair: 33.3

■ Percentage of men developing a mental disorder this year: 25

■ Percentage of visits to doctors' offices that last less than 11 minutes: 41

■ Amount that Americans spend annually on surgery to correct benign prostate enlargement: $3 billion to $4 billion

■ Number of colds per year for those 20 or older: 2

■ Number of years spent to develop a new drug: 12

■ Dollar amount spent on developing a new drug: $230 million

EXTREMES

■ Number of leeches sold each year to American surgeons and hospitals by Leeches USA of Westbury, New York: 10,000

■ Odds of dying from falling out of your bed or chair: 1 in 513,142 annually

■ Longest case of the hiccups: patient hiccupped every 1½ seconds for 69 years, 5 months; this case of hiccups began while the patient was slaughtering a hog

■ Longest period of cardiac arrest in which the victim survived: four hours, after a Norwegian fisherman fell overboard into frigid waters

VITAL READING

The Virility Robbers

Avoiding these everyday chemicals could keep your sex life strong and vigorous.

More and more people are peddling herbal remedies, strange drug cocktails and surgical interventions that promise to pump up testosterone levels, improve erections and increase desire—and watching their profits grow at an unprecedented rate. While some of these approaches may be helpful, many are downright dangerous, and most prohibitively expensive. A growing body of research suggests that boosting sexual performance may not depend so much on what you take in as on what you don't take in.

The potency robbers in question are chemicals called organochlorines. These ubiquitous compounds are produced in the manufacture of pesticides, herbicides, petrochemicals, plastics and paper. You're exposed to them every day: eating sprayed produce, fertilizing your lawn, wearing a freshly dry-cleaned suit or breathing too deeply when filling your gas tank. Once in your body, these compounds take up permanent residence in fat deposits.

What happens once these chemicals are in the male body is the subject of fast and furious debate. In the past year, more conferences have been convened on the effects of organochlorines on the male reproductive tract than in the preceding five

decades. In Copenhagen, investigators from Finland, Denmark, France, the United States and Great Britain gathered to analyze the impact of organochlorines on male reproductive health. Closer to home, the Environmental Protection Agency (EPA) brought together folks from government, academia, industry and public-interest groups to hash out the very same issues.

What has them so stirred up? Global reports of increasing declines in men's reproductive health are beginning to multiply exponentially and correspond exactly with the increase in the use of the organochlorines. The latest report, from the Center for the Study of the Conservation of Human Eggs and Sperm, in Paris, has found that sperm counts have dropped an average of 2 percent in the last two decades. In 1973, the average sperm concentration was 89 million per milliliter of semen, compared with 60 million in 1992. The frequency with which the male factor is responsible for a couple's infertility has increased in recent years from about 10 percent to 25 percent, reports the British medical journal *The Lancet*. And testicular cancer rates have tripled since 1950 and doubled in White men since 1973. Prostate cancer has shown a similar alarming increase.

These human developments, in conjunction with the effects of organochlorines in wildlife, have compelled researchers to step up their efforts at exploring the nature of these chemicals' effects on men. "We conclude that these issues taken in toto indicate the need for a vigorous research effort to understand the extent of the problem, its underlying etiology and the development of a strategy for prevention and intervention," write the Copenhagen group of investigators.

Blocking Out Testosterone

In the past, some scientists have focused on organochlorines acting as a kind of corrupted estrogen, possibly triggering breast cancer, for example, by overloading a woman's system with "bad" estrogen.

Increasingly, however, there's speculation that these chemicals may actually block testosterone, and other androgens, much more directly. "As we look more closely at these particular chemicals, we're finding that some may produce feminizing effects, not by mimicking estrogen but rather by blocking the ability of androgens to work," says Penelope Fenner-Crisp, acting deputy director of the Office of Pesticides Programs at the EPA in Washington, D.C.

The demasculinizing phenomena that researchers have observed, such as decreased sperm count and diminished testicular size, may be merely by-products of the organochlorines' direct impact on testosterone levels. "One possibility is that these organochlorines trigger a man's hormonal feedback system, essentially influencing the brain to shut off testosterone production in the testis," says Kenneth Korach, Ph.D., chief of the receptor biology section at the National Institute of Environmental Health Sciences in Research Triangle Park, North Carolina. "The testis may become much less active; sperm production and perhaps size may decrease."

While the organochlorines' possible fertility effects pose a problem for younger men, direct assault on testosterone levels could have the most impact on men in their fifties and sixties. The reduced libido, fatigue, erectile dysfunction, loss of muscle mass and depression that many men consider natural by-products of aging are often symptoms of low testosterone levels. In fact, subnormal testosterone levels are estimated to affect as many as 15 percent of men over the age of 65.

Are Men at Risk?

One of the biggest questions facing researchers is how much exposure to these organochlorines is too much. "Some researchers believe in the threshold effect; that is, very low levels of exposure wouldn't trigger an effect," explains Fenner-Crisp. "Only very large doses would tip the balance out of your favor."

Others, like Ana Soto, M.D., associate professor of anatomy and cell biology at Tufts University School of Medicine in Boston, believe that lots of exposure to very low levels of these chemicals could create a problem: "Estrogenic chemicals may act cumulatively when each is present at subthreshold doses."

But according to the EPA's Dioxin Reassessment report, the average "body burden" of organochlorines in the U.S. population is already high enough to cause harm.

A Pre-emptive Strike

While researchers are trying to figure out what's going on, we may be unwittingly eating or handling certain chemicals that could be impeaching our manhood. "There's a massive research agenda here that's going to take at least a decade," says Devra Lee Davis, Ph.D., senior adviser to the National Cancer Institute and one of the leading researchers in the field of organochlorines and breast cancer. "But it would be unfortunate if precautionary principles were not being developed to try and reduce exposure to suspect agents."

To that end, here's a list of simple ways you can reduce your exposure to organochlorines, and possibly lessen your cancer risk, while boosting your testosterone levels.

Monitor your drinking water. As many as 3.5 million Americans living in the Midwest have been exposed through their tap water to organochlorine weed killers used on corn, reported the Environmental Working Group recently.

And the problem isn't limited to the Midwest: Fifty percent of Americans drink groundwater that may be contaminated with organochlorines draining from family farms, paper manufacturers and other sources.

If you're concerned about your water supply, contact your local water supplier and ask for specifics about the water quality. You can then call EPA's Safe Drinking Water Hot Line at 1-800-426-4791 and ask operators to help you make sense of the data. If your water does turn out to be contaminated, or if you just want to be on the safe side, consider investing in a water filter. Or simply switch to spring water.

Cut back on meat. Researchers refer to organochlorines as bioaccumulative, meaning that they like to stick around for a good long time and become more concentrated as you move up the food chain. So when a cow chows down on grain sprayed with an anti-androgen herbicide, you get a powerful dose. "Food animals already have a toxic load accumulated in their own fat tissue. When a man eats meat, he gets a much larger dose than he would from eating a vegetable containing some pesticide residue," says Frank Falck, M.D., Ph.D., an ophthalmologist-toxicologist and author of a study that found high concentrations of organochlorines in the breast tissue of women who developed cancer.

When you do eat meat, opt for lean cuts—pesticides seek out fat. Better yet, buy your meat from farms and suppliers that feed their livestock with organic grains and don't use growth hormones. One good mail-order source is Walnut Acres, a Pennsylvania-based organic farm that sells hormone-free chicken, beef and eggs. Call them at 1-800-433-3998 for a free catalog.

Take it easy on your lawn. Researchers have found links between use of herbicides and an increased risk of testicular and prostate cancers. A recent study from Denmark also found that organic farmers had unusually high sperm densities. And another study found that children whose lawns were treated with herbicides had four times the risk of certain kinds of cancers as children with untreated lawns.

"I recommend limiting the use of household pesticides and garden chemicals to those that are absolutely necessary," says Dr. Davis, who cautions that men thinking of fathering a child should refrain from using them at all in the four months before trying to reproduce.

Using mulching mowers, making your own compost and aerating soil can help you grow a healthy lawn without resorting to pesticides and chemical fertilizers. Letting grass remain 2½ to 3½ inches tall can also cut down on unwanted weeds, as the extra blade height can shade them into an early demise.

If you do resort to lawn chemicals, be sure to wear protective clothing that covers as much of your skin as possible. Afterward, wash the clothes for three full laundry cycles using warm or hot water and throw out any clothes on which undiluted chemicals have spilled. For more information, call the EPA's toll-free National Pesticide Telecommunications Network at 1-800-858-7378.

Be fishy about fish. Since many freshwater lakes and streams are loaded with organochlorines, so are many freshwater fish, especially if they hail from one of the Great Lakes or the Chesapeake Bay. Some experts recommend choosing smaller fish (short lives mean less exposure to pollutants), cutting off all visible fat before cooking and opting for saltwater fish whenever you can.

Before baiting your own hook, check with your state department of natural resources and find out if your favorite fishing hole is on any pollutants hit list. If so, go ahead and sink your line—just make sure to throw 'em back.

Skip dry cleaning. One of the most potent organochlorines, perchloroethylene, is used routinely by 90 percent of traditional dry cleaners. "Although the EPA regulates dry cleaners so they don't pollute the outside air, the real source of the exposure is the clothes themselves," says Lance Wallace, Ph.D., an environmental scientist with the EPA's Office of Research and Development. During one of four major studies on personal exposure, Dr. Wallace and his colleagues found that levels of the chemical were about 100 times higher indoors than outdoors at homes with recently dry-cleaned clothes stored in closets.

You can cut your exposure by about 20 percent by hanging your clothes on a balcony or porch for a day before you put them in a closet. Or find one of the crop of dry cleaners that use a solvent-free cleaning process like soap-and-steam.

Freshen your house the natural way. Crystals, balls and solid home deodorizers release the organochlorine paraperidichlorobenzene as they "melt." To play it safe, freshen your rooms the old-fashioned way by opening a window. As for mothproofing woolens, opt for cedar or all-natural herbal packets.

Play it safe when fixing up. Methylene chloride (also known as DCM, methylene dichloride and methylene bichloride) is an organochlorine found in everything from paint removers to wood glues, furniture polishes to varnishes. If you're doing any project involving refinishing of wood, you're probably using DCM.

Look for products in your local hardware store labeled "solvent-free." Check out their labels for any of the aliases of methylene chloride as well as another solvent reported to have adverse hormonal effects, toluene. If avoiding these chemicals isn't possible, make sure that you work in a well-ventilated area, set up a fan near your work space to blow fumes out of the room and wear a respirator mask if you're going to be doing fine work that involves bending down close to the wood. Avoid using one solvent right after another, and skip the beer—alcohol may heighten methylene chloride's effects.

Nature's Cure for a Prostate Problem

A centuries-old herbal remedy may be more effective at shrinking enlarged prostates than the best new drugs.

These days you can't pick up a magazine or watch a late-night TV show without being bombarded with images of men kept up at night by the symptoms of their enlarged prostates: urinary urgency and frequency. Equally inescapable are the claims of major American pharmaceutical companies that drugs like Hytrin, Proscar and Cardura can turn back the clock on enlarged prostate, or benign prostatic hyperplasia (BPH).

The trouble is that for many men with mild symptoms, such drugs can cause more problems than they solve, replacing pesky urinary symptoms with things like impotence, dizziness, low libido and breast enlargement. New research suggests that there may be a way out of this overkill: a kinder, gentler, herbal alternative that's as close as your neighborhood drugstore.

The herb in question is the saw palmetto berry, also called *Serenoa repens*. Native to the United States, it was first used hundreds of years ago by the Seminole Indians, who considered it a potent aphrodisiac. Over the past two decades, however, it has gained wide acceptance as a prostate treatment throughout Europe. In fact, most recent available figures indicate that saw palmetto accounts for 38 percent of all medications prescribed for BPH in Italy alone. That's a bigger chunk of the market than any synthetic BPH drug can claim.

And the herb's continental popularity is not just a matter of folk wisdom. Just ask James Duke, Ph.D., former economic botanist for the U.S. Department of Agriculture and author of the *CRC Handbook of Medicinal Herbs*. "I'd bet my prostate on the fact that this stuff works," notes Dr. Duke, who has devoted the last 55 years to the study of edible plants and medicinal herbs. "Not only are there men in Europe and America who swear by it, but I can count a good number of scientific studies done over the last decade that indicate saw palmetto can help relieve symptoms in men with BPH."

A British study of 110 men with BPH showed that saw palmetto extract significantly increased urine flow, decreased the amount of urine left in the bladder after urinating and reduced nighttime trips to the bathroom. And a study conducted in Italy on 40 BPH patients showed similar improvements in symptoms among men taking the herb, as compared with men taking a placebo.

All Roads Lead to Testosterone

Just how does it work? The herb may prevent the breakdown of testosterone into dihydrotestosterone (DHT), a more potent form of the hormone that researchers believe may trigger prostate enlargement, according to research done by Franco diSilverio, M.D., a urologist at the University Bracci in Rome. And while the herb reduces the size of the prostate, it does so without compromising testosterone levels in the blood. Indeed, lab studies of prostate tissue from rats fed saw palmetto reveal that while their testosterone levels are the same as those of rats that didn't receive the herb, their levels of DHT are lower.

With all the evidence that saw palmetto offers a safe, effective and low-cost option for men with BPH symptoms, what's the real reason the American medical machine has ignored it for so long?

The key, says Dr. Duke, is money. The testing necessary to get Food and Drug Administration (FDA) approval for most drugs costs upward of $200 million. Small herbal companies simply don't have that kind of money. And large drug companies aren't going to spend money on

something that may compete with their top products and, in the case of herbs, can't be patented. "So we're stuck in a system where we pay two to three times more for 'approved' drugs, and our doctors won't recommend an herb that's working for men all over Europe," explains Dr. Duke. "We grow it here and ship it to the Europeans so that they can get the benefits. It makes absolutely no sense."

Another point that makes no sense to many experts is that despite saw palmetto's lack of side effects, the FDA outlawed its sale as an over-the-counter prostate treatment in 1990, the same year that the agency approved the prescription drug finasteride. Notes Andrew Weil, M.D., professor of medicine at the University of Arizona College of Medicine in Tucson and author of *Spontaneous Healing*, "It's hard to avoid the suspicion that their decision could have been influenced by the emergence of a new prescription drug."

Saw palmetto can still be sold legally in the United States as a food supplement, although that designation also means, since it's not a drug, it can't be prescribed by a doctor. But that doesn't stop physicians like Dr. Weil from recommending it to their patients. "Patients will come to me with BPH symptoms and say, 'I'm not ready for hardcore drug therapy.' They're looking for a natural alternative. Saw palmetto is ideal for them, because it's so low-risk. There are no side effects, and if it doesn't work, they can always try standard therapy," he says. "They've literally got nothing to lose and a lot to gain."

Exterminating a Pesky Bug

Suppressing stomach acid won't cure an ulcer. Killing the acid-causing bacteria will.

Although researchers have known for more than ten years that a kind of bacterium is the cause of much stomach pain, most men who walk into a doctor's office with an ulcer still walk out with a prescription for drugs that suppress stomach acid without killing the bug that caused it in the first place.

And the situation only promises to get worse as the aisles of drugstores all across America undergo a revolution. Two acid-suppressing quick fixes—Tagamet (cimetidine) and Pepcid AC (famotidine)—have been approved for nonprescription use and have been elbowing their way past pink and blue jugs of antacids in an attempt to win a share of the $4.8 billion gastric-relief stakes. Now you won't need a doctor to prescribe the wrong drug; you can do it yourself.

Unlike antacids, which neutralize stomach acids after they've been secreted, acid suppressors stop the acid from being released by the stomach in the first place. But, despite their proven effectiveness for treating occasional heartburn, acid blockers don't address the underlying problem in men with more chronic gastric distress: the bacterium *Helicobacter pylori*.

Alive and well in at least 50 percent of all American men, this infectious pest disturbs the cell lining in the digestive tract, leaving it more vulnerable to repeated ulceration by stomach acid and, ultimately, gastric cancer. Recent studies have shown that as many as 90 percent of people with duodenal ulcers (the most common type) and 60 percent of those with gastric cancer are infected with *H. pylori*.

"Treating an ulcer by attacking stomach acid cures a given ulcer, but it doesn't cure ulcer disease, since it doesn't wipe out the bacteria," explains David Peura, M.D., associate professor of medicine at the University of Virginia School of Medicine in Charlottesville. As a result, as soon as a man who's had an ulcer stops taking the acid suppressors, he has a 75 percent chance of developing a second ulcer—and spending more money on drugs. A recent study found that the average treatment for ulcer disease with drugs like Tagamet runs over $11,000 for 15 years. Not an over-the-counter habit you want to get into—unless you have very deep pockets.

And a man with an ulcer undergoing such treatment has more to lose than time and money: Acid blockers can suppress erections and hair growth along with stomach acid. Tagamet works as an anti-androgen, meaning that it can thwart testosterone's action in the body, according to a decade's worth of research. The result? Softened erections, swollen male breasts and thinning hair.

There is an easier way. Triple-drug therapy, a combination of two antibiotics (often metronidazole and clarithromycin) and an acid inhibitor (often omeprazole), costs an average of $300, lasts for two to three weeks and completely cures the disease in more than 95 percent of those treated. There's not universal agreement on which three drugs are best, and some regimens require taking as many as 15 pills a day, but once the bugs are gone, they're almost always gone for good.

Given that doctors have access to the drugs used for triple-drug therapy, why aren't they prescribing them? Many are simply unaware of the supporting research. Even though the National Institutes of Health has released a consensus report endorsing triple-drug therapy for the treatment of ulcers and study after study confirms its efficacy, the Food and Drug Administration (FDA) has not yet formally approved the individual drugs for the treatment of ulcers. Since it's often the pharmaceutical representatives that bring new information to the physicians—and they can't make any claims unless the FDA says so—many doctors are still in the dark.

Heartburn or Ulcer?

So what should you do if it seems as if your stomach may have made it onto *H. pylori*'s hit list? First, stay calm: Most men with stomach upset don't have an ulcer.

If you typically suffer from bloating, gas or cramps, you probably have what doctors call nonulcer dyspepsia, a fancy name for upset stomach. The verdict is still out on whether triple-drug therapy may help these kinds of symptoms; sometimes, relief is as simple as eliminating spicy foods or caffeine. Antacids and acid suppressors can also help.

A burning sensation behind the breastbone after a particularly spicy or large meal usually means heartburn. With a little forethought, acid suppressors can stop the discomfort before it starts. Take one before you pop those peppers. Once you start to feel the burn, however, an antacid will probably be a better—or at least a faster—bet.

Should the pain or discomfort lead you to self-medicate daily for more than two weeks, see your doctor. If you also feel a gnawing sensation above the breastbone, you may be grappling with an ulcer. If your doctor runs a barium x-ray or an endoscopy and confirms its presence, talk to him about trying triple-drug therapy right off the bat.

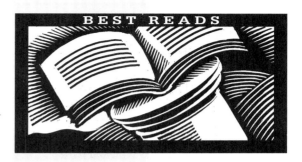

BEST READS

Optimizing Your Healing System

Andrew Weil, M.D., professor of medicine at the University of Arizona College of Medicine in Tucson, certainly has struck a nerve. His book Spontaneous Healing *(Alfred A. Knopf, 1995) has become one of the most well-read health titles of recent years. In it, he describes how the natural power of the mind can play a key role in ridding the body of disease. In this excerpt he introduces several obstacles to proper healing.*

How would you experience optimal efficiency of your healing system? Very likely, you would not be aware of it, because we tend to pay little attention to our health when it is good. You would recover speedily from illness and heal from injuries uneventfully. Ordinary stresses of everyday life might annoy you but would not derange your digestion or blood pressure. Sleep would be restful, sex enjoyable. Aging of your body would occur gradually, allowing you to moderate your activity appropriately and live out a normal life span without undue discomfort. You would not contract heart disease or cancer in middle age, be crippled by arthritis in later life or lose your mind to premature senility.

This scenario is realistic and, I think, worth working for. Actually, the body wants to be healthy, because health represents efficient operation of all of its systems. A useful analogy is the engine of a car. When all components are doing what they should be doing in just the right way, efficiency is maximal, and operation is quiet, producing a "contented" purr that you rarely notice. An engine that calls attention to itself by sounding noisy and rough, knocking and expelling black smoke is not efficient. Since efficiency is the ratio of work done to energy supplied, the sick engine is working harder to accomplish less. In a similar way, it takes less energy to be a healthy person than to be a sick one, and just as a driver may not pay attention to the sound of a well-running engine, people may not be aware of the condition of good health until it breaks down. A program to boost the efficiency of the healing system will not necessarily produce immediately noticeable changes. It is a long-term investment in the future of the body. If you are seeking boundless energy, eternal happiness, an ageless body or immortality, please look elsewhere. I will be writing only of real possibilities, consistent with the findings of medical science.

I propose to introduce this subject by asking you to consider obstacles to healing. If you understand the general kinds of problems that interfere with healing, you will know what kinds of preventive and corrective action you can take.

Lack of Energy

Healing requires energy. Energy is supplied by metabolism, the process of conversion of caloric energy in food to chemical energy that the body can use for its various functions. Malnourished and starving people are not good candidates for spontaneous healing. Even people who eat enough may not metabolize well for one reason or another; despite their caloric intake, they may suffer deficits of energy that impede healing.

A young woman came to me complaining of fatigue; she also had suffered a nonunion of a broken bone in the leg. Over the years, a number of (male) doctors had written her off as a complaining female, but to me the nonunion of a fractured bone and a persistent bruise on a big toe suggested a physical problem; and given her other symptoms and history, I suspected hypothyroidism even though her thyroid function tests were normal. The patient came from a distant city, and I found it very difficult to put her under the care of a physician who was willing to attempt thyroid hormone replacement. When she did start treatment, there was no change in her condition for quite some time. But finally, after ten weeks, her symptoms began to recede. Depression lifted, energy increased and menstruation and digestion improved as metabolism slowly returned to normal. With these changes, her healing ability returned as well.

Hypothyroidism provides a clear illustration of the dependence of the healing system on the availability of energy from metabolism. More common reasons for insufficient metabolic energy are inadequate diets, impaired digestion and improper breathing, all of which are within your control.

An adequate diet means one that provides not only enough calories but also all the nutrients necessary for efficient metabolism without any excesses that promote disease.

The term *impaired digestion* covers a wide range of ailments, from esophageal reflux to hemorrhoids, with a variety of stomach and intestinal complaints in between. But, until proved otherwise, most digestive problems should be assumed to be rooted in stress, because the mind has an unlimited capacity to interfere with normal operation of the gastrointestinal system by disturbing the balance of the autonomic (involuntary) nerves that regulate it.

When I say that improper breathing can lead to deficits of metabolic energy, I have a picture in mind of an extreme example: a man I know in his late forties who suffers from emphysema and lifelong bronchitis and asthma. Despite a healthy appetite, he is no more than skin and bones, unable to store up reserves of metabolic energy simply because he cannot take in enough oxygen to burn the fuel he eats. Even in the absence of chronic lung disease, poor breathing can limit metabolism and the amount of energy available for healing.

Finally, I should mention that lack of energy can also result from immoderate expenditure of energy as a result of overwork, overexertion, lack of rest and sleep and addictive use of stimulant drugs. Obviously, these problems are also correctable.

Poor Circulation

The healing system depends on the circulation of blood to bring energy and materials to a malfunctioning or injured area. You can see graphic examples of impaired healing due to poor circulation in persons with diabetes whose arteries are subject to premature and rapid progression of atherosclerosis as a result of their altered metabolism. Diabetics must be careful not to cut or nick their feet, since even a slight break in the skin may turn into a large ulcer that refuses to heal. The body just cannot supply enough nourishment, oxygen and immune activity to the area because of insufficient circulation.

You can maintain your circulatory system in good working order by following a healthy diet, by not smoking and by exercising.

Restricted Breathing

I have already mentioned that restricted breathing can reduce efficiency of the healing system through its dampening effect on metabolism, but I believe that it can interfere in other ways as well. The operations of the brain and the nervous system depend on adequate exchange of oxygen and carbon dioxide, as do those of the

heart and the circulatory system and all organs of the body. Breathing may be the master function of the body, affecting all others. Restrictions in breathing can be the result of past traumas, both physical and emotional. Most of us have never received instruction about breathing and how to take advantage of it as a harmonizer of mind and body.

Impaired Defenses

Spontaneous healing is unlikely to occur if the body's defenses are weak. Defense is the responsibility of the immune system, whose main job is to distinguish between self and not-self and take action against the latter. When immunity is crippled, as in AIDS, it is easy to see how much of a problem this creates for the healing system. When immunity is weakened in more subtle ways, impairment of healing may be less obvious.

There are three main categories of weakening influences on the immune system: (1) persistent or overwhelming infections, (2) toxic injury by certain forms of matter and energy and (3) unhealthy mental states. You can protect yourself against all of these influences and, in addition, learn techniques to enhance immunity through adjustments in diet, exercise and judicious use of vitamins, minerals, and herbs.

Toxins

Toxic overload is one of the commonest reasons for diminished healing responses, but the subject is immensely complicated, emotionally charged and highly political. We take toxins into our body with the food we eat, the water we drink and the air we breathe, as well as in the form of drugs we use, whether we obtain them on medical prescription, buy them over the counter or use them recreationally. I am concerned about toxic forms of energy as well as matter; electromagnetic pollution may be the most significant form of pollution that human activity has produced in this century, all the more dangerous because it is invisible and insensible.

Whether energetic or material, toxins can damage DNA, which contains the information needed for spontaneous healing; disrupt the biological controls on which the healing system depends; weaken defenses and promote the development of cancer and other diseases that already represent failures of healing by the time they make themselves known. Toxic overload may be a significant cause of allergy, autoimmune disease and a variety of degenerative diseases (like Parkinson's disease and ALS, or amyotrophic lateral sclerosis), whose causes now seem obscure.

The medical profession and the scientific research community have been remarkably slow to pay attention to this issue, which I consider to be one of the greatest threats to health and well-being in the world today. You have probably read stories in the press about clusters of leukemia cases in neighborhoods near power lines, about the increasing incidence of lymphoma among farmers who use agricultural chemicals and about a worldwide increase in asthma and bronchitis as air pollution gets worse. Recently, I have followed news stories about a mysterious cluster of lupus cases in the border town of Nogales, Arizona, not far from my home near Tucson. Systemic lupus erythematosus is a potentially serious autoimmune disease not known to be communicable or to have environmental causes. Yet the incidence in Nogales is many times the national average. In 1994 reporters found that a ranching operation on the Mexican side of the border had been dumping pesticides into streams and burning manure contaminated with pesticides because it could not afford to build a proper disposal facility. No causal link is yet established, but I predict that one will be.

If you want to increase the likelihood of spontaneous healing, it is imperative that you learn to guard against toxic injury. That means limiting exposure, protecting your body from the effects of pollution and helping your body eliminate any toxins that do get in.

Age

We assume that age is an obstacle to healing, that old people do not heal as readily as young people and have lowered immunity and resistance in general. Actually, there is little research to support those assumptions, but observation suggests that they are true. It is impressive to watch how quickly children heal from simple surgeries, like hernia repairs and appendectomies. This is not to say that old people are incapable of spontaneous healing, just that it may take more time. Moreover, methods may exist to protect the healing system from the effects of aging as well as to stimulate general resistance and vitality in the elderly.

Traditional Chinese medicine has identified a number of natural substances that act as tonics of this sort. As a group they appear to be nontoxic and effective. Some of them are now available in the United States. I have reviewed the literature on these substances and have tried some of them myself and with patients. You cannot stop the changes of time, but you can modify lifestyle and activity as you age, and it is good to know that help is available to maintain the efficiency of your healing system.

Obstruction by the Mind

Spontaneous healing can be triggered by mental events; it can also be frustrated by habitual ways of using the mind. I have already noted that the mind can depress the immune system and can unbalance the autonomic nervous system, leading to disturbances in digestion, circulation and all other internal functions. You must know how to use the mind in the service of healing.

Spiritual Problems

During my travels throughout the world, I have met many healers who believe that the primary causes of health and illness are not physical but spiritual. They direct their attention toward an invisible world assumed to exist beyond the ordinary world of the senses. In this realm they search for reasons for illness and ways to cure it. Some of these people believe in karmic causes of illness (actions in the past or in past lives); others, in the ability of deceased ancestors to affect one's life and health; others, in possession by spirits; and still others, in the possibility of psychic attack by malevolent shamans. It is impossible to talk to most scientists about an invisible world, since scientific materialism looks only for physical causes of physical events. I have learned not to try to discuss the possibility of nonphysical causation of physical events with most doctors, but I do discuss it with some patients and think about it a lot. Therefore, I would not consider this discussion without noting the spiritual dimension of healing.

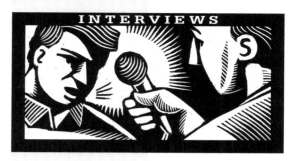

Thomas Platts-Mills on
Asthma Causes and Cures

Anytime Hollywood wants to portray someone as a geek, they have the prop department send over a pair of thick black glasses, a pocket protector, a slide rule and an asthma inhaler. That's not exactly fair to asthma sufferers. After all, many sports stars—including Dominique Wilkins and Jim Ryun—have asthma, too. In fact, asthma affects all types of men and has many different triggers, some easily avoided.

In an interview, Thomas Platts-Mills, M.D., Ph.D., director of the Division of Allergy and Clinical Immunology at the University of Virginia Medical Center in Charlottesville, describes some of the most common causes and treatments for asthma.

How is asthma usually manifesting itself in men between the ages of 25 and 55?

It may show up as a shortage of breath in exercise, coughing and shortness of breath at night or coughing and wheezing during the day. Some of them only have it during exercise.

How quickly will you move to eliminate environmental factors that may be causing the asthma?

If the patient doesn't respond to treatment such as bronchodilators and require inhaled steroids, then it's important to find out what's causing it.

What is the number one environmental cause of asthma among men in this age group?

It's clearly dust mites and indoor animals.

Does that mean you may have to get rid of your dog or cat?

You need to know if they are really causing the problem. We don't recommend getting rid of the cat just because you have asthma. You have to have a positive skin test as well.

Let's say you have a positive skin test to your pet, and asthma?

We would recommend getting rid of the cat. But there are a lot of other steps that you can take. You have to reduce the reservoirs—which is the word that we use for something like a carpet or a sofa that stores allergen from the cat and becomes a major source itself. If you get rid of the carpets and upholstered sofas and cover your mattress and pillow, you can put in an air filter in the house or a room air filter. Probably a HEPA (high-efficiency particulate air) filter. And then the final thing is that you should wash the cat once a week. But it's best to do it yourself instead of having a vet do it.

Suppose someone chose to remove the pet. Would that be the end of their problems?

No. You'd either have to remove the carpet and sofas or aggressively clean them—steam clean them.

Are you familiar with any of the vitamin and mineral therapies that are available today for the treatment of asthma?

They might be helpful in some cases, but when you do controlled trials, you usually can't find an effect.

Do any vitamins or minerals, like magnesium, seem to have more promise?

I think magnesium is interesting, and I don't doubt that some people do better on magnesium, but it's difficult to tell exactly who should receive it.

What about a cup of black coffee?

It's clearly of benefit. That's been known for 100 years.

How long will you have the benefit of asthma symptom reduction after you drink a cup of coffee?

The molecule of caffeine is very similar to the molecule of theophylline, a chemical that is in our asthma medications. It provides relief for about an hour.

Do you believe that foods can bring on asthma?

There's no question about that.

What are the worst offenders, in your opinion?

Eggs, milk and soy can do it. Or any of the major food allergens (shrimp, peanuts and chocolate are others). It's not very common, but it can certainly happen.

Does milk cause mucus?

Yes, or you may simply be allergic to it.

Can you tell me more about the exercise/asthma connection?

Exercise doesn't cause asthma; it triggers asthma. So you can have mild asthma and never see it at all until you exercise, and then it triggers. But exercise isn't the cause. The same thing with cold air. Cold air doesn't cause asthma; it does trigger it.

If you had to recommend anything else for guys suffering from asthma, what would you suggest?

We're seeing patients with asthma in their thirties and forties who have fungal infection on their feet. If they have chronic athlete's foot or fungal infection of their feet, they should ask an allergist whether they think it's contributing to their asthma. And in order to answer that, they need to be skin tested.

What's the connection there?

We think that they are absorbing antigen from the feet, and if you treat the fungal infection on their feet, their asthma often improves. We don't think it's very common. Some of the patients have severe asthma and then they get better on antifungal treatments, so we think it's something that they should think about. In adult males, that is definitely something that they should be aware of.

So the fungal infection shows up first and then the asthma?

Usually, they have known that they had a fungal infection on their feet for years. I've seen people who have known they had fungal infection in their toes and then get sinusitis. They get a little asthma and wheeze, and then they get worse. And when you skin test them, they are allergic to the fungus that causes the infection. It's also quite clear that some of the more severe cases of asthma are associated with sinusitis, but it's difficult to treat sinusitis—a recurrent sinus infection. With the fungal infection of the feet, we think there's something that you can do with it. And that's treat the feet.

Do they have to treat the asthma as well?

We don't ever want to give anyone the impression that they can stop their treatment for asthma just because they've done something else.

Is it true that there's been a doubling of asthma cases over the past decade and, if so, to what would you attribute that?

I don't know, and I'm not sure that it's increased in this age group. It's increased in school-age children, I think. But the big question there is whether it's due to housing conditions. Houses have become tighter and hotter, and more people are spending more time indoors. So that may be important to school-age children; however, there have been many other changes in lifestyle over the past 30 years.

Edward Laskowski on
Knee Pain Causes and Cures

Countless sports greats have been permanently sidelined by knee problems. But it's the sports less-than-greats—your friends, brothers or co-workers—who have the knee problems that scare you. Nothing makes you more sensitive to the slightest twinge of knee pain than losing a tennis buddy for six months to a weekend-warrior injury.

In this interview, Edward Laskowski, M.D., co-director of the Mayo Clinic Sports Medicine Center in Rochester, Minnesota, and a specialist in physical medicine and rehabilitation, details the most common knee problems and some surprisingly simple ways to keep your knees healthy.

What are the most common knee problems?

A sprain or torn ligament. The two most injured ligaments—and the ones we hear most about—are the anterior cruciate ligament (the ACL) and the medial collateral ligament (the MCL). The ACL is one that you hear a lot about in sports—a lot of professional athletes have sustained this injury. It's a significant injury to one of the main stabilizers of the knee—the ligament that controls the forward motion of the lower-leg bone or the tibia. And you don't even have to get hit in the knee to get this injury. Many times it's just an aggressive cutting maneuver—like a soccer player who plants and changes directions quickly. Or a wide receiver. Or a basketball player doing much the same thing.

You may hear a pop during the injury, and most of the time, you're not able to continue your game. Your knee feels like it's buckling or giving way. This is probably what was happening when people used to talk about a "trick knee."

And what about the MCL injury? How does that usually occur?

Someone gets hit on the outside of the leg, and the ligament on the inside gets stretched. A football player might get this if he is running and someone hits him on the outside of the leg. Skiers, too, if they catch an edge wrong.

What should you do if you think that either of these has happened to you?

With an ACL, the best you can do is ice it and then see a doctor. It's an injury that should be x-rayed and evaluated by somebody who has expertise in evaluation of the knee because you can have associated bone fracture and cartilage tears. In addition, in a young athlete who competes in high-impact or rapid cutting or pivoting sports, surgical reconstruction may be considered. An MCL injury is a little different. Grade one injuries are still quite stable. So after you ice it down for a while and get the strength up again, you can really do well with it. The important thing is to do the exercises that are recommended to you. Strengthen that knee.

Some experts recommend walking backward to help rehabilitate a knee injury. Do you ever recommend that?

With backward walking, you're challenging the muscles of your leg in a different way. So if you are a defensive back in football, you really should practice that—backward running and walking—because that's what you're doing in your sport.

That is the principle of "sport-specific" training—you should train your muscle groups in the exact same manner in which you use them in your sport. If, on the other hand, you are a bicycle rider, I don't know if backward walking is really going to add much to your program. I think that you are going to need to train the muscles that are specifically used in biking. Train on the bike more. And work on your strength more in your lower-extremity muscles, along with your aerobic conditioning.

As far as rehabilitation goes, it could be a good tool—depending on what tissue is injured in the lower extremity. It could help you with some hamstring pulls and some other injuries to help you become strong in different motions, but we always go back to what the person is actually going to be doing—either on his job or in his sport—and then we try to train them accordingly.

A tennis player is going to require a lot more lateral and side-to-side movement because he is always cutting across the court and pivoting. You need to train him that way, using, for example, a slide board, something that requires a similar movement.

Slide boards seem dangerous for someone who is worried about his knees. Are they?

Used properly, they're a great aerobic workout, and you're using muscles that you don't normally use when you're just jogging or running. If you're a skater, skier, tennis player or racquetball player and constantly going from side to side, you need your leg muscles strong for that kind of movement. So it's a matter of training the muscles for that kind of activity, and a slide board is a good way to do that.

Some experts suggest placing arch supports or orthotics in your shoes for knee pain. Do you?

It can help. Just because you have flat feet alone doesn't mandate that you are going to have a knee injury or pain. A lot of people have flat feet and don't have any pain at all. But if you have flat feet and do a lot of high-impact exercise like running, you could get something called medial tibia stress syndrome, or shinsplints. And that's because the flatness of the arch concentrates a lot of the force or pressure on the tibia (the lower-leg bone). When you use the arch support, you equalize the force and distribute it more evenly throughout the lower leg. And in the same manner, some people may get more inner knee pain if they do a lot of running and have a significant flat foot. So, yes, sometimes putting in an arch support can help.

Are they expensive?

No, there are some off-the-shelf molds that are good and fairly inexpensive.

Are there other types of knee pain that men need to look out for?

We find patellofemorals pain or anterior knee pain to be a big problem, too. And that's basically a tracking problem of the kneecap.

What causes it?

It can be due to tight muscles on the outside of the upper thigh. That pulls the kneecap to the outside. Tight quadriceps and hamstrings increase the compression forces in the joint where the kneecap meets the knee. Weakness in the inner muscle of the quadriceps can also predispose the kneecap to track improperly, irritating the underlying tissues beneath the kneecap—especially repetitive activities like stair climbing that require knee flexion. Or if you're sitting for a long time at a theater watching a movie—you'll notice some stiffness. Even kneeling or bending for a long time can cause it.

Who seems to have this problem?

It often surfaces when you get into an aggressive exercise program that includes running or impact-loading sports like basketball or volleyball. Usually, these are people who have tight muscles in their lower extremities, especially in that outer band, the iliotibial band, and perhaps in the quadriceps and hamstrings. And they may not do any regular exercises to strengthen the rest of the muscles of the thigh. And sometimes it's just the way that you're made. Some people are just more predisposed with the way their lower extremity bones are aligned to having this kind of pain. People come in and say, "The pain is right here." And they point to their kneecaps.

Will stair climbing bring on this problem?

It can. It's what we call a very flexion-biased exercise. Your knees are always flexed, and you're cranking away at those steps, up and down, up and down. That can bring about the problem. If you work out on a stair-climbing machine properly, it could actually help treat it. But people may notice it for the first time when they start using a stair-climbing machine.

You mentioned people who are born with certain biomechanical problems. How do you treat them for knee pain?

Stretching is key. We really have them work on stretching. A good hamstring stretch, a good quadriceps stretch and a stretch for that tissue located on the outside of the thigh called the iliotibial band. There are very definite, discrete techniques for getting at each of those muscle groups. In combination with that, we like strengthening for the inner part of the quad muscles. *Quad* means "four parts." There's one muscle on the inner thigh of the knee that we want strong because that keeps the kneecap tracking appropriately. And there are some exercises that you can do for that, like squats, leg presses and lunges. Bicycling also tends to work that muscle fairly well.

One of the more severe knee injuries is a meniscal tear. How is that caused?

It usually occurs when your knee is flexed and you are pivoting or changing direction very rapidly—like when you are playing tennis or racquetball. You immediately feel the pain, and you may get swelling that develops over a day. As you get older, there is some wear and tear in the cartilage, and you can also get what's called a degenerative meniscal tear. This is a tear in the cartilage caused by degenerative changes, but it can be made worse by flexing, twisting and rotating your knee and also by impact-loading sports like running.

Why didn't you mention leg extensions?

I really don't like leg extensions. They only work one joint and one muscle. And in no sport do you ever just use that one specific movement. So we like to train a lot of different muscles and a lot of different joints at the same time. That's why we use the squat and the leg press or lunge; they are very similar to sport movements (such as lunging for a tennis ball) and daily-life movements (such as rising up from a chair). We like the exercises to simulate the way people move their limbs in their sport.

Are you suggesting that leg extensions can cause knee problems?

They can. Your leg is a very long lever, and it rotates around your knee. Simple physics says that if you have weight at the end of your foot and you lift that weight, that lever is going to translate a lot of force into the knee. We've done

studies here comparing the leg extension to the squat, lunge and leg press and found that the shear force on the knee is actually less when doing a squat or a lunge than when doing a leg extension. When you do a leg extension, all that you're using is the quad, and all that force is going in one direction. But if you're doing a leg press, you are using the quads, your hamstrings, your calf muscles—all of those contracting at the same time. And that co-contraction is very stabilizing. It protects.

And yet we hear so many terrible things about the squat.

It needs to be done properly, for sure. Technique is very important. But I think that the squat is still a very good exercise, and there are other exercises similar to the squat that certain people may be able to do more comfortably, such as the leg press and the lunge. These are all called closed-chain strengthening exercises, meaning that the foot is planted or attached to something. A leg extension would be an example of an open-chain exercise, meaning that the foot is open and freely movable at the end. We try to focus on these closed-chain exercises because that is how the legs are used in life and sports.

Is this the trend in sports medicine, or is this your own theory?

The idea of closed-chain exercise is one of the more recent advancements in our field, especially for the lower extremities. This is the manner in which our lower extremities are used. We've had recent research that shows the safety of this type of exercise (the co-contraction of muscles reduces shear force), and most physical therapy treatment centers are using these techniques.

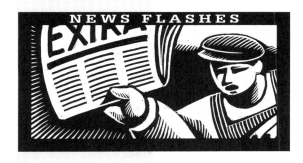

Prostate Cancer Implant Treatment Shows Promise

NEW YORK—Patients with prostate cancer who were treated using implants of tiny radiated "seeds" were just as likely to be free of the disease after five years as were men who opted for surgery to remove the cancer, say researchers at Memorial Sloan-Kettering Cancer Center in New York City.

The participants in the study were men ranging in age from 48 to 80, with the average around 70. The study's long-term results revealed that 60 percent of the subjects showed no evidence of prostate cancer five years after the radiation seed–implants treatment.

With standard external-beam radiation treatment, the prostate is radiated from the outside of the body. Often, normal tissue is damaged along with the cancer. The standard radiation treatment also takes weeks to complete and often causes severe side effects.

In comparison, the implants have to be inserted only once, using ultrasound to guide the placement of tiny rods into the prostate. Each rod is only about the size of a grain of rice, and the insertion can be performed under local anesthesia. Those who undergo the treatment can resume most everyday activities in a few days.

The long-term results from the Memorial Sloan-Kettering study suggest that the seed implants may be a valuable option in the treatment of men with early-stage prostate cancer.

"Vaccine" Treatment for Lymphoma Successful

STANFORD, Calif.—A new technique for creating a vaccine from a patient's own blood shows promise in combating non-Hodgkin's lymphoma, according to researchers at Stanford University.

The study involved four non-Hodgkin's lymphoma patients. In making the vaccine, the researchers harvested the patients' most powerful immune cells—called dendritic cells—from their own blood, primed them to promote an attack on the tumor cells and then put them back into the patients. They primed the cells for the attack by soaking them in a solution that contained a large amount of the tumor's unique cell-surface protein.

After concluding nine months of treatment, the tumors of two of the study's participants had completely regressed. In addition, the third patient's tumor had decreased in size considerably, while the fourth patient's tumor had leveled off after treatment.

The findings demonstrate that the new vaccine procedure was successful at inducing the lymphoma patients to have an immune response. Doctors hope that this technique can be applied to treatments for other types of cancer in the future.

Heel-Nerve Problem often Misdiagnosed

NORFOLK, Va.—Doctors appear to be underdiagnosing a repetitive injury called tarsal tunnel syndrome that mimics heel spur pain, according to a new study done by researchers at the Eastern Virginia Medical School of the Medical College of Hampton Roads in Norfolk.

The researchers worked with 400 subjects who were suffering from heel pain. After treating the participants with standard initial therapies such as arch supports, heel pads and anti-inflammatory drugs, 33 percent of the study group were still unhealed. Typically, foot specialists turn to bone surgery after initial therapies fail. However, the researchers instead tested the nerve response in the feet of these subjects.

The researchers discovered that bone surgery would have given no relief to 70 percent of these subjects because they had tarsal tunnel syndrome instead of heel spurs. This repetitive-strain injury affects many people who make a living on their feet, and it seems to be on the rise. Almost all the subjects in the study were able to gain lasting relief with one of two treatments specific to the syndrome. Approximately half were given special inserts for their shoes and steroid injections, while the remaining half selected surgery that releases pressure on the nerve.

The study's findings suggest that testing for nerve damage should be done before resorting to bone surgery.

Resistance Training May Help Arthritis Sufferers

BOSTON—Weight lifting could be helpful to some sufferers of rheumatoid arthritis, results of a Tufts University School of Medicine study suggest. The findings contradict standard medical ideology, which says that rheumatoid arthritis sufferers should refrain from resistance training to protect their joints.

Researchers from the university compared the effects of resistance training on three different groups of subjects: eight people ages 25 to 65 with rheumatoid arthritis, eight healthy young people and eight healthy elderly people. All the groups participated in resistance-training sessions that were held at two- or three-day intervals.

The researchers found that all three study groups demonstrated significant improvement in strength, compared to a fourth control group that did not participate in the resistance-training sessions. Further, the subjects who had rheumatoid arthritis saw no difference in the number of painful or swollen joints. These subjects also showed significant decreases in pain and fatigue, while they achieved markedly better scores in tests of balance, gait and walking speed.

The study's findings suggest that, contrary to some current medical opinions, resistance training may be helpful for some people plagued with rheumatoid arthritis.

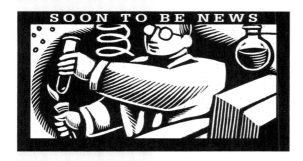

Can a Cold Cure Heart Disease?

Coronary bypass surgery, a common treatment for clogged blood vessels in the heart, could become a less-relied-upon solution if researchers from New York Hospital–Cornell Medical Center in New York City have continued success with a new therapy that uses a common cold virus to trigger the growth of healthy new blood vessels.

This new "bio-bypass" therapy involves infecting the patient's heart muscle with a cold virus that has been modified by the researchers to carry the gene that promotes the growth of new blood vessels. Once the virus is worked into the heart either by direct injection or through a catheter, it has a few days to lay the seeds for vessel growth before the infection is ultimately killed by the immune system.

In early studies using rats and dogs, the researchers have succeeded in promoting the growth of new blood vessels using the modified cold virus. *According to the researchers, human trials could begin sometime in the next two years.*

A New Cure for Baldness?

A team of researchers in California is searching for the specific genes that promote hair growth and reverse graying. The goal is to use gene therapy to cure baldness and graying.

Already, the team from AntiCancer, a biotechnology company in San Diego, has per-

fected a technique for introducing DNA into the cells of hair follicles. The next step is to find the actual genes that will restore hair growth and affect hair color.

While it is currently unknown which genes might induce hair to grow, the researchers speculate that the genes that could "cure" age-related balding may very well be different from the genes that control the temporary hair loss associated with chemotherapy treatments.

The researchers have a few more clues about the genes that regulate graying. They know, for instance, of a gene that regulates an enzyme necessary to hair pigmentation. This gene ultimately could lead the researchers to their goal of influencing hair color through gene therapy. *The researchers have set no timetable but are optimistic that they will identify the genes that they are seeking.*

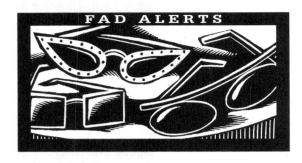

Chromium

 It exploded onto the supplement scene with the kind of promises only an election-year nutrient dare make: increased muscle mass and faster fat loss. It was also just what we wanted to hear. Once an obscure trace mineral that puts the shine on car bumpers, chromium (and its cousin chromium picolinate) became overnight best-sellers.

Some researchers and devotees contend that chromium has lived up to those promises—even if a few studies demonstrate otherwise. But when the final chapter is written, chromium may be better known for helping those with diabetes and hypoglycemia than for building buff biceps.

Why? When you eat simple sugars like candy, cake or even a bagel, your blood glucose levels spike dramatically. To counter this imbalance, your body rushes insulin to the scene by drawing on your chromium stores. The problem is that most people get only about half the chromium they need each day. (The Daily Value is 120 micrograms.) And as if that's not enough to keep your chromium stores in the basement, stress and exercise are thought to remove chromium from your body.

"Once chromium is used, it's lost in the urine. And you need to replenish it, but unfortunately, most people don't get enough," says Richard A. Anderson, Ph.D., lead mineral scientist at the U.S. Department of Agriculture's Human Research Center in Beltsville, Maryland.

It's even worse for those suffering with diabetes. But when Chinese diabetes sufferers participating in a joint United States/China health study were given 200 or 1,000 micrograms of chromium a day for four months, their symptoms and conditions dramatically improved. "They went from a very diabetic range to near normal—a very significant effect," says Dr. Anderson. "There are literally 16 million people with diabetes in the United States and a much larger number who are glucose-intolerant and don't know it. If we're right, these findings could potentially help 40 million to 50 million people in the United States alone."

Some of the foods that deliver the most chromium per serving are eggs, cheese, beef and whole-grain wheat. Ask your doctor before taking supplements; many doctors still believe that it isn't safe to exceed the government-set Daily Value.

Natural Healing

Maybe it's the failed health-reform movement in Washington, D.C., a few years back. Maybe it's the ever-escalating amount of high-tech equipment and high-risk synthetic medications that make up health care as we know it today. Maybe we all yearn for something simpler. But for whatever reason, natural healing methods—cures and preventive actions based on natural ingredients and often-ancient medical practices—have become all the rage.

For a time, natural healing approaches (some call it alternative medicine or complementary therapies, in the belief that they should be paired up with more modern, scientific approaches) were scoffed at by those in the health care mainstream. No longer. The 1996 World Congress on Complementary Therapies in Medicine was attended by many of the nation's most respected doctors in search of new techniques, and the opening speech was made by former Surgeon General C. Everett Koop.

There are dozens of natural healing approaches. Some are as simple as using herbs and spices in place of medicines. *Ayurveda* is a Hindu system of medicine rooted in texts more than 5,000 years old and is based on the premise that people are the product of their environment. *Homeopathy* is the practice of using minute amounts of herbs, minerals and other substances to stimulate a person's natural defenses and help the body heal itself. *Reflexology* is the ancient Chinese science of foot and hand massage; its premise is that you can soothe troubles throughout the body by massaging remote trigger points.

A true sign that natural healing is a major trend is the huge number of books on the topic now hitting store shelves. While many doctors still scoff at many of these "natural" concepts, expect more to be willing to use them in conjunction with more standard medical techniques, particularly if the patient feels strongly about it.

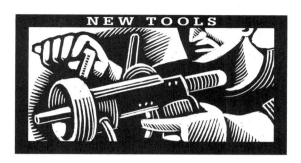

NEW TOOLS

Faster Healing

Hyperbaric Chambers

Sprained your ankle? Twisted your shoulder? You can spend several weeks sidelined with an injury that's slow to heal. Or you can slip into a hyperbaric chamber and cut your recovery time in half.

That's what professional sports teams and a few sports medicine centers are doing. They're using a hyperbaric chamber developed by HYOX Systems in Aberdeen, Scotland. Inside the tiny cockpitlike chamber, injured athletes are exposed to twice the normal levels of oxygen found in the atmosphere.

"The more oxygen certain injuries are exposed to, the faster they heal," especially in cases of sprains, strains and bruises, says Russell Peterson, Ph.D., a Philadelphia physiologist and hyperbaric expert. Sports teams ranging from the NFL's New York Giants to the NBA's Seattle Supersonics already use hyperbaric therapy and say that their injured athletes recover faster when breathing hyperbaric levels of oxygen while in the chamber.

There's only one problem: "Some of those big guys do feel a little claustrophobic in that tiny chamber," says Dr. Peterson. Some who are claustrophobic even refuse to go in them. And although some high-end clubs are beginning to offer hyperbaric therapy, don't go looking for a home model—a hyperbaric chamber will run you $85,000.

Rubbing Out Wrinkles

Renova Skin Cream

To delay the effects of aging and sunlight on your skin, you might try a new cream that may help you smooth emerging wrinkles, brown spots and roughness. Renova, a prescription cream, contains a form of vitamin A called tretinoin. Unlike the prescription Retin-A and over-the-counter alpha hydroxy acids, which work on the skin's surface, Renova is said to work deeper in the skin, where pigment changes occur and fine wrinkling begins. In studies, 65 percent of patients showed a reduction of fine wrinkling and brown spots. Bad news for Clint Eastwood look-alikes, though: The cream can't fix deeply wrinkled skin.

Better Athlete's Foot Relief

Miconazole

Sometimes the burning itch of athlete's foot is so bad that you want to hoof it to your doctor for relief. Before you do this, go shopping. For most people, over-the-counter athlete's foot products that contain miconazole work as effectively as prescription medicines, according to a study comparing remedies at the Veterans Affairs Medical Center in Cleveland. Your cheapest fix will be a store-brand generic powder or spray containing miconazole as the active ingredient, says lead investigator Margaret Chren, M.D. Just be sure to use it daily for four weeks to wipe out the fungus. Products with miconazole are available for about $6.

More Effective Headache Help

Biofeedback Therapy

When tension headaches ignore your aspirin assault, you may find relief at your local biofeedback therapist. John Arena, Ph.D., director of pain evaluation and intervention at the Veterans Affairs Medical Center in Augusta, Georgia, and professor of psychiatry and health behavior at the Medical College of Georgia School of Medicine, also in Augusta, found that biofeedback can teach you to relax your neck muscles and reduce headache symptoms by at least 50 percent. During this type of biofeedback, a doctor places sensors on your neck and shoulders, then directs you to a graph that tracks muscle relaxation. Eventually, you'll learn exactly when and how to relieve the muscle tension that may be causing your headaches.

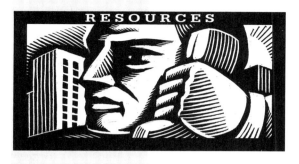

Prostate Information

Prostate Pointers

http://rattler.cameron.edu/prostate/
prostate.html

This is a resource-packed Web site for information on all types of prostate problems, with an emphasis on cancer. The site is run by Gary Huckabay, Ph.D., a mathematics professor at Cameron University in Lawton, Oklahoma. He doesn't dispense any medical advice; he only provides the latest news and research. The Web site offers lots of abstracts from medical journals and conferences. In addition, it provides information from the nonmedical perspective and gives briefs on all the latest news affecting patients. The best thing about this site is that you can get a state-by-state listing of patients in informal support groups, with actual phone numbers instead of e-mail addresses.

Chronic Fatigue Syndrome

Chronic Fatigue and Immune

Dysfunction Syndrome Association

of America

1-800-442-3437

Anyone plagued with or interested in chronic fatigue syndrome can now receive an informational package with just a phone call. The association, which calls itself the leading charitable organization dedicated to conquering this syndrome, will send you a list of support groups in your state and a free packet of information on chronic fatigue syndrome. The message machine can take your call 24 hours a day. The bulk of the association's support comes from individual donations.

Foot Problems

Foot and Ankle Web Index

http://www.footandankle.com

If you've been having foot or ankle problems, have we got a Web site for you. Just log in here and you'll discover information on everything from sports injuries to warts to foot odor. "Ask the Foot Doctor" will e-mail you information concerning your particular foot trouble, along with a guide to licensed podiatrists in your area. The site is a product of Account Mark, a national marketing firm, and it is maintained by Robert Wunderlich, D.P.M. It's for educational purposes only and not for dispensing professional or medical advice. Numerous companies do advertise their products on this site, and ordering information is available.

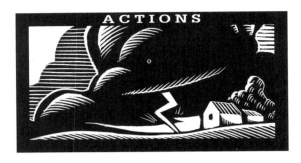

Gentlemen, in case you've forgotten: War is hell, love is a battlefield (thank you and good-bye, Pat Benatar) and life itself . . . is a lot of military metaphors rolled up into one. Since it's never clear what health disaster will befall you—maybe a gas attack during your daughter's piano recital, heart palpitations in the heat of battle or even just high cholesterol—we've compiled this list of handy health cures, based on recent findings and writings, given in no particular order. Take a look and give them a try. And be careful out there.

1. **Flax yourself.** At least one study shows that eating bread made with flaxseed will help reduce high cholesterol levels. During the study, 20 volunteers ate six slices of the bread a day for six weeks. At the end of the study, researchers found that bad, or LDL (low-density lipoprotein), cholesterol levels had dropped on average by 30 points.

"Wouldn't you rather take your medicine as a slice of toast with preserves or orange marmalade?" asks Tom Watkins, Ph.D., laboratory director of the Kenneth Jordan Heart Research Foundation in Montclair, New Jersey. "It sounds a lot better, doesn't it?"

A natural blood thinner, flaxseed apparently helps combat thickening of the blood that occurs as we age. "You need some antifreeze, you know, to thin things down a bit. And it just so happens that flaxseed is a good source of substances that will thin it down," says Dr. Watkins. Ready-to-eat

breakfast cereal made from flax can be found in your neighborhood health food store.

2. **Frolic with folic acid.** Canadian research has shown that 30 percent of all heart disease may be caused by a high amount of homocysteine, a chemical that narrows vital arteries that carry blood within the heart and to the brain. Researchers speculate that a high folic acid concentration in the blood helps to keep homocysteine levels low. Folic acid is called folate in its natural form in food and can be found in those dark green leafy vegetables you probably haven't eaten since you last dined at your mom's house—broccoli, romaine lettuce and spinach—as well as beans, chickpeas and lentils. The Daily Value of folic acid is 400 micrograms; however, 88 percent of Americans usually fall short of getting that amount from their diet. The downside to folic acid: Supplemental folic acid has been known to hide B_{12} deficiencies.

3. **Forgo the fling.** If faithfulness to the one you love isn't enough to keep you out of the arms of another, consider embarrassment. Bedding that beautiful stranger is far more likely to end in impotence than in sexual conquest.

"This happens more often than we might realize," says Wayne Hellstrom, M.D., associate professor of urology at Tulane Medical Center in New Orleans. "It's usually attributed to having too much to drink or being a little nervous, but we know better."

A lurid rendezvous has a way of subconsciously activating the body's fight-or-flight response. This diverts blood from your penis to your muscles and often leaves you limp, he says.

4. **Treat your butt better.** Rather than torture yourself with that bargain-basement toilet paper you usually buy—and consequently increase the risk of irritating your hemorrhoids—spring for a softer bathroom tissue, says Jorge Herrera, M.D., associate professor of medicine at the University of South Alabama in Mobile. But be wary of those made with dyes or perfumes: They can cause itching and swelling if you happen to be allergic to them.

5. **Keep your shoes on.** Friends have told you this to save their noses; our experts tell us that it can help prevent swelling and decrease healing time of a sprained ankle. "Trust me. If you took the shoe off, a sprained ankle would puff up, and you would not get the shoe back on. But if you keep it on, at least until you get to a place where you can treat it, it will keep the swelling down," says Garry Sherman, D.P.M., a former team physician for World Team Tennis now in private practice in Cedar Knolls, New Jersey.

6. **Do a little power lounging.** Normally associated with munching chips or hanging out at the beach, the official power lounging position—in a chair, feet up, knees slightly bent, back tilted at a 20- to 30-degree angle—is the best way to relax while your sore back mends. "Of all the positions, this takes the stress off the low back the best, even better than being flat on your back," says Peter Slabaugh, M.D., spokesperson for the American Academy of Orthopedic Surgeons based in Chicago and an orthopedic surgeon in Oakland, California.

7. **Munch on magnesium.** Long known for its ability to relax the muscles lining our breathing passages, research shows that magnesium may even help fend off an asthma attack. In a British study, researchers exposed more than 2,500 adults to a chemical that triggers airway constriction in asthma patients. As it turns out, those with the least magnesium in their diets were twice as likely to experience an asthmatic reaction as those with the highest magnesium diets. The Daily Value for magnesium is 400 milligrams. Some of the best sources include beans, nuts, whole-grain bread and dark green vegetables such as spinach and broccoli.

8. **Lose your love handles.** Carrying just 15 percent more weight on your frame increases your likelihood of heartburn, but toting a potbelly really seals the deal. "When you're lying down, the fat presses on your stomach, sometimes with enough force to overcome the esophageal sphincter, allowing the acid to seep in," says Gary A. Green, M.D., clinical professor of family practice and associate team physician of intercollegiate athletics at the University of California, Los Angeles. (And until you lose the weight, lose those tight clothes. They can cause stomach pressure, too.)

9. **Take a lunch break.** Barking directives to your staff while gnawing on a sandwich not only makes you look like some Third World potentate but also is a common cause of belching. "You need to just slow down for a few minutes, take time to eat and then go back to what you're doing," says Colin Howden, M.D., professor of medicine at the University of South Carolina School of Medicine in Columbia.

10. **Fiber up.** The experts agree: Eating 20 to 30 grams of fiber a day is a good way to help you avoid constipation. "Probably the easiest way to get that in the diet is to eat salads and fresh fruits with the peels on them, like apples and pears. Also, choose breads with fiber, like wheat or oat bran," says Dr. Herrera. (And no cutting off the crusts like Mom used to do for you when you lived at home.) Some of the most fibrous foods include broccoli, cabbage, carrots and brussels sprouts—all the stuff you never eat.

11. **Chew on this one.** Does your sugarless chewing gum contain sorbitol? It could be causing your diarrhea. When bacteria in your colon sink their teeth into sorbitol, they break it down, creating lots of gas and causing water to flow into your stools. The result is pain and diarrhea.

12. **Banish the milk cow blues.** Remember that government-funded study a few years back? The one where they were trying to figure out if cows were poking holes in the ozone layer by passing too much gas? They would have been better off looking into what happens when humans digest products that come from those cows.

After you drink milk or eat dairy products, enzymes in your intestine called lactase are supposed to digest a sugar in the milk called lactose. The problem is that some people are what doctors call lactase-deficient, meaning that they no longer have the enzyme. The result is lots of gas. If you're one of those, fear not. Lactase tablets or capsules or lactose-free milk, like Lactaid, should solve the problem. Or just don't drink milk.

13. **Brace yourself.** For about $20, you can buy the Nirschl Counter Force brace (available by calling Medical Sports at 1-800-783-2240) or a similar model to help reduce elbow pain—regardless of whether you play tennis. "Worn on the forearm, it helps prevent the pull against the muscle from reaching the tendon," says Robert P. Nirschl, M.D., director of the Virginia Sports Medicine and Rehabilitation Institute in Arlington and creator of the brace. More expensive straps feature fluid- or gel-filled pads, he says.

14. **Try vitamin C and see.** In addition to a quart of orange juice a day, Earl Dawson, Ph.D., associate professor in the Department of Obstetrics and Gynecology at the University of Texas Medical Branch in Galveston, recommends 500 milligrams of vitamin C both in the morning and with dinner to help treat male infertility. A water-soluble vitamin—which simply means that you'll urinate it away once the body has enough—vitamin C apparently protects sperm against toxins like lead and nicotine. In one study, Dr. Dawson divided 75 young male smok-

ers into three groups. One group got a placebo, another got 200 milligrams of vitamin C daily for a month and the third took 1,000 milligrams of vitamin C each day for a month. The higher the men's vitamin C levels rose, the greater the protection they received against the sperm-damaging effects of nicotine.

15. **Mind your minerals.** When it comes to keeping your heart's complex electrical system firing on time, few minerals are as important as potassium and magnesium. "If it's just a matter of an occasional skipped beat and you've been reassured that it's not a potentially dangerous rhythm problem, you may find that it gets better if you supplement with these," says Lou-Anne Beauregard, M.D., a cardiologist at CentraState Medical Center in Freehold, New Jersey, and an electrophysiologist at Robert Wood Johnson Medical Center in New Brunswick, New Jersey. The Daily Value for potassium is 3,500 milligrams. Have an eight-ounce glass of orange juice, a banana and a baked potato, and you're halfway there. For magnesium, an ounce of cashews and a three-ounce serving of halibut gives you almost half of what you need.

16. **Ask for the real thing.** Defizzed Coke works so well for nausea that there's an over-the-counter product on the market called Emetrol that is made of very similar ingredients. "It's basically a high-fructose, sweet, syrupy medicine that is very similar to Coke. I'm not sure how it works, but it must get the job done, because it's something that people have been using for years, and a typical dose is one to two ounces," says Malcolm Robinson, M.D., founder and director of the Oklahoma Foundation for Digestive Research and clinical professor of medicine at the University of Oklahoma College of Medicine in Oklahoma City. You can make your own anti-nausea drink by simply opening a Coke and stirring it for a few minutes until it's flat.

SLEEP

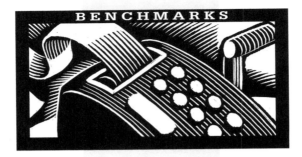

BENCHMARKS

AVERAGES

- Number of hours a man sleeps each night: 7.5

- Percentage of men who sleep with three or more pillows: 14

- Number of Americans who suffer from insomnia at some point in their lives: 56 million

- Percentage of adults who read to help them fall asleep: 20

- Percentage of adults who take a sleeping pill or sleeping aid: 17

- Annual number of injuries involving beds, mattresses and pillows: 360,000

- Percentage of men who have fallen asleep while driving: 27

- Times of day when you are at the greatest risk for being hit by a sleepy driver:
  2:00 A.M., 6:00 A.M. and 4:00 P.M.

- Percentage of Americans who "catch up" on lost sleep over the weekend: 27

- Number of bedrooms in the United States: 260,387,000

- Percentage of men who say that they sleep in the nude: 26

- Percentage of women who say that they sleep in the nude: 6

- Percentage of Americans who say that they are at their best in the morning: 56

- Number of dreams an adult has in a year: 1,600

- Number of nightmares an adult has in a year: 1.5

EXTREMES

- Loudest snore on record: 119 decibels, by Barry Langdon of London

- Longest continuous sleep session: 64 hours

- Longest interval without sleep: 6 days, 4 hours

- Most expensive pillow: ostrich feather–filled, $345

The Importance of a Good Bed

Choosing the right bedding may be the key to banishing back and joint pain forever.

According to a nationwide study of orthopedic surgeons, the single most important tool for preventing back pain is the right mattress. "During sleep, muscles are able to relax and rejuvenate. A poor sleep surface prevents this from happening, and places painful stress on the back," says Stephen Elsasser, M.D., a fellow at the American College for Advancement in Medicine in Laguna Hills, California. Since one-third of our lives is spent in bed, it only makes sense: Poor nighttime posture can equal chronic back pain.

But that may be only the tip of the iceberg. As we get older, the substance that eases movement of the joints diminishes, leaving us more susceptible to both arthritic and general aches and pains. "I see a great number of people with musculoskeletal aches and pains—sore necks, sore hips, sore knees—and one of their frequent comments is that they can't get a good night's sleep," says James H. Wheeler, M.D., an orthopedic surgeon in North Carolina. In fact, even the Arthritis Foundation has named worn-out mattresses as a major player in creating and maintaining joint pain.

So how do you know if it's time to trade in your mattress? The Better Sleep Council recommends asking the following questions.

- Has your sleep set been in nightly use for more than eight years?
- Can you feel or see uneven or sagging areas?
- Do you and your partner both tend to roll toward the middle?
- Is the cover soiled or torn?
- When you wake up, are your muscles sore? Do you still feel tired?

If you answered "yes" to any of those questions, it's probably time that you ventured into the confusing, pressured world of retail bedding.

Big Business

The American bedding business generates $4.5 billion in revenue every year—and that kind of money can generate a lot of smoke without much fire. We heard nonspecific spiel after nonspecific spiel from retailers—lots of medical-sounding words with very little concrete information to back them up.

The basic sales strategy seems to be to get you to lie on the most expensive mattress and ask you how it feels. Well, if you've been sleeping on Uncle Harry's hand-me-down for the last ten years, anything's going to feel like paradise. As soon as you say, "Pretty good," they're all over you like a bad cold. We found that when we asked salespeople for hardware specifics, they tended to look at us blankly and say, in essence, "If it feels good, just buy it." No wonder a sales training kit from one major mattress manufacturer emphasized that most customers (sitting ducks?) make a major bedding purchase at one of the first three stores they visit.

Many of the experts are just as evasive. Calls to untold numbers of sleep-center directors, physicians, physical therapists and researchers yielded surprisingly little concrete information.

"You may talk to a lot of physicians and they'll tell you what they think is the best sleep environment for people with certain conditions such as arthritis or back pain, but the truth is that no one has studied mattress surface characteristics as they pertain to any given disease state," says Mark Mahowald, M.D., director of the Minnesota Regional Sleep Disorders Center in Minneapolis.

A Happy Medium

The critical element in determining the best mattress for you is the interplay between firmness and conformity. "A good mattress has to be firm enough to support your back but soft enough not to create pressure points," explains Dr. Wheeler. If a mattress is too soft, has too much "give," your hips and shoulders will sink, placing a tremendous strain on your lower back.

On the other hand, if a mattress is too firm, the points of contact, or pressure points, which include your head, shoulders, hips, knees and ankles, will be pushed up, creating additional stress both on the points themselves and on your back. In essence, you want something perfectly poised between a beanbag chair and a board lined with telephone books.

One of the reasons that generalized recommendations are tricky is that body weight is obviously a tremendous factor: What supports and conforms well to the body of a 130-pound woman may sag horribly for a 185-pound man. Admittedly, though, you're going to be hard-pressed to make a solid determination just lying on a bunch of mattresses for ten minutes each. That's why you need to talk specifics that will give you a sense of the overall quality and adaptability of a sleep set, stuff like coil numbers, connections and diameters.

Mattress Details

An innerspring mattress consists of a bunch of coiled wires sandwiched between layers of cushioning. The foundation also has coil springs (or a version of them called torsion bars) attached to a wood or steel foundation.

The most important number governing the durability, firmness and conformability of the mattress is the coil count. To simplify things, it's best to compare the number of coils in a full-size mattress, as the mattress manufacturers do, so as not to get muddled when trying to calculate proportionally up to, say, a king.

Basically, the more coils, the more specifically the mattress responds to the differing pressures of your body, dipping here for an elbow, raising there for a small of the back. Don't even think of buying a mattress with a coil count of less than 300, no matter what it feels like in the showroom. A Sealy Posturepedic, for example, has 660 in each full mattress.

Another key factor is the way the coils are linked. It doesn't matter how many coils you have if they're linked in such a way that when one is pressed down, its neighbors crouch down, too, like so many kids playing London Bridge. Be sure to ask your salesman exactly how the coils are interconnected (he should have a little cross-section he can show you). Simmons, for example, sinks its Beautyrest coils into separate fabric pockets and attaches the pockets to each other, avoiding any metal-to-metal contact.

As for the diameter of the coils, the smaller the number, the firmer and more long-lasting the coil. High-end mattresses generally have coil diameters between $12\frac{3}{4}$ and 14.

One feature that you may want to pass by is the "pillow" or "plush" top that most manufacturers offer. "Generally, I would recommend against the top-of-the-line mattresses with the extra tufting on top," says James Cable, M.D., an orthopedic physician at the Texas Back Institute in Dallas. "They take several feet of fiber fill and compress it down to two to three inches. That can get too fluffy and defeat the purpose, in terms of back support, of all those springs," he says.

But no matter which mattress you select, make sure that you rotate and flip it every other week for the first six months. This keeps a "body impression" from forming, which can shorten the life and diminish the comfort of the mattress. After the break-in period, you need to flip and turn only every couple of months.

The Latest in Bedding

Despite the current popularity of innerspring mattresses, the trend seems to be toward fairly expensive, high-quality foam and air alternatives. Two manufacturers, Tempur-Pedic and Comfort Air, are dominating what is currently a largely mail-order market but which promises to be coming to a store near you very soon.

Float on air. The Select Comfort adjustable firmness mattress is a hybrid of old-fashioned waterbeds and camping air mattresses. Using individual air chambers for support, this slim, light mattress offers a handheld control that can adjust firmness (that is, pump up or let air out) to accommodate varying weight and body types. One unique feature in the queen and king beds is a dual adjustability option that lets each partner determine the firmness level of his or her side of the bed. This could be a real plus for couples with widely varying weights.

A recent preliminary study has suggested that spinal misalignments are as much as 40 percent higher on innerspring mattresses as on the Select Comfort, a difference that the manufacturer attributes to the extreme conformability and compressibility of air. It helps, too, that the mattress is light: Turning and rotating an innerspring can be tough on your back.

But with queen sets starting at over $1,000 (more for a "pillow top"), these fancy air bags aren't for the faint of wallet. They do come with a 20-year warranty and a 90-night no-questions-asked refund option. For more information, call Select Comfort at 1-800-535-2337 and they'll send you a free video and brochure.

Swedish luxury. The Tempur-Pedic Swedish mattress is made from a specially developed material originally designed to ease the G-forces astronauts feel after liftoff. Some tough foam. Relatively thin and light, Tempur-Pedic boasts the ultimate in comfort and conformability, relieving tension on pressure points, resulting in good spinal alignment and relief from the pain of arthritis and/or bedsores.

In the research arsenal, Tempur-Pedic also has only one store. A study at the Institution for Clinical and Physiological Research at Lillhagen Hospital in Göteborg, Sweden, determined that sleepers turned over an average of 17 times on the Tempur-Pedic compared with 80 to 100 times on a conventional innerspring, suggesting that sleepers had more restful nights.

Like the Select Comfort, Tempur-Pedic is lightweight, and it doesn't require turning. It's also hypoallergenic and resistant to all sorts of molds and mildews and comes with a nonprorated ten-year guarantee. But it is the priciest of the bunch: A queen mattress with a foundation and shipping will set you back a good $1,450. For a free video and brochure, call Tempur-Pedic's American headquarters at 1-800-886-6466.

American concoction. Simmons recently introduced its new BackCare mattress line. These traditional innersprings are topped by a special foam layer, made with two "support zones," which hold up your lower back and upper thighs, and three "comfort zones" to reduce pressure on the shoulders, hips and knees. In the BackCare Ultimate queen and king sets, you can choose two different firmness levels to accommodate different size sleepers. For more information about the BackCare line and the location of a dealer near you, call Simmons at 1-800-555-2225.

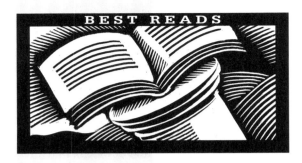

What Your Dreams May Be Telling You

Dreams are surreal, puzzling, enthralling, terrifying. They are also thoroughly your own. Only you can know what your brain is telling you, and why, with dreams. Most people don't bother to find out. In The Dream Sourcebook: A Guide to the Theory and Interpretation of Dreams *(Lowell House, 1995), authors Phyllis Koch-Sheras, Ph.D., and Amy Lemley reveal practical secrets about understanding your mind's nighttime wanderings. In this excerpt, they give an overview of the types of dreams we experience.*

"I am in some kind of prison, aware that my fellow prisoners are being flogged with a large rubber spider. The guards all look like mummies with their faces and bodies covered by layers of tattered cloth. I know they can see, yet they have no eyes."

Is this a "good" dream or a "bad" one? Prison, spiders, mummies—these dream images do not suggest a very restful sleep. But as we've said, there are no bad dreams. So what can be good about a scary dream? Does it contain a message? Is there a hidden meaning? How can you understand what your dreams are trying to tell you?

The dreamer of this dream was curious about what it meant. After thinking about the circumstances of her life at the time, she began to construct an interpretation—an explanation of the meaning of the dream story—that made sense to her. Because the dream occurred during a time when she was working day and night to complete a writing project, she interpreted the dream as a comment on the creative process and how it was working, or not working, for her. How did she come to understand the dream? By breaking down the various elements or symbols of the dream—the prison, the spider, the mummy jailers—and considering the meaning of each one individually. A symbol is defined as an image that stands for something to which it has some distant resemblance; often, it unites several ideas together, adding layers of meaning.

For this dreamer, in this dream, the spider was not a menacing presence, but rather a symbol of creativity, related to the intricate webs spiders spin. The mummies in the dream, unable to speak, restricting the comings and goings of their captives, symbolized the dreamer's own obsession with her work in recent weeks, work that kept her "jailed" as she pursued the difficult task of putting ideas to paper. Would spiders mean the same thing to every dreamer? Not always. To understand a symbol's meaning, you have to consider the dream in context—in relation to your own life, the culture in which you live and even the universal experiences we all share. Only then can you accurately interpret the meaning of the symbols in your dreams. In doing so, you will no doubt find many different meanings even for a single symbol over time. A spider may represent creativity in one dream, restlessness (on eight legs!) in another, mystery and hidden danger in still another dream. Only you, as the director of your personal dream movie, can determine what a dream really means for you.

A lot of people enjoy reading dream dictionaries, those thick-volumed books that list hundreds of symbols, from automobile to zoo, in alphabetical order, with a few specific interpretations down in black-and-white. These dictionaries can offer useful suggestions, but don't look to them for the final word on what your dreams mean. Only you can interpret what a particular symbol means in your individual dreamworld. A dog, for instance, might symbolize a fierce and menacing presence in the dream of someone who had grown up with a fear of the animal but appear as a friend and guide in the dream of a true animal lover. Again, it all depends on the context.

Although no two dreamers will derive the exact same meaning for every symbol, experimental dream research in this century has given us a way of dividing dream symbols into different categories along with some guidelines that will help you to recognize what these symbols mean in your particular dreamworld. Your dreaming mind, as director of several nightly movies, including a slightly longer "feature film" during the final stage of REM (rapid eye movement) sleep, selects characters (and actors), dialogue, plot and setting for a particular effect. The waking mind can then work backward, from the effect or emotion the dream contains to an analysis of each symbol and how it plays into the overall effect. In dreams, you'll find tragedy, comedy and everything in between.

You may ask why, then, dreams can be so bizarre and difficult to figure out at times. For a moment, imagine that you are in another country, where the culture and language are unknown to you. Things look familiar, but the customs surrounding them are totally different. This is the situation in your dreamworld. Words sound the same but can have different meanings. The people you meet, the places you go, the things you see all appear familiar but may, in fact, symbolize or represent other things, people or emotions. You have your own individual dream language, devised by your subconscious to tell you stories that have special meaning to you.

Dreams are valuable life experiences, and, like an anthropologist exploring a unique culture, you can observe them, learn from them, enjoy them and even come to participate more actively in them.

Valuable Dream Areas to Explore

What can we gain from our dream travels? Here are some different types of dreams, with some suggestions about what they have to offer.

Nightmares are frightening dreams that reveal a fear we need to confront or acknowledge. Remembered more often than pleasant dreams, nightmares are defined by the intense feelings they cause, whatever the story line. But don't think of them as bad dreams. Although they bring up negative thoughts and images, they are a positive force in clearing up conflicts. Like the spider dream, a nightmare usually has an important message to convey, even if it may be so scary that a part of you wishes to forget it.

Message dreams are dreams that convey some information you need about your current social, emotional or physical life. These are teaching dreams in which someone is usually there to tell you something important directly: a teacher, a news announcer or clergyman giving you new information to apply to your waking life. At times, a message dream will come in the form of a disembodied voice (with no accompanying visual image); the dreamer may perceive this voice as a voice of the spirit or soul, or of God or an angel.

Healing dreams are message dreams that point the way to better health, sometimes even "diagnosing" a previously unidentified medical condition. How is this possible? True, it may seem like a premonition, but a healing dream is more likely the result of the subliminal perceptions we make throughout our days: our own physical health (or the physical condition of someone close to us, if the dream is about that person), information we've read, advertisements we've seen and so forth. So a dream of rotting teeth that suggests the dreamer is due for a trip to the dentist could be the result of many things drawn from the dreamer's life: a dentist's appointment card found in a pocket, a commercial for fluoride rinse, a subtle pain in a back tooth. Only you, the dreamer, can decide whether the dream is offering a healing message. After all, rotting teeth could symbolize something else entirely. It all depends on you and what the symbol means in your life and in your unique dream language.

Problem-solving and creative dreams offer a new way to look at a situation. Because your dreams take place within your own mind, you are free as a dreamer to sort through all the information and feelings surrounding a conflict or challenge, without the usual distractions of daily life. Your dreaming mind can go where it must to make connections with past experiences, imagine various scenarios or even depict for you the real truth about an issue. There can be real value in "sleeping on it." Problem-solving dreams are the dreams that come after you ask your dreams to help you solve specific problems. They can also arrive spontaneously, as many creative dreams do, in response to your thinking about a difficult problem or perplexing issue the night of the dream. Many significant discoveries and new creations have arisen from this kind of dream.

Mystical, visionary or "high" dreams go beyond dealing with everyday events and concerns to access the dreamer's spirituality. The Tibetan Buddhists call them dreams of clarity. These dreams often include exotic characters who have some universal meaning that is generally understood by all cultures—a bird, a wise old woman, a monster. These archetypes, as Carl Jung called them, often have supernatural qualities and are believed to represent the powerful parts of the dreamer's personality. We call these characters dream helpers—beings who step in to show you the way or offer some new insight. It is quite rare for a dream to take on the added spiritual or mystical dimension of a visionary dream, but when it does happen, it will be clear to you that something special has transpired.

Completion dreams are another way to "sleep on it," serving to sort out the unfinished thoughts and emotions from the previous day or two. After a completion dream, you will wake up feeling resolved and refreshed, as though things are more in order than they were the night before. Sometimes, a recurring nightmare can become a completion dream if you are able to think about the content and pay attention to its meaning; you won't "need" the dream anymore once you have completed the thought, emotion or experience that lay behind it.

Recurring dreams repeat themselves with little variation in story or theme. They can be positive, as with an archetypal visionary dream, but they are more often nightmares, perhaps because nightmares depict a conflict that is unresolved; also, nightmares are more frequently remembered than other dreams.

Lucid dreams are dreams in which the dreamer is aware of dreaming while the dream is occurring and sometimes is able to make choices or otherwise influence the dream's outcome without awakening. These are very special dreams that occur spontaneously for some people but that can be cultivated in others. The Senoi people of Malaysia encourage children to become lucid dreamers from a very young age.

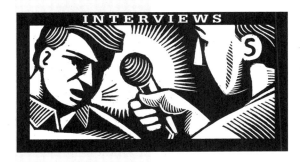

Alex Clerk and Jack Coleman on
Apnea and Snoring

So they call you Buzz Saw? The neighbors complain about your snoring and threaten to have you arrested for disturbing the peace? Doesn't bother you—you sleep through it, right?

Our experts—sleep doctors Alex Clerk and Jack Coleman—say that snoring is nothing to snort at. It can damage the heart and sometimes is a symptom of a more serious malady, sleep apnea. Apnea means "without breath," and that's exactly what happens. Men with this condition stop breathing dozens or even hundreds of times a night, often because of blockages in the throat. Each time, they partially awaken as the body struggles for air.

Clerk is a medical doctor and director of the sleep clinic at Stanford University. Coleman, also a medical doctor, is chairman of the Sleep Disorders Committee for the American Academy of Otolaryngology-Head and Neck Surgery. Dr. Coleman specializes in surgeries that correct the obstructions that cause snoring and apneas.

Below are excerpts from separate interviews with both.

What are the factors that contribute to snoring?

Dr. Clerk: The factors are anatomic: One is fat in your throat. There are also people who don't have a lot of fat there, but because of the way that their jaws are structured, they can still have obstruction of the upper airway. The jaw may be structured in such a way that the tongue can be pushed to the back. This sometimes happens when there is a huge overbite. So a very slim person's tongue can get pushed back, and that person can have sleep apnea, even though he doesn't have fat deposits causing an obstruction.

The second reason is that any time you fall asleep, your muscles relax. So while you may not have a lot of fat or a huge overbite, you can get so relaxed when you sleep that you quit holding the airway open. This is common if you are on (sedative or muscle-relaxing) medications. They can relax the airway muscles.

Why do men snore more than women?

Dr. Clerk: There's a difference in where fat is positioned in men and women. Women, when they gain weight, put it on their hips, but men put the weight mostly in the abdomen and in the neck. So that is one basic reason why that happens. You get more neck and upper airway deposition of fat in men. Also, there may be some hormonal factors. The female hormone progesterone is thought to also protect women a little bit longer against sleep apnea.

So does losing weight work? Is there any fitness routine that will build up those air passage muscles?

Dr. Clerk: Dieting will help you lose the fat. Exercising has been studied but not clearly been shown to help firm up the particular tissues involved.

It is true that you can reduce the number of sleep apneas by losing weight. However, a lot of people who lose weight gain it back. So while we recommend that patients lose weight, we don't rely on that alone as a treatment. It is a good recommendation and can make the other treatments more effective.

Why is laser surgery—in which the offending obstruction is delicately trimmed—good for normal snoring but not for sleep apnea?

Dr. Clerk: Laser surgery is useful only around the little floating tissue in the middle of the top of the throat called the uvula. That can help people who snore, but much more extensive surgery is needed in most cases of apnea.

Continuous positive airway pressure (CPAP—in which you wear a mask that runs a tube through the nose and blows enough air into the throat to keep the passage open) is the immediate option for apnea. Surgery is also a good option. In cases of severe sleep apnea, it's advisable to get CPAP before surgery, because the tissues will swell up after surgery and you'll have worse sleep apnea until they settle down.

The specialists agree that CPAP is the most effective immediate treatment for apnea. But we also hear that many patients won't use CPAP regularly because they find the device so cumbersome and uncomfortable. What are their options?

Dr. Coleman: There are masks of a different design that they can use. There are nasal pillows that just fit in the nostrils rather than over the face. We have different types of machines that offer the same basic treatment as CPAP that some people find more comfortable.

Because I'm a surgeon, I see all the failures. The most common reasons for failure are because it's uncomfortable to wear, they are turning at night and it comes loose and they take it off during sleep.

What can someone who snores or seems to suffer from apnea do to lessen the problem?

Dr. Clerk: For mild snoring, there *are* a few things you can do.
- Use dental devices (mouthpieces of the sort dentists prescribe to protect your teeth from nocturnal clenching and grinding).
- Elevate your upper body in bed.
- Sleep on your side.

Those things will help, but they won't control everything completely. They will lessen snoring and reduce the number of apneas.

Do you see any problem with experimenting with home remedies?

Dr. Coleman: If the problem is only snoring—not apnea—and traditional methods don't work very well, then you have a lot of leeway. But if you have significant apnea, that's a definite medical problem. In that kind of situation, it's probably not a good idea to spend a lot of time trying different remedies. You want to get the patient into some kind of treatment that you know is going to work, even if it's going to be temporary. CPAP is the thing.

Apnea is really bad for the heart. But what about snoring? Does it hurt anything besides your spouse's ears?

Dr. Clerk: That has been looked at, and there is some correlation that snoring, alone, can strain the heart and that people may slowly develop heart disease because of that. Yes, snoring does have some effect on the cardiovascular system.

If you opt for surgery for apnea, what are you getting into?

Dr. Coleman: Some of the surgery is pretty involved, and treatment can be long. Bad facial skeletal structure with dental problems requires orthodontic treatment first and then surgery. It can take two years to get the teeth and dental arch taken care of. If it's just a simple problem involving the palate, then we do a palatoplasty. That involves an overnight stay in the hospital and heals in two to three weeks. What is involved, how much restructuring and how much surgery is needed depends upon each patient's anatomy and the extent of the obstruction.

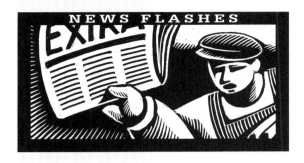

Sleeping Together a Mixed Blessing, Study Shows

BRIGHTON, England—While sharing a bed may increase intimacy, it doesn't guarantee a restful night. A British study found that couples actually sleep better when they sleep alone.

Researchers monitored the sleep of 56 volunteers on two nights—one night when their partners were out of town. When they had the bed to themselves, sleepers moved less during the night, ensuring a smoother night's rest.

Nonetheless, the couples preferred sleeping with their partners, even though they were getting poorer sleep, researchers report. They concluded that the mental benefits of sleeping together outweighed poorer sleep quality.

When asked, women confided that sleeping with a partner made them feel secure. Men said they liked it because it was a habit.

Lost Sleep Can Hurt Immunity

SAN DIEGO—Losing even a few hours of sleep could disarm your immune system and set you up for colds and illnesses, a new study shows.

Twenty-three healthy men ages 22 to 61 spent four consecutive nights in a sleep lab. On the third night, they were denied sleep between 3:00 and 7:00 A.M. Their natural killer-cell activity, a key measure of immune-system strength, dropped 30 percent, researchers reported. That kind of drop can make you easy prey to the common cold and, over time, increase your risk of an even more serious disease.

On the final morning of the study, after the men had returned to uninterrupted sleep, natural killer cells bounced back to their former vitality. Researchers concluded that getting just one good night's sleep will boost your immune cells up to fighting strength once more.

Lavender Oil as Effective as Sleeping Pills

LEICESTER, England—Lavender has long been a folk remedy for sleeplessness. Now, research confirms it.

Early pharmacological and animal trials in aromatherapy have shown that the main components of lavender oil can have a light sedative effect. In the most recent experiment, conducted by David D. Stretch, Ph.D., a lecturer at the University of Leicester and a consultant in research design and statistics, the hours of sleep of each of four nursing home residents were measured for six weeks. Three of the four men were taking sedatives for sleep problems. After two weeks of measurement, all sedative medications were removed. For the final two weeks of the trial period, lavender oil was introduced into the ward with an odor diffuser.

For the three men who had been taking sedatives, the amount of time spent asleep was greatly reduced after withdrawal of medication. But with the introduction of the odor of lavender, sleep returned to the same level as under medication. The fourth man, who hadn't been taking sedatives, slept better with the lavender. All four men were also reported to be less restless during sleep.

Dr. Stretch says that researchers don't yet know whether the lavender oil worked like a drug, altering brain chemistry, or whether its effect was simply like a placebo. He does suggest that lavender oil might be used as temporary relief from long-term medication for insomnia.

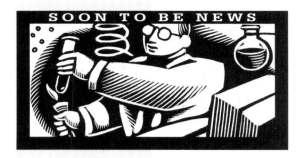

Nap Rooms in the Workplace?

Grabbing 40 winks at work sounds like a great idea to a lot of people, but most employers have yet to appreciate napping's rejuvenating effects. Now, snooze fans, backed by a growing body of research on the benefits of napping, are nudging the once-taboo subject onto the job site.

Studies at Stanford University's Sleep Center suggest that napping is a preprogrammed part of our circadian rhythms, which are regular recurrences of certain activities such as waking and sleeping times. The rhythms peak and ebb in regular cycles, and one of the gateways to never-never land is typically between 2:00 P.M. and 5:00 P.M.

Studies support the added benefits of napping—improvement of mood, alertness and job performance. Instead of putting on another pot of coffee to push you through that slump, consider the European siesta—a short 20- to 30-minute nap. *Look for the marketing of napping "gadgets" like executive recliners and combination desk/beds for the office.*

Will We Be Able to "Switch On" Sleep?

A "slumber switch" buried in the brain slips an alert mind into deep and restful sleep, according to preliminary research by Harvard scientists. The discovery puts scientists on track to make a bigger finding: determining the specific chemicals that cause the switch to put the brain to sleep.

In recent experiments with rats, brain researchers found that during sleep, most of the nerve cells of the brain are turned off by some signal sent out by a small group of cells in the hypothalamus. (The hypothalamus is a structure at the core of the brain that regulates drives like eating, drinking, sex, and now, apparently, sleep.) By tracing the signals, the researchers found that a neuron group called the ventrolateral preoptic area, or VLPO, acts as a slumber switch by turning out the lights in the brain and letting it go to sleep.

If drugs could be found to activate the VLPO, then normal sleep could be prompted with pills that have no hangover effects, unlike some prescription sleeping pills. *Because sleep has phases involving different parts of the brain, extensive research continues at Harvard Medical School and the Scripps Research Institute in La Jolla, California, on the slumber switch and other chemicals involved.*

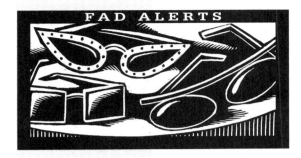

Power Naps

 The concept may not be sweeping the work world by storm, but early afternoon naps seem to improve productivity.

"When I am home, I like to curl up on the floor of my study with my pillow, with the sun streaming in," says Michael D. Myers, M.D., a family physician and obesity specialist in Los Alamitos, California, who often treats patients with sleep disorders. "In the office, if I've had a difficult morning with multiple, complicated patients, I may try a short nap. It's sort of like pushing the reset button on the computer. I wake refreshed and ready for whatever comes in the afternoon. It helps me to function better as a physician, and subsequently, that helps my patients."

To get any real benefit, most people will require at least a half-hour snooze, researchers say. Less sleep leaves them foggy and groggy. And the optimum time for napping is early afternoon, reports sleep researcher and psychologist Timothy Roehrs, Ph.D., director of research at the Henry Ford Hospital Sleep Disorders and Research Center in Detroit.

Napping's not for everyone, though. Some sleep researchers warn that if you consistently have trouble sleeping at night and find yourself regularly nodding off in the daytime, your body clock may need to be reset. To help do that, they advise that you lay off the daytime naps for a while.

Waterbeds

 The term *flotation systems* is headed downstream, but waterbed sales remain afloat after a major washout in the early 1990s, reports Steve Califano, vice-president of Capitol Mattress and Waterbed Warehouse in Latham, New York, which he says is one of New York state's largest bedding stores.

The term *waterbed* is back, says Califano, "because 20 million people have slept on a waterbed in the past and they know what a waterbed is. They may be confused by the term *flotation system*."

Annual sales of waterbeds, after their introduction in the late 1960s, peaked at $1.3 billion in the mid-1980s, says Califano. Now it's about $800 million to $900 million. The industry took quite a hit in the early 1990s. "There was an industry shakeout, and 50 percent of the manufacturers and 35 percent of the retailers went out of business."

Today's waterbeds don't look like waterbeds. They have soft sides, numerous smaller chambers of water (which sometimes are adjustable) and plush, thick, tufted mattress padding. "They look so much like a conventional bed that they sit right alongside the Simmons stuff in the showroom," says Califano. The average waterbed sells for $750, he said.

Today, he said, waterbeds account for "about 18 percent of the bedding market."

Sleep Systems

 Maybe the hottest new development in mattresses is an expensive, highly sophisticated innovation the industry calls a sleep system—a new breed of air mattress.

These aren't for campers. They sell for $1,000 on average, says Califano. Most have tufted padding and look like regular mattresses, but beneath the padding are rubber air chambers hooked to an electric pump. The sleeper, at the push of a button, can adjust the firmness from side to side and sometimes in various zones of the bed. You can find them in independent sleep shops, mall stores and through TV and mail order.

One manufacturer of air mattresses, Select Comfort, cites a study done at the University of Memphis in Tennessee that shows that its mattresses are more effective in maintaining the spine's natural alignment than other mattresses. The manufacturer also claims that the Select Comfort Mattress also more evenly distributes body weight and reduces pressure points.

Califano also cites studies that found adjustable air mattresses superior to other styles of mattresses in evenly distributing body weight.

Industry surveys show that sleep systems comprise about 5 percent of the bedding market, Califano says.

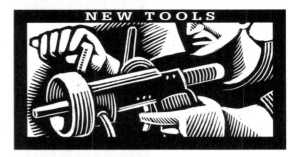

NEW TOOLS

Sounder Sleeping on the Road

Willson Sound Silencer Plus Foam Earplugs

Forty-six percent of business travelers have trouble sleeping while away from home, and noise is the biggest single problem for most, according to a survey commissioned by the National Sleep Foundation and Hilton Hotels. The small, easy-to-insert foam earplugs block out a lot of noise (27 decibels, if that means anything to you) and are easy to fit into an overnight bag or briefcase. $2.99 for four pairs.

Putting a Stop to Snoring

SnorBan

Oral appliances that move the lower jaw forward a bit to reduce snoring work for most people, according to an American Sleep Disorders Association review of 21 studies. SnorBan is one such appliance, available over the counter, that you adjust yourself for a custom fit. It resembles a soft-plastic athletic mouthguard and fits over the teeth, holding the lower jaw slightly forward of its normal position, thus opening the throat airway.

Snoring Relief Labs, the manufacturer, makes no medical claims regarding apnea, a sleep disorder in which breathing stops for frequent and prolonged episodes, but the device has won rave reviews from users (and their spouses) as a tool to stop snoring and has won the endorsement of medical doctors, says inventor Dave Snyder. Michael D. Myers, M.D., a family physician and obesity specialist in Los Alamitos, California, who often treats patients with sleep disorders, saw no problem with trying SnorBan for mild snoring but warned that people should not try to self-treat apnea with Snor-Ban or any other device. Available in drugstores or by calling 1-800-431-8849. $25.95 plus $4 shipping and handling.

Waking Up the Natural Way

sunRIZR Dawn/Dusk Simulator

This computerized alarm clock of sorts slowly brightens your room beginning at a time you specify, simulating a natural dawn—even on a dark December morning. Plugged into a regular or halogen lamp, the sunRIZR Dawn/Dusk Simulator slowly brightens the light over a 45-minute period with up to 400 watts of light. Another model, the sunUP, offers a variable dawn or dusk, from one minute to three hours. Most people, says inventor Blaine Shaffer, prefer around three-quarters of an hour. Shaffer offers a 30-day money-back trial. Order from Pi Square at 1-800-786-3296. sunRIZR, $129, and the sunUP, $198 plus shipping.

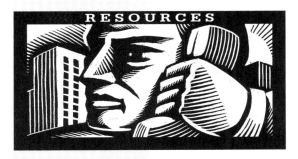

Sleep Apnea/Snoring

American Sleep Apnea Association
2025 Pennsylvania Avenue NW
Suite 905
Washington, DC 20006

This association publishes a bimonthly newsletter, *Wake-Up Call: The Wellness Letter for Snoring and Apnea*, produces patient education videos and maintains a list of patient self-help groups that meet in communities throughout the country. Individuals who join the association (annual fee: $25) receive the newsletter and a MedicAlert bracelet. The association accepts no advertising for the newsletter, so you don't have to worry about ads that tout the latest "miracle cures" for snoring.

Sleep Deprivation

National Sleep Foundation
Department E, Suite 200
1367 Connecticut Avenue NW
Washington, DC 20036

Sleep deprivation has become a national epidemic. In an effort to turn the tide, this foundation works to improve the quality of life of people suffering from sleep disorders and to prevent accidents related to sleep disorders. Its purpose is to educate health care professionals and the public about the treatment of sleep disorders. The foundation promotes patient services, community resources and support groups. It sponsors educational and research programs and gives grants and scholarships in the field of sleep disorders. The foundation provides free booklets to consumers on request.

Sleep Disorders

Mount Sinai Center for Ear, Nose,

Throat and Facial Surgery

Nasal Sinus Center

26900 Cedar Road

Suite 22N

Cleveland, OH 44122

1-800-24-SINUS

This specialty center, associated with Mount Sinai Medical Center, is a worthy resource for information on sleep disorders, especially the relationship of smoking to sleeping problems. Callers can receive free brochures on sleeping disorders, have questions answered by professionals and can be referred to staff specialists for testing and diagnostic procedures.

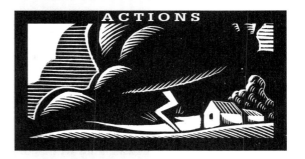

One-third of us experience insomnia from time to time. All of us, as we get older, tend to get less refreshing, rejuvenating deep sleep. It's important that we do get good sleep, because it is during deep slumber that our bodies release and distribute the hormones that repair daily cellular damage and gird our immune systems for battle.

How can you get your best night's sleep ever? Put these concepts to work.

1. Get all worked up. Exercise at least three times a week, preferably in the afternoons, says Michael V. Vitiello, Ph.D., professor of psychiatry and associate director of the Sleep and Aging Research Program at the University of Washington in Seattle. The dramatic effect of exercise on sleep was demonstrated in a study at the University of Washington. One group of seniors exercised aerobically in the afternoons for 45 minutes, three times a week. Another group spent the same time doing stretches. Sleep lab tests after six months of the routine showed that the aerobics group was getting a third more deep sleep than at the outset and was producing 30 percent more human growth hormone (HGH), the chemical that leads the recharging of your batteries when you sleep. The stretching group showed no improvement.

The scientists speculated that this may be because muscle needs more HGH than fat does, so a fit body demands more deep sleep. Or it may be because the warming effect of exercise actually induces deeper sleep. Afternoon exercise slightly raises body temperature and keeps it raised until bedtime.

Don't exercise too close to bedtime, though, or it can interfere with sleep. Try to allow at least three hours to cool down, advises the National Sleep Foundation.

2. **Get in the hot tub before bed.** Or draw a warm bath, advises Michael D. Myers, M.D., a family physician and obesity specialist in Los Alamitos, California, who frequently treats patients with sleep disorders. A nice, long soak in a warm bath appears to bring on the Sandman.

As with many sleep rituals and routines, timing is important. "Take the bath 2 hours before bedtime so that you have 1½ hours to do quiet things when you come out," says Rosalind Cartwright, Ph.D., director of the Sleep Disorder Service and Research Center at Rush–Presbyterian–St. Luke's Medical Center in Chicago. "Use bath oil. It floats on the surface of the water and retains the water's heat. Relax in the tub for 20 to 30 minutes. That relaxes your muscles, too. And when you come out, you're limp as a noodle."

3. **Calendar it.** Schedule enough time for the amount of sleep you regularly need and try to stick to the schedule, even on weekends and holidays, says Dr. Myers.

4. **Dance the night away.** Some people are naturally short sleepers. They can get by on six or fewer hours of sleep, like Winston Churchill and John F. Kennedy were reported to do. If you fall into that category, don't punish yourself and believe that you must lie in bed tossing and turning just because everyone else is in bed. Get the sleep you need and enjoy all the extra free time, says Dr. Myers. Sleep needs vary. Most healthy

adults need seven to nine hours. Some get by on less, some need more.

5. **Make it routine.** Develop a regular, relaxing bedtime routine to unwind and signal your brain that it's time to sleep, advises Dr. Myers.

6. **Play mind games.** You can slip on headphones and listen to relaxation tapes and guided visualizations, but it's better if you learn how to create your own relaxing visualization, says Dr. Myers. "Vivid, relaxing imagery can help people fall asleep. I can sleep on planes because I pretend that the jet engine noise is the sound of a boat engine and that I'm riding out to Catalina Island on a warm, sunny day, the sun beaming down on me—which, for me, is a very relaxing image. People should develop their own relaxing scenarios, envision scenes they find very pleasant and peaceful and relaxing."

7. **Give it a break.** If you can't fall asleep within 30 minutes, don't toss and turn. Get up. "Involve yourself in a relaxing activity, such as listening to soothing music or reading, until you feel sleepy," advises the National Sleep Foundation in its booklet "The ABCs of ZZZs." "Remember: Try to clear your mind; don't use this time to solve your daily problems."

8. **Sleep well on the road.** Bring comfort items from home, such as your own pillow and your coffee mug, to increase your sense of familiarity. Upon arrival at your hotel, arrange for voice mail. Earplugs and a blindfold take up little suitcase room and can save an otherwise impossible night. These suggestions come from a free brochure, "Sleep and the Traveler," published by the National Sleep Foundation. For a free copy of these brochures, write "Sleep and the Traveler," National Sleep Foundation, 1367

Connecticut Avenue NW, Suite 200, Washington, DC 20036.

9. **Declare its purpose.** Make your bed off-limits for anything but sex and sleep, advises Dr. Myers. People who work in bed, read in bed and watch TV in bed will find that their minds don't automatically enter sleepy-time mode, and they may have trouble "going out like a light" when they hit the mattress, notes Dr. Myers.

10. **Seek treatment.** If you consistently wake up tired or are sleepy in the day or if your bed partner tells you that you snore, gasp or stop breathing a lot in your sleep, ask your doctor for a sleep lab assessment, advises Dr. Myers. Sleep disorders can be life-threatening, and the treatment may be relatively simple.

9

HEALTH
MANAGEMENT

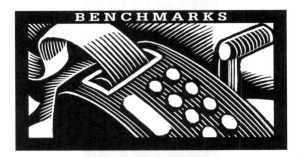

AVERAGES

- Percentage of men who feel younger than their actual age: 53

- Percentage of 2,316 heart attack victims studied who waited more than 20 minutes before seeking medical care: 68

- Number of annual injuries caused by stumbles on stairs, ramps, landings and floors: 1.8 million

- Percentage of workplaces that have been the site of an act of violence: 33.3

- Number of U.S. factories that pose a "high risk" of cancer to nearby residents: 149

- Percentage of doctors practicing in the United States who graduated from a foreign medical school: 16.7

- Day of the week a man is most likely to suffer a stroke: Monday

- Safest day for driving: Tuesday

- You are almost twice as likely to be killed while walking with your back to traffic as you are when facing traffic

- Odds of having a fire in your home, annually: 1 in 4

- Percentage of the time that children's car seats are improperly installed and used: 50

- Percentage of Americans under the age of 65 who have no health insurance: 14.3

EXTREMES

- Number of Britons seeking medical care each year for injuries sustained while attempting to open cans of corned beef: 8,000

- Estimated number of mosquito bites required to drain all the blood from an American adult: 1,120,000

- Number of people injured during a cheese-rolling competition in Cheltenham, England: 18

- Most professional patient: Diagnosed with Munchausen syndrome
(illness where one habitually seeks medical treatment for no medically sound reason), this patient cost Britain's National Health Service an estimated $4 million over a 50-year period. His career as a hospital patient included 400 major and minor operations, and he stayed at 100 different hospitals.

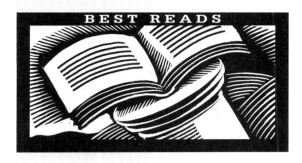

Facing the Facts

Andrew Kimbrell is on a crusade on behalf of the men of America. He believes that the current socioeconomic structure of the United States is oppressive to men and that the miserable state of health that so many men are in is just one of the urgent signs. It is a controversial stance, and his book The Masculine Mystique: The Politics of Masculinity *(Ballantine Books, 1995) is equally pot-stirring. You need not agree with his strident call for action, but it is hard not to be stunned by the statistics that he cites in this opening chapter from the book.*

For several years I have been involved in litigation and lobbying on what are termed men's issues. In addition I have often written about and lectured on the urgent need for a national men's movement. During this time, both in the public media and personally, I have repeatedly met with confusion and consternation over the very concept of "men's issues." Most men and women I encounter respond to the idea that men are experiencing oppression with surprise, humor and sometimes even outrage. The questions tend to be the same: "Why are you writing (talking) about men's issues?" "Why are men whining?" "Why are men angry?" "What is this discussion of a masculine mystique?" "After all," they ask, "aren't men the privileged half of our society?" "Isn't calling for a men's movement as meaningless and ironic as calling for White Power?"

I confess to a lingering frustration over these routine responses. Virtually every statistic on health or survival, and most on economic well-being, show that despite rumors and myths to the contrary, the vast majority of men are being devastated by our socioeconomic system. Though American society continues to empower a small percentage of men and a smaller but increasing percentage of women, it is causing significant confusion and anguish for most men.

This work was written to address the growing crisis for men and masculinity and to provide a blueprint for a transformational political movement for men. However, for the many Americans who see no need for such a movement (or book), clearly a preliminary task is in order. They need to face the facts about men. We begin therefore with an overview of the grim condition of the American male—for many, a long-overdue glimpse into a hidden crisis.

Though few are aware of it, men's life expectancy has dropped dramatically as compared with women's over the last several decades. Due to a variety of causes, including accident, suicide, disease and stress, far too many men are dying ahead of their time. Through 1920 the life expectancy of males and females was roughly the same. Since that time, and increasingly in the 1970s and 1980s, the gap between the genders has widened. Now women are expected to outlive men by approximately 7 years. Currently African-American men have the lowest life expectancy of any population group (64.6 years). White males have a lower life expectancy (72.9 years) than do African-American women (73.8 years) or white women (79.6 years). During the last 30 years, the ratio of male mortality to female mortality has increased in every age category.

Annual statistics show that America's leading fatal diseases target men far more often than women. Heart, lung and liver disease, cancer and hypertension remain inordinately higher for men than for women. For men between the ages of 25 and 65, the death rate from heart disease is about three times that of women in the same age group. Though heart attacks are also the number one killer of women, almost three-quarters of women who die of heart attacks are 75 or older. By this time the average man has been dead for over two years.

Men are also at an increased risk over women of developing and dying of cancer. Over the last 30 years the overall cancer death rate for men has increased 21 percent, while the rate for women has remained about the same. Each year over 55,000 more men than women develop cancer, and 30,000 more men than women die of cancer. In every age group, men's probability of developing invasive cancers is greater than women's. Overall men have a one in two chance of developing cancer, while women have a one in three chance.

Male-specific cancers (e.g., prostate and testicular) have reached epidemic proportions. Each year an estimated 200,000 men are diagnosed with prostate cancer, and about 38,000 will die of it.

Men also suffer disproportionately from a number of potentially life-threatening stress-related diseases, including hypertension and peptic ulcers. Men are, of course, the primary victims of the growing AIDS pandemic.

Men are the primary victims of crime, violence and murder. Rates of violent crimes and theft victimizations remain significantly higher for men than for women. Black men are at the greatest risk of becoming victims of crime, White men have the second-greatest risk, then Black women, and finally White women. A 1994 Department of Justice study found that though violence against women is increasing, men were being victimized by violent crime at a 63 percent higher rate than women. Moreover, since 1976 the rate of murders for men has increased by about 10 percent, while remaining virtually unchanged for

women. As of 1992, men were about 3½ times more likely to be victims of murder than women.

Men comprise the vast majority of those killed or seriously injured on the job. Men represent 55 percent of the workforce but 93 percent of all job-related deaths. Further, over two-thirds of all serious workplace injuries and diseases happen to men. Part of the accident toll is due to our nation's hazardous workplaces. Men still represent approximately 98 percent of the workforce in the nation's most dangerous professions. Thousands of men are killed on the job each year. Every day almost as many American men are killed at work as were killed during an average day in the Vietnam War.

America's men are far more likely than its women to suffer from alcohol or drug addiction. It is estimated that close to 75 percent of all alcoholics are men, and 50 percent more men are regular users of illicit drugs than women. Men also represent close to 90 percent of all those charged with drunkenness, 80 percent of liquor law violators and over 86 percent of those arrested for driving under the influence of alcohol. Men also are about 84 percent of those charged with drug-abuse violations.

Studies show that men are chronically underdiagnosed for depression and other mental diseases. Men are far less likely to be diagnosed for depression than women when the same symptoms are present. A 1991 report indicated that clinicians failed to diagnose depression in two-thirds of male patients who were suffering from well-recognized symptoms of the illness. Additionally, private psychotherapeutic professionals often avoid men, who are perceived as threatening. As a result, men are more likely than women to be transferred away from private care and to public mental health clinics, which are generally understaffed and underfunded.

Males in the United States are the suicide sex. While suicide rates for women have been stable over the last 20 years, among men they have increased rapidly. Overall, men commit suicide at four times the rate of women. Approximately 25,000 men take their own lives each year.

The health and violence crisis for African-American men is especially acute. African-American males have the lowest life expectancy of any segment of the American population. They are especially at risk for cancer. The cancer-death rates for African-American men is significantly higher than that for White males. Black males also suffer from mental disorders at a far higher rate than Black females or Whites. National statistics on inpatient admissions to state and county hospitals show that Black males are institutionalized at more than twice the rate of White males or Black females and over four times more than White females.

Black males also have the highest rate of violent crime victimization. They suffer 60 percent more violent crime than White males or Black females, and more than 150 percent more than White females. Black males ages 16 to 19 are particularly at risk; their violent crime victimization rate is almost double the rate for White males and three times that for White females in the same age-group. Additionally, Black males ages 12 to 24 are almost 14 times as likely to be homicide victims as are members of the general public.

Boys in the United States are diagnosed and treated for a variety of behavioral and mental disorders far more frequently than girls. Boys are twice as likely as girls to suffer from autism and eight times more likely to be diagnosed and medicated for hyperkinesis (hyperactivity). Over 700,000 boys are being drugged for this "disorder" every year. Boys stutter more and are diagnosed as dyslexic four to nine times as often as girls. Young boys are admitted to mental hospitals and juvenile institutions about seven times more frequently than girls of similar age and socioeconomic background.

America's young men (ages 15 to 24) are far more likely than women of the same age group to commit suicide or become addicted to alcohol and drugs. Young men in this age group die at a rate more than three times that of women of the same age. They take their own lives about five times as often as women in the same age group. They suffer alcohol dependency and serious drug addiction at many times the rate of women of the same age group.

Hundreds of thousands of young men are taking steroids and growth hormones. Approximately 500,000 young men are regularly taking dangerous and toxic "body-enhancing" substances, including anabolic steroids and genetically engineered human growth hormone, in an attempt to fulfill the current stereotype of the male body or to enhance their performance in sports.

Men are suffering an epidemic of sexual dysfunction. Studies show that more and more men are experiencing a variety of sexual problems. So-called impotence has become especially prevalent, now affecting more than 20 million American men. Each year there are approximately half a million outpatient visits and 30,000 hospitalizations for "impotence," at a cost of about $150 million. Causes include increases in prostate cancer, psychological stress, abuse of alcohol and drugs and the impacts of environmental toxins.

Despite the view that boys are favored in the classroom, boys are faring far worse than girls in our nation's schools. Those punished and rejected by our school systems are overwhelmingly boys—incidents of corporal punishment and suspension are far more common with boys. Boys consistently represent a disproportionate number of those with low grades at virtually all primary- and secondary-school levels. Eighth-grade boys are 50 percent more likely to be held back a grade than girls. And according to the

U.S. Department of Education, eighth-grade girls are twice as likely as boys to aspire to a professional, business or managerial career. In high school, two-thirds of special education students are boys. Over 60 percent of high school dropouts are boys.

Men are now less likely than women to attend college and less likely to graduate from college. Currently, 46 percent of men attend college versus 54 percent of women. Forty-five percent of men graduate from college, whereas 55 percent of women graduate. Women also represent 59 percent of all master's-degree candidates.

This generation has witnessed a dramatic drop in real wages for the average working man, while that of women has increased. Men in the unskilled-labor market have seen their wages drop over 25 percent over the last decade. Real wages for men under 25 have experienced an even more precipitous decline. Over the last two years, wages paid male high school graduates were 26.5 percent less than in 1979. The recent drop in wages has not been limited to the young or undereducated. College-educated men over 45 have also seen their yearly pay descend by 18 percent over the last five years. In each of these categories women have experienced an increase in annual real wages.

Recent economic trends have left millions of men permanently unemployed or underemployed. The United States has transformed itself into a postindustrial society over the last 20 years. As America's economy becomes ever more high-technology and service-oriented, traditional blue-collar male jobs (that is, factory, construction and transportation) have become scarce. During the 1980s the number of men (22 to 58 years of age) who were working full-time, year-round, declined by over 10 percent. By 1991 the number of men working full-time, year-round (50 to 52 weeks), was declining by 1.2 million each year, while the number of women working full-time was increasing by 800,000. Agricultural work for men has also declined. Over 600,000 farmers have lost their land in the last decade (79 percent of farmers are male).

Male heads of household now have less net worth than women who head households. Due to increasing male unemployment and the demands of child and alimony support, there has been a dramatic decline in the income of male-headed households. According to the U.S. Census Bureau, women who are heads of households now have a net worth 23 percent greater than that of men who are heads of households.

The economic and social crisis for men is especially dire for African-American men. African-American men suffer unemployment rates twice as high as those of White men. Moreover, they are far more likely to be jailed and far less likely to gain an education than African-American women. One out of four African-American men between the ages of 20 and 29 is either in jail, on probation or on parole—ten times the proportion for African-American women of the same age range. Also, more African-American men are in jail than in college, and there are 40 percent more African-American women than men studying in our nation's colleges and universities. Even Black males who succeed in becoming college graduates suffer economically. Their salaries are far less than White male college graduates' and less than both White and Black female college graduates'. By contrast, Black female college graduates now make slightly more than White female college graduates.

The millions of American male veterans who have returned home from war with broken bodies or minds have been grossly neglected. One in three American men is a veteran. The toll of war and our national neglect of these men has been high. Fifty thousand Vietnam War veterans are blind, and 33,000 are paralyzed. It is estimated that nearly 100,000 Vietnam veterans have committed suicide since the end of the war, almost twice the number of men killed in battle. Researchers also estimate that 20 percent of all Vietnam veterans and 60 percent of combat veterans were "psychological casualties." Within the first decade after the war, a presidential review found that 400,000 Vietnam veterans were either in prison, on parole, on probation or awaiting trial. Now 25 percent of the men in prison are Vietnam veterans. Furthermore, on any given night an estimated 271,000 of the nation's veterans are homeless. Adding insult to injury, government reports show a shocking lack of adequate hospitalization and mental health facilities for veterans.

The problem of homelessness is primarily a problem of single adult men. Homelessness is often perceived as a problem primarily of women and children. About 10 percent of our homeless are children, another 10 percent are adults with children (a majority of whom are women). The rest, approximately 80 percent, are single adults. Out of that total, about 80 percent are single men. From these statistics a picture of the homeless emerges that is different from that usually portrayed. Of all the homeless adults, single or with families, 70 percent are men. And of all homeless people—adults or children—men represent 58 percent of the total, and boys 7 percent.

Millions of fathers have lost meaningful contact with their children as family courts discriminate against men in child custody decisions. Throughout the United States, divorce is reaching epidemic proportions. One recent estimate is that two-thirds of all first marriages will end in separation or divorce. Slightly more than half of all divorced couples have children 18 years of age or younger at the time of their separation. Each year there are approximately one million divorces which affect one million children. Fathers and children have been the biggest losers in divorce and custody wars. Mothers initiate divorce actions at over twice the rate of

men, while, in many jurisdictions, men receive physical custody of children in only about 10 percent of all contested divorce cases.

Discrimination against fathers by custody court judges and lawyers is a major factor in fathers losing custody of their children. A New York State Task Force survey revealed that nearly three-quarters of attorneys surveyed believed that child custody awards are "often" or "sometimes" based on the assumption that children belong with their mothers rather than on independent facts. Over half of the attorneys believed that judges "always" or "often" employed a maternal preference in custody awards, and 24 percent of attorneys believed that judges "rarely" or "never" gave fair and serious consideration to fathers seeking physical custody of their children. Statistics for 1992 on child-support awards show the result of the discrimination practiced against fathers in New York State courts. The courts issued 65,536 support awards involving 94,788 children; only 3,537 (3.7 percent) were given primary residence with their fathers.

Approximately six million American fathers are now divorced "visiting" fathers. The plight of these men and their children is virtually ignored. Due in part to custody orders, move-away mothers, psychological stress, denied visitation by the mother, remarriage and relocation, about 40 percent of children see their nonresident father once a year or not at all.

The toll on the mental health of fathers is high. The suicide rate for divorced men is four times that of divorced women and higher than that of other men. Divorced men also have higher rates of drug and alcohol abuse and depression than single or married men or single, married or divorced women.

Men are increasingly torn between the necessities of their job and their desire to have time for their families. In a 1993 poll, fathers were asked what part of their lives they would "most like to change." Almost three-quarters of those polled said, "I'd spend more time with my children." This represented a nearly 20 percent increase in this response since 1984. Fathers' conflict over spending more time with their children is exacerbated by their continual role as the primary breadwinner. In 1991, among married couples with preschool children, 77 percent of all fathers were employed full-time, year-round, compared to only 28 percent of all mothers.

Men face serious discrimination in the criminal justice system. Overall, 94 percent of those incarcerated in U.S. prisons are men. The male incarceration rate is more than 16 times higher than the female incarceration rate, though females are charged with nearly 20 percent of all crimes. Men are less likely than women to receive a plea bargain. They routinely receive longer prison sentences than women for the same offense. Men also comprise virtually 100 percent of those executed in the United States each year.

The increasing number of men now heading single-parent households are given virtually no social or government support. Fathers now head over 1,300,000 single-parent households. This is the fastest-growing trend in parenting in the United States. Many of these new single-parent fathers need support in order to cope with their new financial and personal responsibilities. While numerous government and private programs have been designed for the single mother, programs to aid the single father are almost nonexistent.

As life in the workplace "harness" undermines men's health and their ability to parent, it also makes men obsolete after they retire. Older men, with the exception of the tiny minority who are part of the power elite, are viewed as little more than useless when they can no longer fulfill their primary role as productive workers. Of course, old age in our society too often means obsolescence, vulnerability and alienation regardless

of gender. However, it is especially cruel for men. Due to the stresses of their lives, fewer men reach old age than women. However, for those who do, it is often traumatic. America's elderly men commit suicide over five times more often than women of the same age. Their health is often far poorer than that of their female counterparts. They are twice as susceptible to cancer and more vulnerable to other chronic illnesses. Furthermore, men over 65 are twice as likely to be victims of violent crime as women in their age group and almost four times as likely to be hospitalized for alcohol-related medical problems.

As society begins to face the hidden crisis for men—a reality marked by disease, premature death, suicide, addiction, homelessness, violence, the increasing stresses of work and divorce, and obsolescence in old age—perhaps it will come to better understand the need for men to address this increasing tragic toll on men and boys. Perhaps men and women alike will no longer view the idea of men's issues with humor or surprise but rather with empathy and understanding. Perhaps those confused by the concept of a men's movement will see its importance and understand its vital role in addressing this hidden crisis.

Choosing Your Doctor

Men will search the world over for the perfect mechanic, the guy who always knows where that annoying squeak is coming from, will talk to you like you're another mechanic and won't try to pass off used parts. Why, then, won't men do the same for their bodies? Choosing the right doctor is one of the most important things that you can do for yourself, and in this excerpt from Symptom Solver: Understanding—And Treating—The Most Common Male Health Concerns *(Rodale Press, 1996), authors Alisa Bauman and Brian Paul Kaufman tell you how to do it.*

On the surface, doctors all look the same. They wear white coats and stethoscopes. They have horrendous handwriting. They have motel-room art, year-old magazines you wouldn't have wanted to read when they were new and syrupy elevator music in the reception area. They have a gatekeeper who wants to see your insurance card before you get your coat off. And they all have various impressive-looking framed documents and diplomas hanging on the walls.

So how do you tell one from another? And does it *really* make a difference who your doctor is?

You bet your life.

It's one of the most important decisions you can make. It's also a decision a lot of guys put off until injury or illness forces their hand. Sure, the National Center for Health Statistics in Washington, D.C., says the average man makes about 2.3 visits to the doctor per year. But that's an average: For every guy who makes four or five trips, there's one who doesn't go at all.

"A man can get to 35 years old and never see a doctor. They sometimes go longer. Sometimes I see men in their fifties, and they tell me they've never been to a doctor," says Bruce K. Lowell, M.D., an internist and geriatrician in Queens, New York, and author of *Body Signals: When to Relax, When to Be Concerned and When to Go to the Doctor Immediately*. "They have a million rationalizations. 'I have to work. I can't afford to take the time off.' But the bottom line is fear and denial."

A Different Kind of Checkup

As we all know, the worst time to go looking for a trustworthy car mechanic is when something's wrong with your car. So why would you wait until something's wrong with your body to find a doctor?

Take the time now to make your choice. Establishing a professional relationship and rap-port with a physician can help you live a longer and more satisfying life, says Dr. Lowell. If you're confused about what to look for, read on. Despite appearances, all doctors aren't the same. Here are some key areas to examine as you make your choice.

Get on board. About two-thirds of U.S. doctors are board-certified. That means the doctor received extra training in a specialty after medical school and then passed a national exam.

"Your odds are better with a board-certified doctor. It's an important thing to look at," says Timothy B. McCall, M.D., a practicing internist in Boston and author of *Examining Your Doctor*. Some doctors claim to be certified in a specialty when, in fact, they are not, Dr. McCall says. You can call their bluff by checking their credentials. Call the American Board of Medical Specialists at 1-800-776-2378 to confirm board certification.

Consider a female physician. You might initially feel skittish the first time you drop your trousers in front of an adult female wearing white. But choosing a woman doctor is something to consider, says M. Robin DiMatteo, Ph.D., professor and chairwoman of the psychology department at the University of California in Riverside.

In various studies women doctors outranked their male counterparts when it came to communication skills. Women doctors also focused more on prevention. They dealt more with psychosocial aspects of health, such as family and work life. They spent more time with their patients. And they even smiled and nodded more often.

"I know several men who, after many years of going to male doctors, eventually switched to women and were a lot more comfortable. They said that the relationship was so supportive and the communication was so good that they didn't feel the least bit embarrassed," Dr. DiMatteo says.

Think young. Admit it. When you think

doctor, the first image that comes to mind is Marcus Welby, M.D. Kindly. Wise. And, well, old. Possibly because new medical school courses are teaching doctors communication skills, younger doctors, on average, tend to be able to relate to patients better, Dr. DiMatteo says. They also tend to include patients more in their health care decisions rather than take an authoritarian role, she adds.

Make it convenient. If you can only go see the doctor during your lunch break and his office is closed at lunch, chances are that you'll never see the doctor. You want visits to the doctor to be convenient. Find out the doctor's office hours, office location, billing procedures, whether testing is done at the office or somewhere else, how long you must wait for an appointment and anything else that would make seeing the doctor more convenient, says Kenneth Goldberg, M.D., director of the Male Health Center in Dallas and author of *How Men Can Live As Long As Women*.

Tune in to general hospital. Hospital quality varies tremendously, Dr. McCall says. For example, the mortality rates in large teaching hospitals tend to be much lower than in small, rural, non-teaching hospitals. Also, some hospitals specialize in treating certain conditions, and they tend to have lower mortality rates for those diseases. For instance, hospitals that do a lot of bypass surgery tend to have lower death rates for that surgery, Dr. McCall says.

"Part of assessing if this is the doctor for you is assessing whether this is the hospital you want to be in," Dr. McCall says. "People look at choosing a doctor, at choosing a health plan and at choosing a hospital as if they are always going to be healthy. You ought at look at doing these things as if you're going to be sick and as if you're really going to have to deal with this person."

You should make sure that the hospital where your doctor will send you is close to home, has a good reputation and has facilities to treat your specific health needs. You can call the Center for the Study of Services in Washington, D.C., at (202) 347-7283 to order a $12 book, *Consumer's Guide to Hospitals*, which contains death rates and other information about 5,500 U.S. hospitals.

Call for backup. Find out who the other M.D.'s are in the practice. Make sure you wouldn't mind being treated by them when your main doctor is unavailable, Dr. Goldberg advises.

Check classroom attendance. You'd think no doctor would ever want to have anything to do with a classroom setting again after all those years of medical school. But doctors who want to keep up with medical advances will take a few continuing medical education courses a year. Ask any prospective doctor whether he takes such courses. If the answer is yes, find out which courses, Dr. Goldberg says.

Interviewing Techniques

It's role-playing time. You're a manager with the power to hire a highly skilled specialist for a position that is absolutely vital to the company's growth. After identifying the leading job candidate by reviewing credentials, what do you do?

Set up an interview. Face-to-face. And that's exactly what you need to do when you hire a medical professional to take care of your health needs. Ask for a few free minutes of the doctor's time. If he won't see you for free, look for another doctor. "I have had people move to town, and they have certain problems and they want to look the medical plan over. I don't think any sensible physician would charge for that," says Rex Daugherty, M.D., a physician in private practice in Pawhuska, Oklahoma.

Interviewing the doctor will help you discover something very important—his personality. And you're looking for two traits in particular.

- An ability to communicate clearly: You want your doctor to be able to explain medical terms—sigmoidoscopy, corpus spongiosum, prostaglandin—in a way that you can understand.
- A willingness to treat you like a partner, not like a child: You don't want a doctor who says, "You have pyogenic granuloma. You need surgery." You want someone who explains your condition and possible treatments and allows you to ask questions, Dr. DiMatteo says.

The doctor's ability to communicate and treat you like a partner will affect how well you respond to medical treatment, she says.

According to Dr. McCall, here are some questions you might want to ask the doctor during your interview.

- How do you feel about second opinions?
- How do you feel about nonmedical treatments?
- What preventive programs would you suggest for someone my age?
- How do you feel about involving patients in decision making?

The doctor may only be able to give you five to ten minutes. So if you have easy questions that any receptionist can answer (do you take my health insurance?), then ask the receptionist.

During the interview, pay attention to whether the doctor is listening to you and whether he is carefully considering the questions. Look for traits that are important to you. For example, if you value a doctor who can look you in the eye when he's talking, watch his eyes.

"I think you can just get a feeling for someone. Sometimes you walk in, and the doctor and his staff are like little Napoleons and you just don't connect. Other times you feel like, 'This is a regular person. I can deal with this person.' Some of it's just a gut feeling," Dr. McCall says.

According to Don R. Powell, Ph.D., presi-dent of the American Institute for Preventive Medicine in Farmington Hills, Michigan, and author of *Self-Care: Your Family Guide to Symptoms and How to Treat Them*, here are some questions you may want to ask yourself after the interview to help decide whether this is the doctor for you.

- Did the doctor listen to me and answer my questions, or was he vague?
- Do I feel comfortable with this person? Could I tell him about something personal? Could I ask something that might sound dumb?
- Is the office staff friendly?
- Could I understand what the doctor was saying?

Working Together

Okay, you're still the manager, and you've hired the employee you want based on a great interview. Now what? At most places, the person you hire comes in on probation so that you can see how he actually performs the job. Once again, the same standard applies to your doctor.

"Ultimately the measure of how well a doctor practices is how well a doctor practices," Dr. McCall says. "So much of the choosing we do in life, whether it's jobs or colleges or relationships, you find out what you have after you've had it for a while."

You don't, however, have to let the doctor dictate your relationship. In fact, you shouldn't. Remember, you are partially in control of how well you and your doctor get along. There are many good reasons to make sure that you establish a good relationship with your doctor. Here are a few.

- You'll more likely get special treatment. If your doctor actually knows you personally, he will be more likely to agree to schedule changes, to make an exception to the rule or arrange for after-hours calls, Dr. Daugherty says.

• You'll listen. About 38 percent of patients don't follow short-term advice from their doctors, and 43 percent don't follow long-term advice. In various studies, Dr. DiMatteo has found that part of the problem is that the patient does not understand what the doctor says and is too timid to ask questions. Having a good relationship with your doctor, where you treat one another as health partners, will help alleviate your shyness, she says.

• You'll get better. Fully discussing the situation with your doctor can make the difference between getting cured and staying sick. In one study, headache sufferers whose symptoms improved the most during a six-month period were the ones who discussed their symptoms the most fully with their doctors at the first visit.

"Patients are less likely to volunteer symptoms if the doctor is trying to act like their parent," says Richard Honaker, M.D., of Carrollton, Texas, where he is the president of Family Medicine Associates of Texas. "But male patients respond better if they feel like the doctor is a business partner. It would be like the doctor and patient were discussing an issue about the business. It happens to revolve around his stomach or his nose or his throat."

So start acting like your doctor is your business partner. If your accountant started throwing around technical terms and mumbo jumbo about numbers, you'd stop him and demand: "What does that mean? What's the bottom line?" Do the same thing with your doctor.

And don't be afraid to take the initiative. You may have read about a nutritional therapy that your doctor doesn't know about. Instead of waiting for him to bring it up, ask him whether eating an apple a day will keep the tennis elbow away. He might answer, "Uh, dunno." Then say you're willing to try it. And ask whether he'd be interested in hearing about your progress, suggests Robert Abel, Jr., M.D., clinical professor of ophthalmology at Thomas Jefferson University in Philadelphia. He is also a key player in Jefferson's Alternative Medicine Program, which is examining the future of healing in the twenty-first century.

"If you are told, 'Inquire wherever you want. Whatever information you can find, I would like to hear about it'—that's the kind of doctor you want to be with," Dr. Abel says.

Getting What You Need

Here are a few ways you can make sure that you stand up for yourself.

See your doctor. The more you do it, the easier it will get, Dr. Honaker says.

Remember who pays the rent. His rent. And the answer is: You do. Remind yourself of this fact. Either you or your health insurance company is forking out a wad of cash every time you see the doctor. This isn't charity work. The doctor needs you and your money, so don't ever feel that you're wasting his time.

"Whether it is a large or small concern, the physician should listen to the patient and see what can be done. I never feel like my time is wasted by any patient," Dr. Daugherty says.

Fly solo. Women have more experience with doctors. So having your spouse in the examining room with you may increase your chances of getting the right questions asked. Then again, some wives take over the visit.

Instead of letting their husbands talk, it's the wives who describe the symptoms. And they tend to exaggerate, Dr. Lowell says. "Wives are getting their information secondhand. And they know their husbands never complain. So they take it for granted that if the husband is complaining, the pain has to be a lot worse than he says it is," Dr. Lowell says. It may sound like good fodder for a sitcom, but Dr. Lowell has actually watched husbands and wives heatedly argue about what type of pain the husband is feeling.

Go to rehearsal. Before you even step into the doctor's office, rehearse what you want to say, Dr. DiMatteo advises. And if it's your first visit, be prepared to talk about the following: your medical history, your dietary habits, your occupation, your sleep habits, any family problems, your lifestyle, your stress level and your attitude toward health.

Make a list. It works for Santa. It can work for you. Write down whatever it is you want to be sure to tell the doctor and bring it with you. When listing symptoms, be as specific as possible. Even write the date and time each one occurred. List what you want to talk about in descending order of importance. Sending the doctor your list ahead of time is even more effective, says Dr. Abel.

Don't feel rushed. It seems like the doctor is always in a hurry. And that hurriedness may make you feel like he doesn't have time for your piddling little question. That's not true.

"I'm going to tell you a secret about medical practice. You know how doctors are always rushing from one room to another? And they seem to be rushing so they can go take care of really sick people or people with emergencies? They really are rushing to the next patient because the more patients they see, the better their income," Dr. DiMatteo says.

Now, if Joe Towe in the next room has an ingrown toenail, then Joe's toe can wait. "You have just as much right to the doctor's time as anybody else," Dr. DiMatteo says.

Be persistent. So you tell the doc, "Hey, don't leave yet. I have an important question." He tells you he has a patient backlog that's 12 days long. And you don't want to push it. Then ask if there's someone else in the practice you can talk to—a nurse, a health educator, a dietitian. Or ask him to refer you to written information. Or a support group. Or make another appointment with the doctor, says Dr. DiMatteo.

"You have to get your questions answered. If the doctor doesn't answer your questions, you're going to end up with a lot of trouble down the road," she says. "Often the doctors don't make those referrals because they think patients don't want them. I think just by being direct the patient gets the doctor's attention."

Follow through. If you leave the office with unanswered questions, send a follow-up letter. In it, you can summarize what the doctor said to make sure that you got it straight as well as question him further. "Believe it or not, anyone who takes the time to write something down gets a response," Dr. Abel says. "But a phone call is random. You may get called back at a time you are not thinking about things. You feel like you've interrupted somebody else's schedule. You are embarrassed. So you hurry. Then you forget to ask something."

Act like a parrot. Repeat what the doctor has told you to do. It will let the doctor know whether you understand, Dr. Powell says in his book.

Speak up. So the doctor's telling you how eating a head of cauliflower every day for a month will get you back in tip-top shape. You're nodding your head, but all you can think is: "I hate cauliflower." Tell the doctor. If you don't, he'll assume you're on that cauliflower diet when you're not. Then when you return a month later and you're still sick, he'll prescribe something stronger—perhaps a head of broccoli to go along with it. Or, worse, he'll think he misdiagnosed you and order up a battery of tests to find out your real problem.

Sweeten him up. In one study, when internists were given small bags of candy as gifts, they performed much better on tests of problem-solving ability than doctors who didn't receive anything. Even simply saying thanks when he helps your ills go away can go a long way toward improving your care. "Acknowledge your doctors' accomplishments and tell them when they're doing good work," says Alice M. Isen, Ph.D., professor of psychology at Cornell University in Ithaca, New York. "Too often we only give feedback when things aren't working."

Tell him off. You don't have to be a bully about it, but if you find your doctor repeatedly doesn't answer your questions, then tell him about it. Give the doctor a chance to change. "Some doctors are willing to change," says Dr. DiMatteo. "Say, 'I don't like a relationship where things are one-sided. I really want to be a participant, and I think I can be a better patient and take better care of myself if you answer my questions and we can talk about different strategies and possibilities for my care.'"

If the doctor doesn't change, that means it's time to find a new doctor, says Dr. DiMatteo. If you find yourself in that position, go back to the top of this chapter and start all over again.

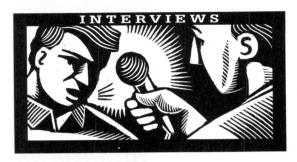

Mike Magee on
A Positive Approach to Medicine

Balancing our physical, mental and social well-being is just as crucial as pumping iron or eating lots of bran flakes, says Mike Magee, M.D., executive director of the Positive Leadership Institute and president of Positive Medicine, in Philadelphia (1-800-PRIDE-13).

Exercise, low-fat eating and other traditional health mantras are an important part of Dr. Magee's approach to health care. But he also believes that to be truly healthy, men should focus more on personal relationships and community involvement. In this interview excerpt, Dr. Magee, a former senior vice-president of Pennsylvania Hospital and current professor of surgery at Jefferson Medical College of Thomas Jefferson University in Philadelphia, talks about getting balance back into your life.

The four things that our readers value are being physically strong, having energy, mental toughness and sexual vigor. How do these things fit into your vision of positive medicine?

To me, the key is energy. If you don't have the energy to do something, you are physically, emotionally and spiritually impotent. What causes you to have that infusion of energy? To me, what causes you to have it is to have a life that is properly balanced. Which means that you're in contact with human beings of all ages and with nature, that you are listening and that you have a passion for what you do, both at work and at home. If you have those things, you can have balance and contentment.

Unfortunately, many men don't know the way back into a balanced life. Trapped in these men's past were balanced lives as children. They have lost the way somehow.

At what age do you think that men lose their balance?

I think when they reach junior high. I think part of it is tied to the chemical changes with reaching puberty.

What does that have to do with anything?

I think that in raising three boys myself and to think back on my own life, it creates a greater sense of isolation. A greater need to prove yourself, a greater tendency toward competitiveness, a loss of free spirit and a comfortable joy of being a child.

What are some things that men can do to manage their health care and get balance back into their lives?

Number one is to listen to women.

Oftentimes their perspective of balance in life is different. They tend to be more humanistic and to see life in the long-term perspective.

A second step would be to be comfortable with the concept of change. I think that change has hit men particularly hard because they are so sensitive to the issue of failure, specifically financial failure. The whole issue of being the bread-winner and their ability to be financially secure causes them—if their job disappears—to really question themselves at the core. So I suggest reading more about change and becoming more comfortable with it.

How does that affect their health?

I certainly believe that stress has a negative impact on health beyond whether it can lead to cancer, raise your blood pressure or cause you to drink. There are general issues about life balance and happiness that are impacted by the depression that comes when you lose your sense of self-worth. So I think to be able to think ahead and imagine what you might do is important.

A third issue would be to consider seriously the issue of pacing. I know many men whose pacing is way off. You can see it in the way they drive their automobiles and their overall sense of urgency.

What do you mean by that?

I get nervous about men whose lives are totally out of balance, figuring that they have it licked if they get on the stair-climbing machine for an hour each day. To me, that is just adding wackiness to wackiness. I believe that the best exercise expands body, mind and soul simultaneously. So I like exercise that brings you in contact with other people. I don't mind exercises in the gym and so forth, but I like it to be something that is not frantic. This pacing issue is very important to me. This running from one thing to another, pursuing exercise as competitively as one would pursue jobs these days—I don't think it is particularly healthy. It may look healthy to people, but I don't think that it is.

So fight off that tendency?

Yes, which brings me to the next point, which would be to develop a sense of closeness to nature, whether it's a flower show in an urban environment or moving to a more rural area.

Or just gardening in your backyard?

Yes, or just gardening in your backyard. That sense of being able to recognize it as a good thing when the birds wake you up at 6:00 in the morning, as opposed to "The damn birds just woke me up."

Does participating in the rearing of your children have an effect on your health?

I think that it helps you to put into perspective what is driving you and what is important. It also cushions any downturns that you may have. So, for example, if I am having a bad day, week or year at work, and yet I can see that my children are finding success, I can live off their success for a while, and that can insulate me and make me feel comfortable.

The other thing is that by watching young children, it allows you to examine your own values. Take time to notice how their lives are balanced, look at their approach to nature and see how much time they invest in playing versus working. Look at their sense of inclusiveness. If you look at when they are near their mother and father, they not only grab for Mom, but grab Dad, too, and pull them together. There are a lot of things that kids can teach us.

What else is important to maintain a balanced life?

Listen better. A lot of times you see conversations going on when there is no conversation. One person is talking and the other person is not listening. Again, we can learn a lot from children by looking at the way they listen. If you are not listening to a child, they will pull on a pant leg until they really get your attention. They don't like it when you play a game of listening when you are not.

So you would suggest practicing intently listening to someone five to ten minutes a day?

Yes. Listen more and talk less. I think that many men feel that they have to tell their whole life story in five minutes to let everybody know

what they have achieved. A let-me-show-you-what-I-have-done-with-my-life type of thing.

So stop making every conversation a job interview?

Exactly. Sit back and actually get to know the person by asking questions like, "What do you do?" "How did you get interested in that?" Everybody likes to talk about what they do. It can be very interesting to be on the listening side of the equation.

What else?

I think that I would recommend editing more. Most men brutalize themselves. The words that go through their heads are not, "Gee, Mike, you are a great guy. Look what you have achieved with your life!" The words that go through are, "You're such a jerk. How could you be such a jerk? Why did you do that? Why are you such a bigmouth?" So it is a useful exercise to spend a week and just write down what is going on in your head, and what you find is that there are five, six or seven phrases that we say to ourselves that degrade us.

One of mine is, "Why are you such a jerk?" Well, now that I am conscious that I say that to myself, if I hear myself say, "Why are you ...," I just stop it. I don't do it anymore. I don't know if that has made me a decidedly better person. But I do know that calling myself a jerk probably doesn't do much good for me.

What does that do to you physically?

I think the questions are out on that stuff because we are still discovering how the brain interacts with the external environment, and we are still discovering what this type of self-degradation does to your immune system. I think that, at the very least, it limits your potential as a human being. It makes it less likely that you will have long-term contentment, success from the standpoint of personal and professional balance. It makes it less likely that you will be successful, have romantic relationships or be a good listener and mentor for your children. All these things mean that, economically and personally, you will be less successful. Whether that affects your immune system remains open to question.

How important is it to have passion for what you do?

From my standpoint, if you have too much time on your hands, you worry yourself to death. I think that a passionate person is an engaged person. He may be passionate about another human being, and if so, he is figuring out how to demonstrate his love. If he is passionate about an idea, he is trying to figure out how to make it a reality. If he is passionate about his profession, he is productive, and he is creating. If he is passionate about nature, he is walking every weekend, or he is engaged politically in trying to protect the environment.

So the worst thing that I can see is passivity, lack of emotion, lack of love of anything. If you have no beliefs or are bored, I think that it is dangerous for society, and it creates a human being that is a drone.

But how does this lack of passion affect your health?

I think that number one, if you look at violence or any dangerous social behavior as a health issue, it makes it more likely that you are going to get dragged into things that can harm you. It creates the setting for greater job instability because those types of people do not continuously improve, and they do not evolve and change with the environment, so they are more likely to be left behind. It creates people who do not develop communication skills. It creates people who are more prone to depression, more prone to be one-dimensional and, therefore,

more prone to stress. Will all of this lead to physical disease? I believe it will.

This is a very untraditional list. The things we were expecting to hear were, "Okay, number one, you need to exercise. Number two, you need to have a good relationship with your doctor. Number three, you don't want to smoke." Where do those fit in?

I think that they are extremely important. They are at the core of some of our success in prevention. But my view of wellness goes beyond that. You have to provide people with enough knowledge to grow.

How do you do that?

Most people would say that the foundation for the pyramid is prevention. Just get them not to smoke, not to drink, not to carry guns, not to do this or that. What that fails to acknowledge is that, to get people not to smoke, not to drink, you have to provide them with a sense of self-esteem that would make them do what is good for them. If you don't care about yourself, why would you do something responsible for yourself? What I am saying is that at the core of health is providing people with enough knowledge to grow, enough conviction to persist, enough imagination to consider their own solutions and enough love to promote self-esteem. Those are the real health issues—knowledge, conviction, love and persistence.

How does that fit in with what men should be doing?

The everyday man in society has grossly underestimated his role as a leader. His role at home, as a leader, is at least as important as his role at work as a leader and in the community as a leader. What is he doing to protect the health of himself and his family? What is he doing to provide knowledge to his family? What is he doing to provide conviction? What is he doing to provide his children with the concept that you have to persist through difficult times that are bound to come? What is he doing to make sure that his child feels love and has self-esteem? I know that these are not traditional views of health, but if you look at health in narrow terms, you will never achieve it. My entire professional life has been about trying to broaden our view of health. In one sense I am an odd duck, but I can tell you that I am becoming less odd as time goes on.

John J. Connolly on
Sorting Out the ABCs of HMOs

Millions of American families have switched their health care coverage to health maintenance organizations, or HMOs. Are you getting the best health care for your dollars? How do you make a wise choice among several different plans? To answer these and other questions, we interviewed John J. Connolly, Ed.D., president and chief executive officer of Castle Connolly Medical, publisher of The ABCs of HMOs *and* Castle Connolly Pocket Guide: How to Find the Best Doctors, Hospitals and HMOs for You and Your Family. *Dr. Connolly is former president of New York Medical College.*

Why are men so behind the eight ball in terms of looking at health care?

For two reasons. In terms of the man's perspective, it is because men grow up with a macho attitude. The male attitude being instilled in them includes denial of pain and toughing things out. So when it comes to health care, they deny their own health care needs. If they get a pain or they get injured, they try to tough it out. It is a value system inculcated into men in our culture.

At the same time, caregiving has traditionally been a woman's role in our society. Women make about 67 percent of the health care decisions in the United States, and they tend to make most of the health care decisions for the family.

Men leave it to women to do this and then deny their own health care needs. It all fits in with our cultural image of maleness and femaleness.

How do you pick an HMO when you are presented with several different plans at work? What should you be looking for? What are some basics?

Too often, when it comes to selecting a managed care plan, men simply look at a list of doctors. If their doctor isn't on it, they just look for a doctor in their area.

What they should be doing is really making the same kind of study of that managed care plan that they would for anything else related to their work or their lives, buying a car or planning a vacation, for example. Choosing a health plan is a very important decision.

They should really look at the coverages, especially as they relate to their needs and their family needs. There are two specific things that I feel are important to mention. One is pre-existing conditions. Be aware that some plans will cover them after a waiting period and other plans will not cover them at all. You don't want to stumble into a plan that doesn't offer coverage for pre-existing conditions that someone in your family may have.

The other issue is the yearly or lifetime cap. A lot of plans have a $1 million lifetime cap. And as we know, $1 million of health care coverage can be eaten up rather quickly if you have a catastrophic illness or accident. There are managed health care plans that don't have caps, and I am a strong advocate of those.

We've heard something about high-option and low-option HMO plans. What are those?

As in almost anything else, the more you pay, typically the more coverage you receive.

In our book *How to Find the Best Doctors, Hospitals and HMOs*, we list examples of what we call high-option and low-option coverages. They tend to be related to the cost of the plan. An HMO, for example, might have a certain limit on a benefit or coverage. Let's suppose that a man is active but gets injured on occasion. The HMO might have a very restrictive limit on rehabilitation services. But another plan might have a much richer limit on those services. The same thing might be true in terms of behavioral or mental health care. There might be a very strict limit in one program and a much higher limit in another. Would you like a couple specific examples out of real plans?

Sure.

For example, let's suppose that it is an older couple and they are concerned about home health care. A higher-end plan, and these are from actual plans that we have examined, might offer 180 visits a year. A lower-end plan might offer only 20 visits per year. In terms of a substance-abuse program on an outpatient basis, some plans you might term the higher option have unlimited coverage. Others might have only 30-day coverage per year. In physical therapy, a high-end plan offers about 60 visits a year. A lower-end plan usually limits you to about 20 visits.

Now, those are just examples, but they demonstrate why it's important for someone to sit down and really look at his needs and how they fit into those distinct coverages.

What about point-of-service plans?

In a point-of-service (POS) plan, if you stay within the network, the HMO basically pays for everything under its normal arrangement. There may be a small co-pay, but the POS plan gives you the option of going outside of the plan and choosing other providers, although you pay a much higher portion of the costs. The insurer might reimburse you 80 percent instead of 100 percent, for example. The question also must be asked, 80 percent of what? Is it 80 percent of the insurer's own fee schedule or 80 percent of what might be called usual, customary and prevailing? If they reimburse you at a lower rate, you may pay a great deal more. POS plans are the fastest-growing kind of managed care plan because they give people more choices and options—if they pay for it.

Is that the best option for most men?

I believe it is. Americans basically want choice, and the POS plan gives them choice when they feel they need it. If they have a special problem that they don't feel will be dealt with, the plan gives them that option to go to any provider, doctor or hospital, in or out of the network, even though it costs more.

Now, once you are in an HMO, how do you get the most out of it? How do you pick a primary care physician, and how do you get past that gatekeeper to the specialist when you need it?

There are a couple basic rules. The first one is really putting a little effort in picking a primary care physician. Don't just pick a name. Find out if he is board-certified and in what year by calling the American Board of Medical Specialties at 1-800-776-2378, or even asking the doctor what medical school, what residencies, what certification he has. I feel that board certification is essential.

Also, if you can, try talking with other people who have been cared for by that doctor. Note what hospital the doctor has an appointment on, because an HMO might have dozens of hospitals. Some of them may be very good; some of them may be not so good. You want to make sure that you select a doctor who is on the staff of a hospital that you think is particularly excellent.

Second, don't do as too many of us do: Choose the doctor and then never bother to see him. Take advantage of his services, because they are already paid for in most cases. Setting up an appointment, getting that baseline physical, establishing a relationship with the doctor and making sure that he is somebody to whom you can relate and whom you feel you can trust is important because that person is going to be your primary care physician, hopefully for many years.

If you don't like the doctor, don't be afraid to change. Virtually all HMO plans allow changes. Now, there might be restrictions. They might say that you can only do it every six months, or something similar, but change if you don't have a good trusting relationship with your primary care doctor.

In terms of getting past the gatekeeper...

I think that is a really good issue. One of the primary concerns people have is referral to specialists. The only answer I have is that you have to be assertive. The squeaky wheel gets greased, and if you are not pressing and making sure that you are demanding everything that you feel you need as a patient, you are going to get what's handed to you. And it may not be the best.

And so in my view it is important to be as educated as possible about your own problems and about what's available through the HMO. Be as demanding as you need to be to get the best care possible!

But as you well know, too many people just take what's handed to them. And they don't get the best care. Being assertive and knowing the rules are two things that you must have in your favor. You really have to know your coverages, you have to know what you can demand and you have to know the appeals process within the HMO.

What are the trends creeping up on us in health care that we may not be aware of, and what can we do about them?

There are some good trends, and I'll try to mention those, but in managed care particularly, there is the issue of physician incentives and compensation. People are really troubled by it. If my doctor is financially rewarded for denying me care in some way or penalized for providing too much care, who is watching out for me in this system? If I can't really trust my doctor to do it, and I certainly can't trust the insurer to do it, it comes back to the patient. People have to be more informed, educated and assertive. Many states are passing a whole range of bills regulating managed care to try to make it more responsive to patients and to protect patients in a managed care environment. But it still is going to come back to patients to protect themselves.

You said that there are a couple of good trends that you wanted to talk about.

Yes. One good trend, and I think particularly supported by managed care, is the development of clinical practice guidelines and outcome studies. Under an indemnity system, hundreds of thousands of doctors were all out there caring for their patients in their offices, in hospitals and doing their own thing. It was impossible to get the data to really see what worked best. However, when you have those hundreds or thousands of doctors in a network where the managed care organization has access to all the patient information—what care is being provided, what medications are being used, what the patient demographics are like—you have tremendous potential to really look at what is happening and to see what works best. I think that is going to be an immense benefit to our health care system and to people in general.

It is now possible, because of that information all being centralized, to really do effective outcomes studies. And then from that, to develop good clinical protocols and say: "Look— we've studied thousands of patients, and this particular approach works on this problem ten times better than our other approaches and costs less," or maybe it costs the same but works a lot better or maybe it costs a little more but works five times as well. I think that is a wonderfully positive contribution that managed care will end up making to the health care system.

And another would be . . .

Well, the other one is controlling costs and cutting out waste. You hear all the horror stories about managed care and issues like denying care and that kind of thing, but one of the things that we forget is that one of the reasons that managed care is there and is becoming such a powerful engine in the health care machine is the fact that it controls costs. And it is cutting a lot of waste out of the system. And if it is doing that without reducing the quality of care, I believe that is a very good thing for our society.

The bottom-line question: What are the five smartest things that a man can do to manage his own health care?

One, have the right attitude that you need to be an informed assertive consumer. Two, recognize that in this new health care system the real responsibility for health care is going to fall to you. Three, seek out the very best practitioners and providers you can, whether it is doctors or hospitals or chiropractors or podiatrists or whoever it is.

I think four would be to really learn the rules of whatever system is caring for you or paying for your care. Learn those rules and work them to your advantage to the maximum degree possible. And last, never be afraid to change if you don't feel that you are getting the care you need.

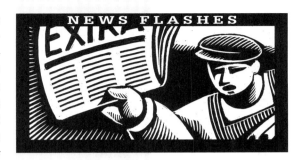

Age a Factor in Doctor-Patient Relationships

COLUMBUS, Ohio—The closer in age a patient is to his doctor, the less chance he might have to give input concerning medical decisions, a new study suggests.

Researchers randomly divided in half a group of 818 medical students, residents and medical school faculty members from Ohio State University in Columbus and the University of Kansas in Kansas City and had each group read a vignette that described the medical condition of a hypothetical patient. One of the groups was told that the hypothetical patient was 25 years old, while the other group was told that the patient was 75 years old. Both groups were then asked to respond to 13 medical care decisions and explain who should make each of the decisions: the doctor only, both the doctor and the hypothetical patient or the hypothetical patient only.

The researchers found that the younger students and resident physicians advocated greater patient input in the medical decisions from the 75-year-old hypothetical patient than they did from the 25-year-old. In a striking contrast, the older, more established physicians of the medical school faculty advocated greater patient input from the 25-year-old hypothetical patient than they did from the 75-year-old.

Overall, it appeared that those in the study generally advocated more decision-making power for older patients than for younger ones. The findings suggest that younger patients may have to be proactive in their relations with their doctors if they want more input in medical decisions, particularly if their physician is also young.

Bad Eating Habits Cause Health Costs to Soar

HIGHLAND PARK, Mich.—There is a high correlation between healthy behaviors and lower medical costs, according to a recent study involving 6,000 Chrysler Corporation employees and their families.

The study kept track of participants for three years. It monitored behaviors that would have a direct impact on health and also tallied the participants' health care costs. The health behaviors that were charted included smoking, weight control, exercise, alcohol use, eating habits, stress, mental health, cholesterol level and blood pressure.

The study showed that people with poor health habits spend more money on health care than people with healthy habits.

The health behavior that accounted for the highest increase in health care costs was eating habits. The study showed a 41 percent difference in the health care costs of those who had poor diets and those who had healthy diets. As for the smokers in the group, the study indicated that they had a 31 percent higher annual claim cost than the nonsmoking participants. Those who were overweight or had high blood pressure paid higher costs because of their tendency to spend more time in the hospital.

Participants who were overweight were hospitalized 143 percent more than their average-weight counterparts, and those with high blood pressure spent 24 percent more days hospitalized than those with normal blood pressure.

New Prostate-Surgery Process Saves Time, Money

CHICAGO—A team of doctors and nurses at the University of Chicago's Louis A. Weiss Memorial Hospital has devised a new process that cuts the hospital stay for patients undergoing radical prostatectomy by more than half without having any negative effects on surgical outcomes or patient satisfaction.

The new process is the culmination of a number of procedural changes that the hospital staff made to their standard surgical routine for prostate removal. The changes included a switch from general to epidural anesthesia, increased patient education prior to surgery, minor alterations in the surgical procedure itself and an accelerated period of recovery in which postoperative narcotics were replaced with less complex pain medications.

The medical group's novel approach ultimately shortened the average surgical patient's hospital stay from 4.6 days to 1.7 days and reduced blood loss by one-third. There was also a one-fourth reduction in operating time. As the result of these decreases, there was a 32 percent reduction in cost for the patient, dropping the average cost from $20,000 to less than $14,000.

Most important, the new process elicited extremely high levels of patient satisfaction, with 92 percent of the patients expressing satisfaction with their pain relief and 96 percent saying that they were satisfied overall.

Doctors Frustrated by Patients Who Don't Listen

BOSTON—While doctors seem to be more confident now about giving their patients advice concerning good health habits, they also feel a deep frustration about their inability to get their patients to act on that advice, say researchers from the Harvard School of Public Health and the Iowa Department of Public Health.

The researchers conducted a survey of 460 Massachusetts primary care physicians that documented the doctors' opinions of and strategies for patient counseling. Of the physicians studied, most believed that it was part of their responsibility to counsel patients about healthier lifestyles and health risk factors. Yet, at the same time, only about a third of the doctors reported being optimistic about their ability to assist patients to change their habits.

The results also showed that many doctors are selective about the type of health advice they will distribute to their patients. Most of the doctors studied were likely to warn patients about the negative health and safety effects of smoking, illegal drug use, alcohol abuse and neglecting to wear seat belts. Yet only half of the doctors counseled their patients about the potential health risks associated with high intakes of saturated fats, being overweight and neglecting to exercise.

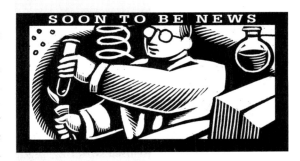

A Vaccine for Herpes?

Researchers are testing several experimental vaccines, and one test that is nearing conclusion is a vaccine for genital herpes.

One out of five people in North America is affected by this sexually transmitted disease, and so there is marked interest in the vaccine's effectiveness on those infected with herpes as well as their uninfected partners.

In the early stages of the clinical trials, the vaccine appeared to promote the development of antibodies to the virus and seemed to be well-tolerated by the patients. In the final-stage clinical trials, which are currently under way, the researchers will try to determine whether the vaccine can protect an individual against contracting herpes from an infected partner. *If this last segment of the trials is successful, the vaccine could be available within five years.*

Health Care in the Air?

In an effort to reduce the number of times that flight plans have to be diverted because a passenger has suddenly become ill, British Airways is working with the University of Edinburgh in Scotland to create a medical diagnostic system that would monitor a flier's vital signs and transmit the information through a satellite link to a doctor on the ground.

In-flight medical emergencies occur once in every 753 flights, costing airlines untold dollars. Many airlines already have doctors on call 24 hours a day, but it can be difficult to converse with them through radio contact because of atmospheric conditions or because of flight paths over remote parts of the globe.

The new diagnostic kit will enable the flight crew to measure a person's pulse and respiration with simple monitors that are attached to the patient's skin. More traditional medical devices like stethoscopes are rendered useless during flight due to the background noise in the airplane. *A prototype of the in-flight diagnostic kit could be in testing in 1997.*

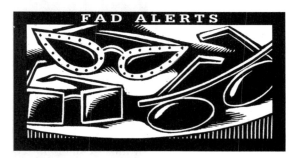

FAD ALERTS

Cigars

Take the cigar off the endangered species list.

Once considered an "absolutely sacred rite" by Winston Churchill, cigar smoking seemed destined for extinction just a few years ago. But it has suddenly regained respectability among the hip, rich and famous from coast to coast, including Arnold Schwarzenegger, Joe Pesci, Christian Slater, Rush Limbaugh, Bill Cosby, David Letterman, Tom Selleck and even President Bill Clinton. Since the mid-1990s, cigar imports have soared 140 percent, according to *Cigar Aficionado* magazine. Demand is so great that an estimated 55 million stogies are on back order. At the same time, more than 100 swank cigar lounges have opened nationwide.

"In the last three to four years, cigar smoking has become very popular. I think that the pendulum has swung so far toward the anti-smoking crowd that there was bound to be a backlash. The more you try to restrict something, the more people seem to be attracted to it," says Robert Langsam, founder and chief smoking officer of the International Association of Cigar Clubs. "But I think it's also because a cigar is a very attainable luxury. It's soothing, flavorful and relaxing. It always has been a symbol of success and the good life. And it just seems that there's a trend toward appreciating those things again," he adds.

Cigars are also appearing in the mouths of

more women, including actress Demi Moore and supermodel Linda Evangelista.

"After 10:00 P.M., 40 to 50 percent of my clientele are women, and a lot of them are single," says Langsam, who is also owner of Heaven, a Naples, Florida, cigar lounge. "It's absolutely a great way to meet women."

And if you really want to make an impression, offer her an Avo, a mild cigar from the Dominican Republic that appeals to many women, says Phillip Dane, owner of Phillip Dane's Cigar Lounge in Beverly Hills, California.

But be prepared to shell out some bucks. A good cigar can cost anywhere from $3 to more than $15, Langsam says. Then if you really get into it, you can spend another $250 to $1,000 for a humidor to keep your cigars fresh.

And what do doctors think about all of this? While it would be foolhardy to endorse or encourage tobacco use in any form, smoking cigars rather than cigarettes is the lesser of two evils, says Alan Blum, M.D., associate professor of family practice at Baylor College of Medicine in Houston. A cigar smoker who inhales, for instance, is three times more likely than a nonsmoker to develop lung cancer. But if you smoke cigarettes, your risk is ten times greater.

"In reality, someone who has a cigar occasionally isn't taking much of a risk. If you savor a cigar once or twice a week, you're probably causing yourself no more harm than having a steak once a week," Dr. Blum says. "But if you smoke ten a day, I have no doubt that you would be at substantial risk for cancer of the mouth, esophagus and kidneys as soon as 20 years down the line." As for chewing tobacco, there's still a high risk for cancer of the mouth in as little as a decade. Besides, what woman doesn't find it a gross habit, he adds.

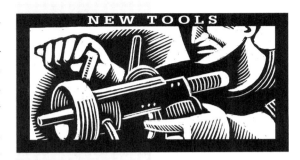

NEW TOOLS

Understanding the Health Care System

Magee's Positive Choice Tools

In the good old days, going to the doctor—that is, if you bothered to go—was simple. You walked in, were examined and listened to him tell you information in a way that emphasized one-way communication. Then you shelled out a few dollars and were gone. It was a no-brainer.

Now there are health maintenance organizations, preferred provider organizations, deductibles, lifetime maximums and other assorted annoyances. Yes, it's a jumble out there, and unless you know what you're doing, it's easy to wind up with sky-high medical bills and little or no care to show for it. But hacking your way through the tangle of confusing medical forms, doctors and services is a lot easier with *Magee's Positive Choice Tools*. Written by Mike Magee, M.D., executive director of the Positive Leadership Institute and president of Positive Medicine, a former senior vice-president of Pennsylvania Hospital and current professor of surgery at Jefferson Medical College of Thomas Jefferson University, all in Philadelphia, this 56-page guide features practical, step-by-step plans for choosing the best doctors, insurance programs and hospitals for you and your family. Each section includes ten insightful questions to ask health care providers that can help you make realistic choices about managing your well-being. Write to: Positive Medicine, Inc., 800 Spruce St., Philadelphia, PA 19107, or call toll-free at 1-800-PRIDE-13. $10.

Using the Best Doctors

Medi-Net

If you sense your physician has more in common with Dr. Demento than C. Everett Koop, you might want to check him out with Medi-Net, a nationwide computer service that maintains records on thousands of physicians who have been disciplined by state medical examination boards.

It's important to be able to access this information, because doctors are often licensed to practice medicine in several states. So it's possible for a physician who has had his license revoked in one state to continue practicing in another, says Richard B. Schiff, director of medical information at Medi-Net. In many states, physicians who have had their licenses suspended or revoked can, when a stay is issued by the court or board, continue practicing while they appeal the medical board's findings. This process can be long and drawn out, lasting sometimes for years.

"We have run across physicians who have been harming their patients for years who still are able to practice in state after state," Schiff says. Medi-Net reports do not make any judgments. The reports merely state the findings of the various agencies involved. But if you examine a physician's disciplinary record and see that he or she has had a number of probations, a license suspension or revocation, or has been found guilty of gross negligence, that should be a clue to you that this may not be the person you want providing your health care. In addition, if the physician you inquire about is disciplined within 12 months of your initial call, Medi-Net

will mail you an update free. Call toll-free, 1-888-275-6334. $15 for the first doctor and $5 each for others requested during the same call (limit of six).

Medical Help away from Home

HotelDocs

Diarrhea in Dallas, sunburn in San Diego or a migraine in Minneapolis are among a business traveler's worst nightmares. But you can have these conditions treated and many other ills without leaving your room if you call HotelDocs at 1-800-468-3537. A dispatcher will take your medical information and send a physician, dentist or specialist to your hotel room within 35 minutes. The doctors supply the medications, so you don't have to hunt for a pharmacy. Hotel-Docs is available 24 hours a day, seven days a week in 130 cities nationwide. $150 per exam, covered by most insurance plans. Check with your insurance company beforehand to ensure that it will provide coverage.

Less Expensive Life Insurance

Zurich Life Insurance of America/
Life of Virginia

Regular exercise and eating well don't count for much at most insurance companies, but a few are beginning to offer discounts to customers who choose healthy lifestyles. Ask your own insurer. If he doesn't know what you are talking about, you can mention this company.

Chicago-based Zurich Life Insurance of America offers a special policy, "Super Select Term," for people who don't smoke or abuse drugs or alcohol and who have normal blood pressure, good driving records and healthy weight. Since these factors reduce policyholders' risks of dying any time soon, they are rewarded with a lower premium. Phone 1-800-269-9669. Savings: Up to 70 percent.

Predicting Future Eye Problems

The Foundation Fighting Blindness Grid Test

If you want a vision of your eyes' future, try this. Order the grid test offered by the Foundation Fighting Blindness. To take the test, simply cover one eye and look at the dot in the center of the grid. If the lines around the dot are straight, you probably won't have macular degeneration, a disease that's projected to rob ten million baby boomers of their sight as they age. (If the lines are wavy or distorted, see your eye doctor for a proper diagnosis.) The disease, which decreases central vision and the eyes' ability to see fine detail, is the leading cause of blindness in people older than 60. While you might not be anywhere near that age, now is the time to adopt some preventive strategies. Wear ultraviolet-blocking sunglasses; eat a diet rich in leafy green vegetables such as spinach, kale and collard greens; don't smoke and give yourself this eye test every once in a while. For a copy of the grid and other information, phone the Foundation Fighting Blindness toll-free at 1-888-394-3937. Free.

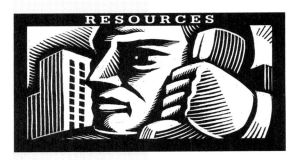

Safe Driving

American Academy of Orthopaedic Surgeons and the National Highway Traffic Safety Administration
1-800-824-2663

Concerned with the large number of injuries and deaths every year from auto accidents? If so, call for your free copy of the brochure "Drive It Safe." This brochure includes information on the proper use of seat belts, head restraints and children's car seats. You can leave your name and address 24 hours a day.

General Health

Harvard Pilgrim Health Care
http://www.hchp.org

This Web site offers easy-to-find and easy-to-read answers to common health, safety and fitness questions. The Health Library is well-stocked and contains information on everything from prostate trouble to eyestrain to knee pain. In the Wellness section, you'll find prevention and diet tips and instructions on how to perform self-exams. A Seasonal Topics page provides health care advice appropriate to each season. The Web site is run by Harvard Pilgrim Health Care, New England's largest nonprofit managed care organization.

Health Maintenance Organizations

Physicians Who Care

10715 Gulfdale, Suite 275

San Antonio, TX 78216

1-800-545-9305

If you are considering joining a health maintenance organization (HMO), you might be interested in a new brochure put out by Physicians Who Care, a doctors' organization that was established to educate the public about health maintenance organizations. The free brochure, titled "Are You Thinking of Joining an HMO," explains what HMOs are, outlines some of the major problems that patients have when part of an HMO and suggests courses of action to avoid these common problems. It also provides you with an "HMO Checklist" by which you can evaluate any HMO. Overall, the brochure is intended to help you determine whether joining an HMO is the best decision for you.

Motorcycle Safety

The Motorcycle Safety Foundation

1-800-833-3995

With over 28 million men riding motorcycles, motorcycle safety has become a public concern. The Motorcycle Safety Foundation offers free information for new, future or experienced bikers including information packets on financing, buying and insuring a motorcycle. The foundation can also tell you where you can take a safe-riding course that's tailored to your skill level and is close to home. The Motorcycle Safety Foundation is funded by the major U.S. motorcycle manufacturers, who united to reduce motorcycle accidents and injuries through operator education, licensing improvement and public information.

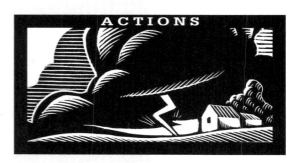

ACTIONS

Some decisions are a cinch. Sunny day. Convertible. Your lover at your side. Top down? Definitely. But the ones involving your health are often a lot less cut-and-dried. Here are 15 ideas that will help you manage your health wisely.

1. **Get a baseline physical.** If you haven't had a physical since you played freshman football, now's the time to do it, says Eric G. Anderson, M.D., a family physician in San Diego. It will give you and your doctor an opportunity to evaluate your overall health and establish a trusting relationship.

2. **Stomp out the smokes.** Nag, nag, nag. We know you've heard this one before, but here's a compelling reason that might even get the Marlboro Man to quit: You'll have better sex. Smoking cuts down on blood flow to the penis, and you know what that means. In fact, smokers were twice as likely as nonsmokers to be impotent in the Massachusetts Male Aging study.

3. **Strangle stress.** Up to 90 percent of all visits to doctors are for stress-related disorders. Robert S. Eliot, M.D., founder of the Institute of Stress Medicine in Jackson Hole, Wyoming, suggests that regular exercise should be a fundamental part of any relaxation program. It can lower anxiety, fend off depression and increase your self-esteem. So try simply walking 15 to 20 minutes a day.

4. **Make farce a habit.** Humor is a powerful ally in your quest for a healthy life. A good laugh strengthens the immune system, decreases the production of stress-related hormones, relaxes tense muscles, keeps your mind engaged and boosts oxygen flow and blood circulation to all parts of the body, says psychiatrist William Fry, M.D., associate clinical professor emeritus at Stanford University School of Medicine.

5. **Let anger go.** Hostility and anger can make your risk of heart disease and other killers increase, researchers say. So do this. Pretend that the world will end tomorrow. What would you do? Get angry and seek revenge against your enemies?

"I know of no one who has ever done this exercise who said that they'd go out and do nasty things," says Redford Williams, M.D., author of *Anger Kills* and director of the Behavioral Medicine Research Center at Duke University Medical Center in Durham, North Carolina. "People usually say that they'd go out and smell the roses or get in touch with family and friends. It's always something positive and upbeat."

Now take a step further. Write down what you'd do and then do it. You'll probably do something constructive with your day, be more tolerant of others and have a more hopeful outlook on life, Dr. Williams says.

6. **Call a close friend.** If you can't name someone off the top of your head whom you can confide in, you may be at greater risk for fatal heart disease than other men. A Duke University study found that, of men with heart disease who weren't married and had no friends or confidants, half died within five years of being diagnosed. In comparison, only 17 percent of similar patients died if they had more social support.

No, you don't have to go out and try to be a social butterfly. But having one good friend—even if it's your wife—makes a big difference in relieving anxiety and depression, Dr. Williams says.

7. **Take your pulse.** First, get a good night's sleep. When you wake up, take your pulse, counting the number of beats in one minute. That's your resting heart rate. The lower it is, the less your heart has to work to pump blood throughout your body. The less it has to work, the longer it's likely to last. If your resting pulse is below 70, that's good, and if it's 45 to 50, that's great—as long as it increases normally with exertion, says Carl Lavie, M.D., medical co-director of cardiac rehabilitation and prevention at Ochsner Heart and Vascular Institute in New Orleans. A resting heart rate above 70 isn't necessarily bad, but if it's consistently high, especially if it's way over 70, your body is probably out of shape. That means that you're at greater risk of a heart attack or stroke. To cut that risk, get out of bed and go for a 30-minute walk. That's all the activity you really need, three or four times a week, according to Harvard researchers.

8. **See how you measure up.** It won't replace a routine physical exam, but here's a quick test you can do right now to determine your risk of heart disease. Measure your waistline at your belly button with a measuring tape (sorry, no sucking in the gut allowed). Now divided that number by your height in inches. If the result is more than 0.46, you could be headed for a weight-related problem, such as heart disease or diabetes. Researchers from Toranomon Hospital in Tokyo found that the waist/height ratio is a better predictor of heart disease than the more commonly used waist/hip ratio. If your number is on the high side, don't be alarmed. But do bring it up at your next checkup. Your doctor will probably suggest that you start a moderate exercise program to trim down.

9. **Flip through your family album.** Many factors that lead to cancer, heart disease and other ailments have genetic links. Take a hard look at your family history. Note the age at which your relatives had heart attacks, strokes or developed cancer, says Paul N. Hopkins, M.D., associate professor of internal medicine at the University of Utah Cardiovascular Genetics Research Center in Salt Lake City. If your family members had these diseases earlier than expected—most strokes, for example, occur after age 70—then you may be at higher risk of early development, too. But in some cases, you may be able to do something about it.

If you have a family history of very high cholesterol, for instance, especially if your high cholesterol was found at a very young age, you may have a problem called familial hypercholesterolemia, an unusually high cholesterol level that, in your case, may be mostly due to genetics. If so, Dr. Hopkins suggests that you may be an immediate candidate for drug treatments in addition to diet and lifestyle changes. The rest of us may get by on just diet and lifestyle changes.

10. **Tally up your HMO.** Tuna, salmon and sturgeon are all fish but they appeal to distinctly different tastes. The same is true of health maintenance organizations (HMOs). But picking the right one for you can be as simple as keeping score, according to Mike Magee, M.D., executive director of the Positive Leadership Institute and president of Positive Medicine (1-800-PRIDE-13), a former senior vice-president of Pennsylvania Hospital and current professor of surgery at Jefferson Medical College of Thomas Jefferson University, all in Philadelphia. Ask yourself ten questions, he says.

Does the plan cover preventive services such as immunizations, regular checkups and colonoscopy? (Give the HMO two points for each service provided.)

If you and your wife are planning to have a family, does this plan cover prenatal care, circumcision, ultrasound, amniocentesis and neonatal and intensive care? (Award two points for each service.)

How many of the following special treatments are covered: liver transplants, bone marrow transplants, laparoscopic hernia repair, outpatient psychiatric treatments and physical therapy? (Award two points for each service.)

What percentage of my prescriptions are covered? (Award one point for 0 to 10 percent, two points for 20 percent, three for 30 percent and so on.)

If I seek emergency care outside my region, what percentage of the cost is covered? (Award one point for 0 to 10 percent, two for 20 percent, three for 30 percent and so on.)

If I decide to have a test or procedure that is not approved, what percentage of the cost is covered? (Award one point for 0 to 10 percent, two for 20 percent, three for 30 percent and so on.)

If I decide to see a doctor outside the plan, what percentage of the cost is covered? (Award one point for 0 to 10 percent, two for 20 percent, three for 30 percent and so on.)

Are patients responsible for the insurance paperwork each time they are seen? (Award ten points if patients aren't responsible for paperwork, one point if they are. If this is unimportant to you, award five points.)

Are patients required to physically have completed paperwork in-hand in order to see another doctor or to have a test or procedure performed? (Award ten points if completed paperwork is unnecessary, one point if it is. If this is unimportant to you, award five points.)

How close is the health plan's hospital to my home? (If within 20 minutes, award ten points; within 30 minutes, seven points; within 40 minutes, five points; within 50 minutes, three points; 60 minutes or more, one point.)

Now add up the numbers. The HMO with the highest score is probably your best bet.

11. **Take a seat.** After you've checked out a doctor's background—education, hospital affiliations and board certifications—make an unannounced visit to his office and just sit in the waiting room for 20 to 30 minutes, Dr. Anderson suggests (if someone asks what you're doing, just say that you're waiting for a friend).

Then just look around. Are patients treated with courtesy? Is the office clean? Are the magazines current? Are waiting times for appointments brief? If not, are apologies and explanations offered? These are signs of a well-run office, Dr. Anderson says.

If you're impressed, take the next step and schedule a get-acquainted visit with the doctor. (Some physicians don't charge for it. Ask the receptionist when you phone for an appointment.)

When you go for this visit, are you seen on time? Are you given a sheet explaining the doctor's fees and services? Does the doctor maintain eye contact? How long can you talk before the doctor interrupts you? Does the doctor give you his full attention, or does he allow phone calls and other distractions to disrupt your visit? Does he encourage questions? Do you feel comfortable with him? If not, find another doctor, Dr. Anderson suggests.

12. **Do your homework.** No, you don't need to know as much as your doctor, but you should know enough about a medical problem so that you can ask good questions. Your library and national organizations like the American Heart Association are good places to start. Computer online services and the Internet, which now carry information from various nonprofit groups, are terrific sources of information, Dr. Anderson says.

The Foundation for Informed Medical Decision Making has videotapes available on topics such as prostate cancer, benign prostate disease, low back pain and mild hypertension. Videotapes cost $49.95, plus shipping. For a brochure and additional information, write to the Foundation for Informed Medical Decision Making, P. O. Box 5457, Hanover, NH 03755-5457, or fax them at (603) 650-1125.

13. **Compare notes with your pharmacist.** Ask both your doctor and pharmacist for a list of side effects and written instructions for your medications, suggests Dr. Anderson.

If there are any discrepancies between the advice you get from your doctor and pharmacist, he advises that you take the information to your doctor, or if you have to start taking the medication immediately, ask your pharmacist to call you doctor for clarification. A good doctor will gladly help you resolve your concerns. If your physician becomes defensive or isn't willing to discuss the subject with you, you may want to consider going elsewhere for your medical care.

Try to buy *all* your medications, including over-the-counter drugs, at one pharmacy. That will help your pharmacist determine if you're at risk for drug interactions, Dr. Anderson says.

14. **Get a second opinion.** "Any doctor worth his salt welcomes someone getting a second opinion. It shouldn't be considered a threat," Dr. Anderson says. "It's in the doctor's as well as the patient's best interest to get second opinions."

If the second opinion differs from the first, don't hesitate to seek the opinion of a third doctor, says John J. Connolly, Ed.D., president and chief executive officer of Castle Connolly Medical, publisher of *Castle Connolly Pocket Guide: How to Find the Best Doctors, Hospitals and HMOs for You and Your Family*, and former president of New York Medical College. Some situations when you shouldn't think twice about getting opinion include (1) before major surgery, (2) when the diagnosis is serious or life-threatening, (3) if you think the number of tests or procedures recommended is excessive, (4) if the treatment is risky or expensive, (5) if a course of treatment isn't working and (6) if you question the doctor's competence.

15. **Scrutinize those bills.** If you do get hospitalized, take a close look at those incoming bills, says Ann Anderson, R.N., managed-care director of Ethix Corporation, a company that audits hospital bills. A misplaced decimal point can easily turn a $25 box of surgical gloves into a $2,500 outrage.

To reduce your chances of paying for an accounting blunder, take these precautions, according to Anderson.

• Prior to being admitted, ask your doctor for the medical name and billing codes for the procedures you'll be receiving. Then contact the hospital's billing department and ask for the procedure's costs along with the daily room rate and hourly charges for operating and recovery rooms.

• Take a notepad during your stay and jot down names and amounts of medication you take and how many hours you spend in the operating and recovery rooms.

• Demand an itemized bill. The standard "summary invoice" you receive from many hospitals isn't detailed enough for you to spot errors. In a practice called bundling, hospitals often charge you for everything, even if it is never touched. You may, for example, be charged for a whole box of surgical gloves that wasn't necessary. Avoid this practice by asking your doctor, as soon as possible, to tell you what he did and did not use. Once you get the bill, compare it to your notes. And be sure to check for clerical errors.

• Request an audit. If you find an error, ask the hospital for an explanation. If that fails to answer your question, send a written request for a formal audit to the hospital's billing department manager. Don't pay your bill, or your portion of it if you're insured, until everything is resolved to your satisfaction.

Credits

Excerpt from *Living Longer Stronger* (page 23) by Ellington Darden, Ph.D. Copyright © 1995 by Ellington Darden, Ph.D. Used by permission of The Berkeley Publishing Group.

Excerpts from *Smart Exercise* (pages 25 and 106) by Covert Bailey. Copyright © 1994 by the Covert Bailey Revocable Trust. Reprinted by permission of Houghton Mifflin Company. All rights reserved.

Excerpt from *Stop Aging Now!* (page 47) by Jean Carper. Copyright © 1995 by Jean Carper. Reprinted by permission of HarperCollins Publishers, Inc.

Excerpt from *Super Nutrition for Men and the Women Who Love Them* (page 53) by Ann Louise Gittleman. Copyright © 1996 by Ann Louise Gittleman. Reprinted by permission of M. Evans and Company, Inc.

"Peak Erotic Experiences" from *The Erotic Mind* (page 76) by Jack Morin, Ph.D. Copyright © 1995 by Jack Morin, Ph.D. Reprinted by permission of HarperCollins Publishers, Inc.

Excerpt from *Protein Power* (page 107) by Michael R. Eades, M.D., and Mary Dan Eades, M.D. Copyright © 1996 by Creative Paradox. Used by permission of Bantam Books, a division of Bantam Doubleday Dell Publishing Group, Inc.

Excerpt from *The 22 (Non-Negotiable) Laws of Wellness* (page 162) by Greg Anderson. Copyright © 1995 by Greg Anderson. Reprinted by permission of HarperCollins Publishers, Inc.

Excerpt from *Spontaneous Healing* (page 189) by Andrew Weil, M.D. Copyright © 1995 by Andrew Weil, M.D. Reprinted by permission of Alfred A. Knopf, Inc.

Excerpt from *The Dream Sourcebook* (page 214) by Phyllis R. Koch-Sheras, Ph.D., and Amy Lemley. Reprinted with permission of The RGA Publishing Group. Copyright © 1995 by The RGA Publishing Group.

Excerpt from *The Masculine Mystique* (page 229) by Andrew Kimbrell. Copyright © 1992 by Andrew Kimbrell. Reprinted by permission of ballantine books, a division of Random House, Inc.

Photographs from part 1 were taken at Main Street Fitness in Manayunk, Pennsylvania.

Index

Note: <u>Underscored</u> page references indicate tables. *Italicized* references indicate photos. **Boldface** references indicate primary discussion of topic.

A

Account Mark, 205
ACE, 46
Achilles tendon injuries, 40
ACL injury, **35**, 195–96
Adultery, 206
Advanced Sports Concepts Big Ball, **37**
Adventure hiking, 39
Aerobics, 26, **34**
African-American men, socioeconomics and, **231**, 232
Age Erasers for Men, **135–38**
Aging, 47, 234. *See also* Longevity
anti-aging drug, **147**
attitude and, **136–37**
brain changes with, **170**
eating less and, **60**
secrets to aging well, 137
sex and, **84–86**
spontaneous healing and, **192**
steps for improving with age, **135–36**
Stop Aging Now!, **47–48**
22 (Non-Negotiable) Laws of Wellness, The, **162–64**
Air filters, asthma and, 194
Ajoene, blood-clot prevention and, 134
Alcohol, 68, 84
addiction, 230–31
beer, **59**, 69, 124
wine, 67, 69, **117**, **154**

Allicin, 133–34
Alprostadil (Caverject), 91
Alternative medicine, **153**, **202–3**
Alzheimer's disease, 178
American Academy of Orthopaedic Surgeons, **253**
American Board of Medical Specialists, 235
American Dietetic Association, 66
American Heart Association, **153**, 257
American Institute for Cancer Research, **65**
American Psychological Association Help Center, **175**
American Sleep Apnea Association, **223**
Amphetamines, 84
Amyotrophic lateral sclerosis, 192
Anger, 161, **255**
Angiotensin-converting enzyme (ACE), 46
Ankle problems, 42, **205**, 207
Anorexia, **122**
Anterior cruciate ligament (ACL) injury, **35**, 195–96
Antibiotics, natural, 127
AntiCancer, 201

Anti-Diet Kit, **120–21**
Antioxidants, 47, 53–54, 134, **141–44**
beta-carotene, **148–49**
coenzyme Q$_{10}$, **149–50**
defense against free radicals, **142**
dietary, 143
melatonin, **148**
quality products, **144**
supplements, **143–44**
water-soluble, 144
Aphrodisiacs, 58, **82–84**
smells, **90–91**
Apnea, **217–18**, 223
Apomorphine, 82
Arch supports, 197
Arm exercises, 15, *15*, 41
Arthritis, **200**
Artificial flavorings, **146**
Artificial insemination, **95**
Aspirin, 146
Asthma, **193–95**, 207
Athlete's foot, **204**
Attitude, **136–37**, **160–61**
Autism, 231
Avocados, 47, 83
Ayurveda, 203

B

BackCare mattresses, **213**
Back problems, 207

Backward walking, knee injuries and, **196**
Bacteria, beneficial, **127–29**, 155
   strategies for attracting, **128–29**
Bacteria-laden food, **129**
Bagels, sports performance bars vs., <u>35</u>
Balance recommendations, 241–42
Bald-Headed Men of America, **174**
Baldness, **201**
Bananas, 35, <u>35</u>
Barbecue sauce, **64**
Barbiturates, 84
Basal cell carcinoma, 146
Basketball, 167
   Advanced Sports Concepts Big Ball, **37**
   ankle protection and, 42
   freestyle jump roping and, 27
   knee pain and, **197**
   tips to improve shooting, **3**
   Zen meditation and, **165–66**
Bathroom tissue, health problems and, 206–7
Baths, warm, sleep disorders and, **225**
Beds, **211–13**, 219
   waterbeds, **221**
Bedtime snacks, **105**
Bee pollen, 68, 83
Beer, **59**, 69, 124
Behavioral disorders, 231
Bench press, **17–18**, *17–18*, 30, 42
Benign prostatic hyperplasia (BPH), **186–87**
Beta-carotene, 55, 143–44, **148–49**
Beta Sweet carrots, **61**
Biceps extensions, 41

Bicycling, 26, **38**, 42
Bifidobacterium bifidum, **127–29**
Bio-bypass therapy, **201**
BioDots, **172–73**
Biofeedback therapy, **204**
Birth control, male, **92**
Black men, socioeconomics and, **231**, 232
Blenheim Ginger Ale, **63–64**
Blood pressure, high. *See also* Hypertension
   salt and, 45, **59–60**
   strength training and, **24–25**
Blood pressure testing, **153–54**
   exercise readings, **32–33**
Blood sugar, **172**
Bodybuilding, **25**. *See also* Exercise; Weight lifting
Boron, 178
BPH, **186–87**
Brainpower, 177–79. *See also* Memory; Mental toughness
   aging-related changes, **170**
   cognition enhancers, **173–74**
Bread
   flaxseed, **206**
Breakfast, **121**, 123, 177
Breast implants, **81–82**
Breasts, **79–82**
   stimulating, **81**
   suckled, **81**
Breathe Right nasal strips, **36**
Breathing
   restricted, 190–91, **191**
Brewer's yeast, chromium and, 131
British Airways, medical diagnostic system and, **249–50**
Bupropion, 82

C

Cabbage soup diet, **119**
Calcium, 129, **130**
Calorie counting, 55–56, 114
Cancer, 229–30, 256. *See also* Prostate cancer; Skin cancer
   American Institute for Cancer Research, **65**
   bacterial prevention of, **128**
   colon, **151**
   death rates, 230
   herbicides and, 185
   lung, 251
   male-specific, 230
   Resources, **152**
   stomach, 155
   testicular, 185, 230
Cancer Information Service (CIS), **152**
Candida Albicans, **128**
Candidiasis, 128
Carbohydrates, **104**, 108
   balancing intake of, **108–10**
   high-protein low-carbohydrate diets, **118**
   low-fat high-carbohydrate diet, **107–10**
Cardura, 186
Caverject, 91
Centerfold syndrome, **77–79**
Center for the Study of Services, 236
Chemical fertilizers, **185**
Chemical virility robbers, **183–86**
Chewing tobacco, **35–36**, 251
Chicago Institute of Neurosurgery and Neuroresearch, **175**
Child custody decisions, **233**
Childrearing, **242**

Note: <u>Underscored</u> page references indicate tables. *Italicized* references indicate photos. **Boldface** references indicate primary discussion of topic.

Chili peppers, sensitivity to, 66–67
Chinese ginseng, **73–74**
Cholesterol, **60**, 103–4
Cholesterol levels, 133–34, 140, **206**
CholesTrak home test kit, **150–51**
Choline, 173
Chromium, 54, **131–32, 202**
Chronic Fatigue and Immune Dysfunction Syndrome Association of America, **205**
Cigars, **250–51**
Cimetidine, 188
Circulation, poor, **191**
CIS, **152**
Clarithromycin, 188
Clif Bar, 35
Cobalt, 54
Cocaine, 84
Coenzyme Q$_{10}$, xii, **149–50**
Coffee, **62**, 178, 194
Cognition enhancers, **173–74**
Coke, defizzed, as nausea remedy, 208
Cold, common, **201**
Colon cancer, **151**
Comfort Air, 213
Condom Country, **96**
Condoms, **96, 98**
Confide HIV testing service, **151–52**
Consumer's Guide to Hospitals, 236
Continuous positive airway pressure (CPAP), **218**
Contraception, male, **92**
Cooking. *See also* Diet(s); Eating; Food(s); Nutrition
  equipment, **48–53**, 57
  knives, **48–50**
  pots and pans, iron, **50–51**

Gourmet in a Box, **64**
healthy, 57
strategies for men, 56–57
Cooking in the Nude: Quickies, **95**
Copper, 54, **132**
Coronary artery disease, **24, 169**
CPAP, **218**
Creative thinking, **177**
CREB, 171
Crew aerobics, **34**
Cross-country skiing, 26
Curls
  barbell, 30
  dumbbell, 21, *21*, 31
  lying dumbbell, 14, *14*
  two-up, one-down leg, 20, *20*
Cybersex, **93**

D

Damiana, as aphrodisiac, 83–84
Dandelion, as cognition enhancer, 173
Death rates, 230
Deborah's Country French Bread, 64
Dehydroepiandrosterone (DHEA), **147**
Depression, **139**, 140–41, 179, 230
DHEA, **147**
Diabetes, **202**
Diarrhea, 207
Diet(s). *See also* Eating; Food(s); Weight loss
  Anti-Diet Kit, **120–21**
  cabbage soup, **119**
  high-fat, 146
  high-protein low-carbohydrate, **118**

low-fat, **59**
low-fat high-carbohydrate, **107–10**
low-salt, **45–46**
repeated dieting, **115**
solo and social dieters, **111–12**
yo-yo dieting, 115
Zone, **103–5**
Diet pills, **117**
Digestion, 127
Digestive problems, **188–89**, 190, 207
Dihydrotestosterone, 187
Discrimination, **233**, 234
Disease(s). *See also* Health; Heart disease; *specific diseases*
  fatal, 229–30
  mind-disease connection, **139–41**
Doctor-patient relationships
  age and, **247–48**
  reasons for establishing, **237–38**
  ways to stand up for yourself, **238–40**
Doctors. *See* Physicians
Dogs, **171**, 194
Do It Sports, **38**
Dream dictionaries, 214–15
Dreams, **214–16**
  sexual, **99**
  for success, 176
Dream Sourcebook, The, **214–16**
Drinking water, 39, **184–85**
Drinks, smart, **173–74**
DriOn, 95
"Drive It Safe" brochure, 253
Drug addiction, 230–31
Drugs
  anti-aging, **147**
  diet pills, **117**
  memory-boosting, 172

Note: Underscored page references indicate tables. *Italicized* references indicate photos. **Boldface** references indicate primary discussion of topic.

Drugs *(continued)*
  prosexual, 83
  recreational, 84
  side effects, 257
Dumbbell curls, 31
  calf raises with dumbbells
    on knees, 21, *21*
  lying, 14, *14*
Dyslexia, 231
Dyspepsia, nonulcer, 189

E

Earplugs, **222**
Eating, **43–69**. *See also* Diet(s);
    Food(s)
  Actions, **66–69**
  adventurous, **64–65**
  aging and, **60**
  Benchmarks, **44**
  Best Reads, **47–55**
  before drinking, 68
  eat-late gain-weight theory,
    115
  exercise after, 67
  Fad Alerts, **61–63**
  goals, **124**
  health costs and, **248**
  Interviews, **55–58**
  News Flashes, **59–60**
  New Tools, **63–65**
  Resources, **65–66**
  romantic dinners, **57–58**
  sex and, 58
  Soon to Be News, **60–61**
  strategies for men, **55–57**
  taking time for, 207
  30-second rule, 69
  travel and, **121**
  Vital Reading, **45–46**
Eating disorders, **122**
Eating plan, 124
Eat-late gain-weight theory, **115**

Effleurage, 98
Ejaculations, premature, **94**
Ejaculatory fluids, 99
Elbow pain, 208
Elderly men, 162, 234. *See also*
    Aging
Electric Press, 96
Emetrol, 208
Emotional pain, 161, **168–69**
Emotions, **159–60**
  Best Reads, **159–62**
  dealing with, **161–62**
  strategy for bouncing back,
    177
Energy, lack of. *See* Fatigue
Environmental toxins, 231
Erections, 86
  herbs for, **73–74**
  numbing creams to prolong,
    94
Ergometers, for exercise warm-
    up, 29
Erogenous zones, 88–89
Erotic experiences, peak, **76–79**
Erotic Mind, The, **76–79**
Escherichia coli, **127–28**
Essential fatty acids, 55
Exercise, 123–24. *See also* Exer-
    cises, specific; *specific
    activities*
  in afternoon, 41
  after-workout meals, 42, 104
  asthma and, 194
  benefits of, 161, 207
  blood pressure readings
    and, **32–33**
  closed-chain, 198
  effects on sleep, **224–25**
  faster better workouts, **29–31**
  goals, **124**
  immunity and, **154**
  insulin resistance and, **105**
  intense, 124
  leisure-time activities and,
    33

mental, 178
month-per-year formula
    for, 124
after overeating, 67
pain during, **24**
sensate-focus, **97**
Smart Exercise, **25–26**, **106–7**
strength-training myths,
    23–25
technique for commitment
    to, **114**
time management for, 123
working out with wife, 40
Exercise machines, **32**, 123
  leg machines, 40–41
  Precor M9.45 treadmill, **120**
  Reebok Sky Walker, **37**
  sizing, 40
  slide boards, 196
Exercises, specific
  arm, 41
  back squat, 16, *16*
  bench press, **17–18**, *17–18*, 42
  boredom busters, **13–16**
  compound, **7**
  with fast benefits, **25–26**
  freestyle jump roping,
    27–28
  incline one-arm lateral
    raises, 15, *15*
  kneeling close-grip triceps
    extensions, 15, *15*
  leg, **18–22**, 40–41, 198
  limbering up fast, **4–6**
  low pulley cable fly, 13, *13*
  lying dumbbell curls, 14, *14*
  order of, **32**
  power clean and press, 8, *8*
  power lunge, 9–10, *9–10*
  push-ups on knuckles, 41
  squats, 198
  standing single-knee raise,
    16, *16*
  standing straight-bar
    pulldown, 14, *14*

Note: <u>Underscored</u> page references indicate tables. *Italicized* references indicate photos.
Boldface references indicate primary discussion of topic.

total-body, **7–12**
visual acuity, 41
Exercise shoes, 41–42, 197
Eye problems. *See* Vision
EZ-Detect test, **151**
EZ Gard Shock Doctor, **36–37**

F

Falk Library of the Health
    Services, University
    of Pittsburgh, **153**
Familial hypercholesterolemia,
    256
Family history, **255–56**
Famotidine, 188
Fast food, **59**
Fat, **106**, 108
    balancing intake of, **108–10**
    burning, **103–4**
    energy, **106–7**
    high-fat diets, 146
    low-fat food, 59, 61
    low-fat high-carbohydrate
        diet, **107–10**
    obsession with, **106–7**
    strategies for trimming, 56,
        67–68
Fathers, 233–34
Fatigue, **190–91**
    chronic fatigue syndrome,
        205
    salt depletion and, **46**
Fat-stimulating products, **119**
Fatty acids, essential, 55
Feelings. *See* Emotions
Fenfluramine, 82
Fiber, 54, 207
Fig bars, 35, *35*
Fish, 68–69, **185**
Fitness, **1–42**. *See also* Exercise
    Actions, **39–42**
    Benchmarks, **2**

Best Reads, **23–26**
Fad Alerts, **35–36**
Interviews, **27–31**
month-per-year formula
    for, 124
News Flashes, **32–33**
New Tools, **36–38**
Resources, **38–39**
Soon to Be News, **34**
strength-training myths,
    23–25
Vital Reading, **3–22**
Flavonoids, 59
Flavorings, artificial, **146**
Flaxseed bread, **206**
Flirting, 96
Flotation systems, **221**
Flour, refined, **54**
Focus, **177**, 179
Folic acid, **144**, 206
Food(s), **108**. *See also* Diet(s);
    Eating
    after-workout meals, 42
    aphrodisiacs, 58, **82–84**,
        90–91
    asthma and, 194
    bacteria-laden, 129
    bedtime snacks, **105**
    coffee and tea products, **62**
    convenience, **62**
    fast, **59**
    fat-stimulating products,
        119
    filling, 122–23
    freezing, 52
    fruits, vegetables, grains and
        seeds, **155**
    functional, **121**
    glycemic index of, **104**, 104
    healthy snacking, 65
    high in fructo-
        oligosaccharides,
        129
    low-fat, **61**
    Nutrition Hot Line, **66**

prepackaged prepared, 112
quality, **53–55**
refined, **53–55**, 54
refrigerating, 52
serving size, 124
SnackWell's Toaster Pastries,
    121
specialty, **62**
sports performance bars, 35
storing, 52
*Super Nutrition for Men and
    the Women Who Love
    Them*, **53–55**
tea, 59, **62**
Food poisoning, **127–28**
Food processors, 51
Food safety, **65–66**
*Food Smart: A Man's Plan to
    Fuel Up for Peak
    Performance*, **48–53**
Foot and Ankle Web Index,
    205
Foot problems, **205**, 207
Foreplay, **87–89**
Foundation Fighting
    Blindness, 253
Foundation for Informed
    Medical Decision
    Making, 257
Free radicals, 53–54, 134, **142**
FreeStyle Roping, **27–28**
Freezers, storing food in, 52
Fructooligosaccharides, bacte-
    ria and, 129
Fruits, 47–48, 68, **155**
Fungal infections, 195, **204**

G

Garlic, 83, **133–34**
Genetics
    baldness and, **201**
    history, **255–56**

Note: Underscored page references indicate tables. *Italicized* references indicate photos.
Boldface references indicate primary discussion of topic.

Genetics *(continued)*
  infertility and, **145**
  memory and, **171–72**
Genital herpes vaccine, **249**
Ginkgo biloba, **73**, 83, **93–94**,
  173
Ginseng, **73–74**, 173
Glycemic index of foods, **104**,
  104
Glycerin, 76
Go Ask Alice service, **96**
Golf, 3, 39, 40
Good Health Web site, **152**
Good Vibrations Catalog,
  96
Gourmet in a Box, **64**
Grains, disease prevention and,
  155
Granola bars, sports
  performance bars vs.,
  35, 35
Graying hair, gene therapy
  and, **201**
Growth, Law of Lifetime,
  162–64
Growth hormone, 224, 231
Gum, sugarless, as cause of
  diarrhea, 207

H

Harvard Pilgrim Health Care,
  253
HDL, 103
Headache, biofeedback and,
  204
Healing
  with hyperbaric chambers,
  203
  natural, **153**, **202–3**
  Spontaneous Healing,
  189–93
Healing dreams, 215–16

Health. *See also* Mental toughness; Sexual health
  mind-disease connection,
  139–41
  psychology of, 76–77
Health care
  health maintenance organizations (HMOs),
  244–47, 254, 256
  in-flight, **249–50**
  *Magee's Positive Choice
  Tools*, **251–52**
  trends in, **246–47**
Health Center for Better
  Living, 84
Health costs, **248**, 258
Health maintenance organizations (HMOs),
  244–47, 254
  choosing, 244, 256
  high-option vs. low-option
  plans, 244–45
  point-of-service plans, 245
Health management, **227–58**
  Actions, **254–58**
  Benchmarks, **228**
  Best Reads, **229–40**
  Fad Alerts, **250–51**
  Interviews, **240–47**
  News Flashes, **247–49**
  New Tools, **251–53**
  recommendations for, **241**
  Resources, **152–53**, **253–54**
  Soon To Be News, **249–50**
Heart attacks, 256
  artificial flavorings and,
  146
  exercise blood pressure
  readings and, **32–33**
  sex and, **90**
Heartburn, **188–89**
Heart disease, 229–30
  beer and, **59**
  bio-bypass therapy, **201**
  death rate, 230

  depression and, **139**
  folic acid and, **145**, 206
  garlic and prevention of, 134
  minerals and prevention of,
  129–31
  recommendations to
  prevent, **103–4**
  Resources, **153**
  snoring and, 218
  strength training and, **24**
  stress reactions and, **169**
  tea and, **59**
  vitamins and prevention of,
  128
  waist/height ratio test, 255
Heart rate, 255
Heart Smart Restaurants International, **121**
Heel pain, **199–200**
Helicobacter pylori, 188
Helmets, **38**
HEPA filters, asthma and, 194
Herbicides, **185**
Herbs
  as aphrodisiacs, 83
  for better erections, **73–74**
  for enlarged prostate,
  186–87
Herpes vaccine, **249**
HGH, exercise and, 224
High blood pressure. *See also*
  Hypertension
  salt and, 45, **59–60**
  strength training and,
  24–25
High-carbohydrate diets, low-
  fat, **107–10**
High cholesterol levels, 133–34
High-density lipoprotein
  (HDL)
  home test kits, **150–51**
  insulin and, 103
High-efficiency particulate air
  (HEPA) filters, asthma
  and, 194

Note: <u>Underscored</u> page references indicate tables. *Italicized* references indicate photos.
Boldface references indicate primary discussion of topic.

High-fat diets, 146
High-protein low-
    carbohydrate diets,
    118
HIS 'n' HER motion-activated
    night-lights, **95**
HIV Confide testing service,
    151–52
HMOs. *See* Health
    maintenance organiza-
    tions
Homeopathy, 203
Home test kits
    for cholesterol levels,
    150–51
    for colon cancer, **151**
    Confide HIV testing service,
    151–52
Homocysteine, folic acid and,
    for heart disease
    prevention, 145
Hospital bills, detecting errors
    in, **258**
Hospitals, assessing quality of,
    236
HotelDocs, **252**
Human growth hormone
    (HGH), exercise and,
    224
Humor, health benefits of, 123,
    254–55
HUMOR Project, **175**
Hyperbaric chambers, injury
    recovery and, **203**
Hypercholesterolemia,
    familial, 256
Hyperkinesis, 231
Hypertension, 140, 229–30
    salt and, 45, **59–60**
    strength training and, **24–25**
Hypoglycemia, **202**
Hypotension, neurally medi-
    ated, 45, **46**
Hypothyroidism, 190
Hytrin, 186

I

IFIC, **65–66**
Immunity
    exercise and, **154**
    impaired, **191**
    marital spats and, **170**
    natural, 127
    sleep deprivation and, **219**
    weakening influences on,
    191
Implants
    breast, **81–82**
    Norplant, 80
    prostate cancer treatment
    and, **199**
Impotence, **91–92**, 206, 231
Infections
    candidiasis, **128**
    fungal, 195, **204**
Infertility, **145**
Injury
    Achilles tendon, 40
    anterior cruciate ligament,
    35, 195–96
    knee-injury repairs, **35**
    staying in shape and, 166
    toxic, **191–92**
    workplace, 230
In-line skating, 26, 42, **119–20**
Insemination, artificial, **95**
Insomnia, 219
Insulin, diet and, **110**, 118
Insulin resistance, 103, **105**,
    155
Intercourse. *See* Sex
International Food
    Information Council
    (IFIC), **65–66**
In vitro fertilization, **95**
Iron, diet and, 54
Iron pots and pans, cooking
    and, **50–51**
IvyBlock, **152**

J

Jalapeño peppers, sensitivity to
    hotness and, 66–67
Jody Maroni's Sausage
    Kingdom, **64–65**
Jump roping, freestyle, **27–28**

K

Kefir, bacteria and, 129
Kitchen
    how to stock, **48–53**
    mapping out, **51–53**
    organizing, 56
    tools for, **51**
Knee-injury repairs, **35**
Knee pain, **195–98**
Knee raises, 16, *16*
Knives, kitchen, **48–50**
Kola nut
    as aphrodisiac, 83
    cognition enhancers and, 173
K2 Four Super-Sidecut skis,
    37–38
K-Y jelly, condoms and, 98

L

Lactaid, 208
Lactase, digestion of diary
    products and, 208
Lactobacillus acidophilus,
    127–29
Lactose, digestion of diary
    products and, 208
Laughter, 123, 254–55
    HUMOR Project, **175**
Lavender oil, sedative effect of,
    219

Note: <u>Underscored</u> page references indicate tables. *Italicized* references indicate photos.
Boldface references indicate primary discussion of topic.

Law of Lifetime Growth,
   162–64
LDL. *See* Low-density lipoprotein
L-dopa, aphrodisiac effect of,
   82
LEARN weight-control
   program, 111
Lecithin
   memory and, 177–78
   refined foods and, 55
Leg exercises, **18–22**, 40–41
   calf raises with dumbbells,
      21, *21*
   leg extensions, 19, *19*, 29–30,
      198
   leg press, 19, *19*
   standing toe raises, 22, *22*
   step-ups, 21, *21*
   stiff-leg dead lifts, 20, *20*
   two-up, one-down leg curls,
      20, *20*
Leisure-time activities, **33**
Leukemia, 192
Licorice root, as aphrodisiac, 83
Life expectancy, **137–38**, 229.
      See also Longevity
Life insurance, **252–53**
Lifetime Growth, Law of,
   162–64
Limbering up stretches, 4–6
Lipase, refined foods and, 55
Lipoprotein
   high-density, 103, **150–51**
   low-density, 104, 134,
      150–51
Liver disease, 229–30
Living Longer Stronger, **23–25**
Longevity, 229. *See also* Aging
   life expectancy quiz, **137–38**
   Living Longer Stronger,
      23–25
   secrets to, 137
Long johns, polyester, perspi-
   ration and, **95**

Love and Romance Home
   Page, The, **96**
Love making. *See* Sex
Love potions, 84
Low-density lipoprotein
   (LDL), 104, 134
   home test kits, **150–51**
Low-fat foods
   fast foods, **59**
   tasty, **61**
Low-fat high-carbohydrate
   diet, **107–10**
Low-salt diets, **45–46**
Lubricants, 96
   choosing, **76**
   condoms and, **98**
   personal, **74–76**
   rules for using, 76
Lubrin inserts, 98
Lung cancer, 251
Lung disease, 229–30
Lunge, 5, *5*
   power, 9–10, *9–10*
Lycopene, 146
Lymphoma, 192, **199**

M

Macronutrients, **108–10**
Magee's Positive Choice Tools,
   251–52
Magnesium, 54, **130**, 194,
   207–8
Male Body, The, **159–62**
Manganese, refined foods and,
   54
Manta Ray, **37**
Marijuana, sexual problems
   and, 84
Marriage, immunity and, 167,
   170
Masculine Mystique, The,
   229–34

Massage, 88, **175**
Massage oils, **98**
Masturbation, 90, **97**
Mattresses, 211, **212–13**
   Select Comfort, 222
   sleep systems, **221–22**
   waterbeds, **221**
MCL injury, 195–96
Meat, **185**
   safety test, 66
Medial collateral ligament
   (MCL) injury, 195–96
Medical emergencies, in-flight,
   249–50
Medical help. *See also* Physicians
   researching, **257**
   while traveling, **252**
Medical Sports, 208
Medications, pharmacists and,
   257
Medicine
   alternative, **153**, **202–3**
   positive, **240–44**
Medi-Net, **252**
Meditation, **165–66**, 167, **179**
Melanoma
   ABCD rule, **133**
   guide to stopping, **132–33**
Melatonin, xii, **148**
Memory. *See also* Mental
      toughness
   blood sugar and, **172**
   genetic manipulation and,
      171–72
   vitamin B benefits and,
      170–71
Memory-boosting drugs, 172
Meniscal tears, 198
Menopause, lubrication and,
   75–76
Menstrual cycle, lubrication
   and, **75**
Mental disorders, 230–31
   depression, **139**, **140–41**,
      179, 230

Note: <u>Underscored</u> page references indicate tables. *Italicized* references indicate photos.
Boldface references indicate primary discussion of topic.

Mental stress. *See* Stress
Mental toughness, **157–79**
  Actions, **176–79**
  aging-related changes, **170**
  Benchmarks, **158**
  Best Reads, **159–64**
  blood sugar and, **172**
  building, **165–67**
  cognition enhancers and, **173–74**
  creative thinking and, **177**
  exercises for, **167–69**, 178
  Fad Alerts, **172–74**
  genetic manipulation and, **171–72**
  Interviews, **165–69**
  memory-boosting drugs and, 172
  News Flashes, **169–71**
  repeated dieting and, **115**
  Resources, **175**
  Soon To Be News, **171–72**
  stress and, **168**, 169
  vitamin B benefits and, **170–71**
Merrell Hiking Center, **39**
Methylene chloride, sexual problems and, 186
Methylparaben, lubricants and, 76
Metronidazole, ulcer treatment and, 188
Met-Rx bar, 35
Miconazole, athlete's foot relief and, **204**
Milk
  asthma and, 194
  bacteria and, 129
  digestion problems and, 208
Mind-body connection, 169
  in disease, **139–41**
  psychology of health, 76–77
  in spontaneous healing, **192**
Minerals, 108, **131–32**, 194, 208

heart-helping, **129–31**
lost in refined foods, 53–54, 54
Molybdenum, erections and, **132**
Motion-activated night-lights, 95
Motorcycle Safety Foundation, **254**
Mount Sinai Center for Ear, Nose, Throat and Facial Surgery Nasal Sinus Center, **224**
Mouth guards, **36–37**
Muscle relief, **175**
Music therapy, 178

N

Naps, **220–221**
Nasal Sinus Center, Mount Sinai Center for Ear, Nose, Throat and Facial Surgery, **224**
Nasal strips, breathing and, **36**
National Association of Anorexia Nervosa and Associated Disorders, **122**
National Cancer Institute, **152**
National Certification Board for Therapeutic Massage and Bodywork, **175**
National Highway Traffic Safety Administration, **253**
National In-Line Basketball League, 120
National Sleep Foundation, **223–24**
Natural healing, 127, **153**, **202–3**

Nausea, Coke as remedy for, 208
Neurally mediated hypotension (NMH), dietary salt and, 45, **46**
Night-lights, **95**
Nirschl Counter Force brace, 208
NMH, dietary salt and, 45, **46**
Non-Hodgkin's lymphoma, **199**
Nonoxynol-9, lubricants and, 76
Norplant, mammary gland fluid and, 80
Not Just Johns, 95
Numbing creams, premature ejaculation prevention and, **94**
Nutrition. *See also* Cooking; Diet(s); Eating; Food(s)
  Stop Aging Now!, **47–48**
  Super Nutrition for Men and the Women Who Love Them, 53–55
Nutrition Hot Line, **66**

O

Oil(s)
  massage, **98**
  olive, **62–63**
Old age, 162, 234. *See also* Aging
Olestra, 61, **119**
Olive oil, **62–63**
Omeprazole, ulcer treatment and, 188
Onions, 48, 83
Optimism, **136–37**
Organochlorines, **183–86**
  ways to reduce exposure to, **184–86**

Note: Underscored page references indicate tables. *Italicized* references indicate photos.
Boldface references indicate primary discussion of topic.

Orthotics, 197
Os-Cal, 130
Outercourse, **87–89**
Oxygen chambers, injury
    recovery and, **203**

P

Pain
    emotional, 161, **168–69**
    during exercise, **24**
    knee, **195–98**
Paraperidichlorobenzene,
    home deodorizers and,
    186
Parkinson's disease, 192
Penis rings, erections and, **74**
Pepcid AC (famotidine), 188
Peppers
    chili, hotness of, 66–67
    sweet, red vs. green, 69
Perchloroethylene, dry
    cleaning and, **185–86**
Performance. *See also* Sports
    performance
    in school, 231–32
Performance anxiety, 40
Pesticides, **185**
Physical examinations, 254
Physical fitness. *See* Fitness
Physicians, **234–40**
    board-certified, **235**
    checking out, **256–57**
    choosing, **234–40**
    doctor-patient relationships,
        237–38, **247–48**
    HotelDocs, **252**
    listening to, 239, **248–49**
    Medi-Net, **252**
    second opinions, **257**
    techniques for interviewing,
        236–37
Physicians Who Care, 254

Pi Square, 223
Point-of-service (POS) plans,
    245
Poison ivy, **152**
Poison oak, **152**
Polyester long johns, perspira-
    tion and, **95**
Positive medicine, **240–44**
Positive Medicine, Inc., 240,
    252
Positive thinking, **160–61**,
    251–52
POS plans, 245
Potassium, health benefits of,
    130–31, 208
Pots and pans, iron, **50–51**
Powerbars, carbohydrates in,
    35, 35
Power moves, 7–12
    power clean and press exer-
        cise, 8, 8
    power lunge, 9–10, *9–10*
Power naps, **221**
PR Bar, carbohydrates in, 35
Precor M9.45 treadmill, **120**
Premature ejaculation, **94**
Press. *See also* Bench press
    power clean and, 8, 8
Propylparaben, lubricants and,
    76
Proscar, enlarged prostate and,
    186
Prosexual drugs, 83
ProstaScint test, prostate can-
    cer and, **147**
Prostate cancer, 133, 185,
    230–31
    garlic and, **134**
    implant treatment, **199**
    ProstaScint test for, **147**
    risk factors, **145–46**
    tomatoes and, **145–46**
Prostatectomy, radical, **248**
Prostate Pointers Web site, **205**
Prostate problems, 133, **186–87**

Prostate surgery, **248**
Prostatitis, 128
Protein, **105**, 108, 178
    balancing intake of,
        108–10
    high-protein low-carbohy-
        drate diets, **118**
Protein Power, **107–10**
Pumpkin pie smells, as aphro-
    disiac, **90–91**
Push-ups, on knuckles, 41

R

Race walking, 26
Rapid eye movement (REM)
    sleep, dreams and, 215
Red clover, as aphrodisiac, 83
Red peppers, vitamin content
    of, 69
Reebok Sky Walker, **37**
Refined foods, **53–55**
    minerals lost in, 54
Reflexology, 203
Refrigeration, length of food
    preservation and, 52
Rehabilitation
    knee, **196**
    month-per-year formula
        for, 124
Relaxing visualization, 225
REM (rapid eye movement)
    sleep, dreams and, 215
Renin, heart attack risk and,
    45–46
Renova skin cream, **204**
Resistance training, 23–25. *See
    also* Exercise; Strength
    training; Weight lifting
    for arthritis, **200**
Retirement, problems during,
    234
Rheumatoid arthritis, **200**

Note: Underscored page references indicate tables. *Italicized* references indicate photos.
Boldface references indicate primary discussion of topic.

Rice, refined, nutritional value of, 54–55
Romantic dinners, **57–58**
Rowing, 26
Runner's World Online, **38–39**
Running, **38–39**, 42
Running shoes, 41–42

S

Safer-sex supplies, 96
Safety
 food, **65–66**
 meat test, 66
 motorcycle, **254**
Salicylates, heart attack risk and, 146
Salt, **45–46**
 fatigue and, **46**
 high blood pressure and, 45, **59–60**
Sarsaparilla, as aphrodisiac, 83
Saw palmetto berries
 as aphrodisiac, 83
 enlarged prostate and, **92**, **186–87**
Scents, as aphrodisiacs, **90–91**
Select Comfort Mattress, **213**, 222
Selenium
 disease prevention and, 144
 refining process and loss of, 53
Semen, odor of, **99**
Sensate-focus exercises, improving sex and, **97**
Sensor Products, **95**
Sex, **71–99**
 Actions, **97–99**
 age and, **84–86**
 Benchmarks, **72**
 Best Reads, **76–84**
 cybersex, **93**

eating and, 58
 Fad Alerts, **92–94**
 foreplay, **87–89**
 heart attacks and, **90**
 Interviews, **84–89**
 lubrication and, **74–76**
 News Flashes, **90–91**
 New Tools, **94–95**
 peak erotic experiences, **76–79**
 Resources, **96**
 Soon To Be News, **91–92**
 before sports, **93**
 vision loss during, **90**
 Vital Reading, **73–76**
Sex: A Man's Guide, **79–82**, **82–84**
Sex drive, 85
Sex toys, 96
Sexual arousal, **80–81**
Sexual desire, **77–79**, 84–85
Sexual dreams, **99**
Sexual dysfunction, 231
Sexual health
 C. Albicans infections, **128**
 Resources, **96**
Shoes, 207
 exercise, 41–42, 197
Sildenafil (Viagra), impotence and, 91–92
Silicon, health benefits of, **132**
Single-parent households, 234
Skating, in-line, 26, 42, **119–20**
Skiing, 26, **37–38**
Skin cancer
 ABCD rule, **133**, 154
 guide to stopping, **132–33**
 protection against, **146**
Skin creams
 IvyBlock, **152**
 numbing, **94**
 Renova, **204**
Sleep, **209–26**
 Actions, **224–26**
 Benchmarks, **210**

Best Reads, **214–16**
Fad Alerts, **221–22**
Interviews, **217–18**
needs, 225
News Flashes, **219**
New Tools, **222–23**
with partner, **219**
rapid eye movement (REM), 215
Resources, **223–24**
"slumber switch" and, **220**
Soon To Be News, **220**
traveling and, 225–26
Vital Reading, **211–13**
Willson Sound Silencer Plus Foam Earplugs for, **222**
Sleep deprivation, **219**, 223–24
Sleep disorders, **224**
Sleep lab assessments, 226
Sleep systems, **221–22**
Slide boards, strengthening leg muscles and, 196
"Slumber switch," 220
Smart drinks, **173–74**
Smart Exercise, **25–26**, **106–7**
Smells, as aphrodisiacs, **90–91**
Smoking, 39–40, 155–56, 254
 cigar, **250–51**
Snacks. *See also* Food(s)
 after-workout, 42, 104
 bedtime, **105**
 healthy, **65**
SnackWell's Toaster Pastries, **121**
SnorBan, **222–23**
Snoring, **217–18**
 factors that contribute to, **217**
 laser surgery for, **218**
 recommendations to lessen, 218
Wake-Up Call: The Wellness Letter for Snoring and Apnea, 223
Snoring Relief Labs, 222–23

Note: <u>Underscored</u> page references indicate tables. *Italicized* references indicate photos.
Boldface references indicate primary discussion of topic.

Socioeconomics, oppression of men and, **229–34**
Sociology of weight loss, **111–13**
Sodium, heart attack risk and, 130, **131**
Solo dieters, 112
Solvent-free products, **186**
Sony Bryan's Smokehouse, **64**
Sorbitol, as cause of diarrhea, 207
Spanish fly, myths about, **83**
Specialty foods, 62
Specialty Sauces, 62
Spontaneous Healing, **189–93**
Sports, **38**. *See also specific sports*
Sports performance, 27, 40–41, 176
  improving, **3**
  sex and, **93**
Sports performance bars, carbohydrates and, **35**, 35
Sports vision, 41
Spouse
  doctor visits and, 238
  exercising with, 40
  stress relief and, **171**
Squamous cell carcinoma, 146
Squats, 31, 198
  back squat, 16, *16*
  Manta Ray device for, **37**
  super squat, 11–12, *11–12*
Stairclimbing, 26, 29, 197
Step aerobics, 26
Step-ups, 21, *21*
Steroids, 231
Stomach, shrinking, weight loss and, 122
Stomach acid, myths about ulcers and, **187–89**
Stomach cancer, 155
Stomach ulcers, 128, **187–89**
Stomach upset, **188–89**, 207
Stop Aging Now!, **47–48**

Strength training, 42. *See also* Exercise; Weight lifting
  boredom busters, **13–16**
  Manta Ray device for, **37**
  myths, **23–25**
  workouts, **29–31**
Stress, 231
  marital, **170**
  mental toughness and, **168**, 169
  reactions, **169**
Stress management, 58, **140**, 166–67, 176, 254
  American Psychological Association's Help Center, **175**
  BioDots for, **172–73**
  disease and, **139–40**
  dogs and, **171**
  music and, 178
Stretches, **4–6**
  great divide, 6, *6*
  for knee pain, 197–98
  lunge, 5, *5*
  quad-buster, 5, *5*
  triangle, 4, *4*
Stripping, as foreplay, **98–99**
Stroke, family history and, 256
Sucrose, lubricants and, 76
Sugar(s)
  blood, **172**
  refined, **54**
  special, **129**
Suicide, 230–31, 234
Sulfur, disease prevention and, **132**
SunRIZR Dawn/Dusk Simulator, **223**
Super Nutrition for Men and the Women Who Love Them, **53–55**
Surgery
  laser, **218**
  prostate, **248**

Swimming, 26, **36**
Symptom Solver, **234–40**

T

Tagamet (cimetidine), 188
Tarsal tunnel syndrome, **199–200**
Tea, **62**
  heart disease prevention and, **59**
  stroke prevention and, 67
Tempur-Pedic mattress, **213**
Tennis, **3**, 40
Testicular cancer, 185, 230
Testosterone
  organochlorines and, 183–84
  prostate enlargement and, 187
Time management
  for doctor visits, 236
  for eating, 207
  for exercise, 123
  for fathers, 233–34
  lunch breaks, 207
  for sleeping, 225
Tobacco products
  chewing tobacco, **35–36**, 251
  cigars, **250–51**
Toilet paper, health problems and, 206–7
Tomatoes, 48, 67, 83, **145–46**
Tools, kitchen, **51**
Toxins, 128, **191–92**, 231
Toys, sex, **96**
Trace minerals, 108, **131–32**
Travel
  eating and, **121**
  HotelDocs, **252**
  sleeping and, 225–26
Trazodone, 82
Treadmills, **32**, 120

Note: <u>Underscored</u> page references indicate tables. *Italicized* references indicate photos.
Boldface references indicate primary discussion of topic.

Trek Lunar helmets, **38**
Tretinoin, wrinkle prevention and, 204
Triceps extensions, 30–31, 41
    kneeling close-grip, 15, *15*
Tums, calcium supplementation and, 130
22 (Non-Negotiable) Laws of Wellness, The, **162–64**

U

Ulcers, 128, **187–89**
United States Golf Association, **39**
University of Illinois Functional Foods for Health Web site, **121**
University of Pittsburgh Falk Library of the Health Services, **153**

V

Vaccines
    for herpes, **249**
    for lymphoma, **199**
Valsalva retinopathy, 90
Vaseline Intensive Care lotion, condoms and, 98
Veterans, socioeconomics and, 232–33
Viagra, impotence and, 91–92
Vietnam War veterans, socioeconomics and, 232–33
Virility, 85, **183–86**
Vision
    exercises for, 41
    Foundation Fighting Blindness grid test, **253**
    loss during sex, **90**

Visualization, relaxing, 225
Vitamin A, 53
Vitamin B, 53, **170–71**, 179
Vitamin B$_6$, 128, 173
Vitamin C, 53, 144, 173, 208
Vitamin E, 53, 55, 142–44
Vitamins, 67, 108
    for asthma, 194
    heart-helping, 128
    supplements, 119
    water-soluble, 144
Volleyball, 197

W

Waist/height ratio, heart disease risk and, 255
Waist/hip ratio, heart disease risk and, 255
Wakeboarding, **34**
Wake-Up Call: The Wellness Letter for Snoring and Apnea, 223
Walking, **25–26**, 40, 154–55
    backward, **196**
    race, 26
Water, 108
    exercise performance and, 39
    pollution and, **184–85**
Waterbeds, 221
Water sports, **34**
Weight lifting, 7, 42. *See also* Exercise
    boredom busters, **13–16**
    Manta Ray device, **37**
    strength-training myths, **23–25**
    workouts, **29–31**
Weight loss, **101–24**. *See also* Diet(s); Eating; Food(s)
    Actions, **122–24**
    for apnea, **217**

Benchmarks, **102**
Best Reads, **106–10**
Fad Alerts, **118–19**
families and, **112**
indications for, 111
Interviews, **111–14**
LEARN program, 111
News Flashes, **115–16**
New Tools, **120–21**
Resources, **121–22**
sociology of, **111–13**
Soon To Be News, **117**
tools for, **115–16**
Vital Reading, **103–5**
at work, 123
Weight management, **113–14**
    Anti-Diet Kit, **120–21**
    eat-late gain-weight theory, **115**
    "ideal" weight and, **116**
    technique for commitment to, **114**
Wellness
    22 (Non-Negotiable) Laws of Wellness, The, **162–64**
    Wake-Up Call: The Wellness Letter for Snoring and Apnea, 223
Wet suits, swimming performance and, **36**
Wheat, refined, nutrition and, 55
Wild yams, as aphrodisiac, **83–84**
Willson Sound Silencer Plus Foam Earplugs, **222**
Wine, 67, 69, **117**, 154
Women. *See also* Spouse
    menopause and, **75–76**
    menstrual cycle and, **75**
    physicians, 235
    postpartum period and, **75**
Workouts
    after-workout food and, 42, 104

Note: <u>Underscored</u> page references indicate tables. *Italicized* references indicate photos.
Boldface references indicate primary discussion of topic.

Workouts *(continued)*
    efficient, **120**
    faster better, **29–31**
    with wife, 40
Workplace injury, 230
World Congress on
    Complementary Ther-
    apies in Medicine,
    202–3
Wrinkles, **204**

Y

Yahoo! Sexuality Guide, **96**
Yams, wild, as aphrodisiac,
    83–84
Yogurt, cultures and, **129**
Yohimbine, as aphrodisiac, **74**,
    82
Yo-yo dieting, 115

Z

Zen meditation, **165–66**, 179
Zinc, 53–54, 132
Zone, The, **103–5**
Zone diet, **103–5**
Zurich Life Insurance of
    America/Life of
    Virginia, **252–53**

Note: <u>Underscored</u> page references indicate tables. *Italicized* references indicate photos.
Boldface references indicate primary discussion of topic.